Handbook of Angiography

Handbook of Angiography

Editor: Tom Anniston

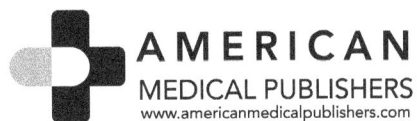

AMERICAN
MEDICAL PUBLISHERS
www.americanmedicalpublishers.com

AMERICAN
MEDICAL PUBLISHERS
www.americanmedicalpublishers.com

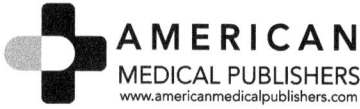

Cataloging-in-Publication Data

Handbook of angiography / edited by Tom Anniston.
    p. cm.
Includes bibliographical references and index.
ISBN 978-1-63927-072-9
1. Angiography. 2. Diagnosis, Radioscopic. 3. Radiography, Medical. I. Anniston, Tom.
RC691.6.A53 H36 2022
616.130 754 8--dc23

American Medical Publishers,
41 Flatbush Avenue,
1st Floor, New York,
NY 11217, USA

ISBN 978-1-63927-072-9 (Hardback)

Contents

Permissions

List of Contributors

Index

Preface

The medical imaging technique that is used to visualize the lumen of blood vessels and organs of the body is known as angiography. It majorly examines arteries, veins and the heart chambers. This technique is used by injecting a radio-opaque contrast agent into the blood vessel and imaging using X-ray based techniques. Coronary angiography, fluorescein angiography, microangiography, neurovascular angiography and peripheral angiography are some examples of angiography techniques. Coronary angiography is one of the most common angiograms which are performed to visualize the blood in the coronary arteries. Cerebral angiography can lead to complications like stroke, allergic reaction, thrombosis and embolism formation. Medical procedure in which a fluorescent dye is injected into the bloodstream falls under the domain of fluorescein angiography. This book provides comprehensive insights into the field of angiography. It provides significant information of this discipline to help develop a good understanding of this field. This book will serve as a valuable source of reference for graduate and postgraduate students.

Significant researches are present in this book. Intensive efforts have been employed by authors to make this book an outstanding discourse. This book contains the enlightening chapters which have been written on the basis of significant researches done by the experts.

Finally, I would also like to thank all the members involved in this book for being a team and meeting all the deadlines for the submission of their respective works. I would also like to thank my friends and family for being supportive in my efforts.

Editor

Cardiac gating calibration by the Septal Scout for magnetic resonance coronary angiography

Garry Liu[*†] and Graham A Wright[†]

Abstract

Background: Electrocardiogram (ECG) gating is commonly used to synchronize imaging windows to diastasis periods over multiple heartbeats in magnetic resonance (MR) coronary angiography. Calibration of the ECG gating parameters is typically based on a cine cardiovascular MR (CMR) video of the beating heart. Insufficient temporal resolution in the cine-CMR method, however, may produce gating errors and motion artifacts.

It was previously shown that tissue Doppler echocardiography (TDE) can identify accurate diastasis window timings by observing the movement of the interventricular septum (IVS). We present a new CMR technique, the Septal Scout, for measuring IVS motion. We demonstrate that cardiac gating windows determined by the Septal Scout produce sharper coronary MR angiography images than windows determined by cine-CMR.

Methods: 9 healthy volunteers were scanned on a GE Optima 450w 1.5T MR system. Cine-CMR was acquired and used to identify the start and end times of the diastasis window (W_{cine}).

The Septal Scout employs a one-dimensional steady-state free precession (SSFP) readout along the ventricular septum prescribed from the 4-chamber view. The Septal Scout data is processed to produce a septal velocity function, from which the diastasis window was determined (W_{sep}).

Non-contrast-enhanced MR angiography was performed twice for each volunteer: once gated to W_{cine}, once to W_{sep}. Vessel sharpness was assessed subjectively by two experienced observers, and quantitatively by full width half maximum (FWHM) measurements of cross-sectional vessel profiles.

In addition, TDE was performed on a subcohort of 6 volunteers where diastasis windows (W_{TDE}) were determined from the IVS velocity measured in the 4-chamber view. W_{sep} and W_{TDE} were compared using Pearson's correlation.

Results: MRA acquisitions were successful in all volunteers. Vessel segments produced smaller FWHM measurements and were deemed sharper when imaged during the Septal Scout gating windows ($p < 0.05$). Subjective assessment of sharpness also improved for the Septal Scout-gated scans ($p < 0.01$ for both observers). Lastly, W_{sep} and W_{TDE} were highly correlated ($R > 0.98$, $p < 0.001$).

Conclusions: The MR Septal Scout technique was introduced and demonstrated to be more accurate at determining cardiac gating windows than cine-CMR, yielding sharper coronary MR angiography images.

Keywords: Cardiac gating, Magnetic resonance coronary angiography, Septal scout

* Correspondence: garry.liu@swri.ca
†Equal contributors
Department of Medical Biophysics, University of Toronto, Toronto, ON, Canada

Background

Magnetic resonance coronary angiography (MRCA) is a potential diagnostic tool for coronary artery disease (CAD). Compared to the current gold standard, x-ray angiography, benefits of MRCA include three-dimensional visualization of coronary vessel lumens, and not subjecting patients to the risks associated with catheterization [1,2] and ionizing radiation [3]. MRCA, however, requires long acquisition times that span multiple heartbeats. Cardiac motion is particularly problematic for MRCA because high spatial resolution is required for diagnosing CAD.

Prospective cardiac gating remains the most effective tool for reducing cardiac motion artifacts in MRCA. The general principle behind cardiac gating is to synchronize, for each heartbeat, the imaging window with the diastasis period. Shechter et al. and Johnson et al. have measured coronary artery velocities during diastasis to be on the order of 10 mm/s [4,5]. Several authors have also estimated imaging window durations within diastasis that will limit blur artifacts to within sub-millimetre pixels. Their estimates include: 66 to 330 ms with a mean of 187 ms for the entire coronary tree [4]; 66 to 220 ms with a mean of 120 ms for the right coronary artery (RCA) [6]; and, 65 ± 42 ms for the mid-RCA [7].

Cardiac gating is most commonly facilitated by the use of (1) the electrocardiogram (ECG) for monitoring ventricular systole onset, and (2) a cine cardiovascular MR (CMR) video of a heartbeat obtained prior to the MRCA scan for finding the timing of diastasis relative to the ECG. Yet, the use of cine-CMR to determine ventricular diastasis may produce cardiac gating errors due to insufficient temporal resolution of the cine-CMR method.

The temporal resolution of a conventional cine acquisition depends on the number of k-space lines acquired per segment (of k-space) per heart beat, herein denoted lines per segment (LPS), multiplied by the acquisition time of each k-space line, commonly known as the repetition time (TR). The number of segments used to complete k-space coverage dictates the number of heartbeats required for the total scan duration. For example, consider the cine parameters: heartbeat duration, 960 ms; field of view (FOV), 35 cm; number of frames, 30; TR, 4 ms; partial Fourier acquisition matrix size, 160 × 256; and LPS, 16. The cine acquisition would span 10 heartbeats, have a true temporal resolution of 64 ms. Extending this example with approximate motion parameters, a mid right coronary artery moving at a peak velocity of 12 cm/s during rapid filling and decelerating constantly over 100 ms toward rest during diastasis will traverse 1.5 mm in the 50 ms preceding diastasis. The reverse motion may be observed transitioning from diastasis to atrial contraction. Therefore, during transitional cardiac phases pertinent to ECG gating, the conventional cine acquisition may not provide the sufficient frame rate to resolve the motion of an RCA

segment. In addition to inadequate temporal resolution, cine acquisitions are susceptible to temporal data-mixing if the subject's heart rate varies during the scan duration.

In this paper, we present a new CMR technique, the Septal Scout, for determining the timing of the diastasis period. The Septal Scout measures ventricular septal motion. We demonstrate that cardiac gating windows determined by the Septal Scout produce sharper MRCA images than windows determined by cine-CMR. To facilitate a user-independent assessment of the diastasis period from cine-CMR data, an empirical approach was chosen based on identifying a plateau period of high frame-to-frame correlations during diastole [8].

Methods

Study subjects

This study was approved by the Research Ethics Board at Sunnybrook Health Sciences Centre, and all volunteer subjects provided written informed consent prior to participation in the study. We studied 9 healthy male volunteers of age 30 ± 4 years. Each volunteer performed a series of breath holds for 15 to 20 heartbeats, during which non-contrast-enhanced MRA was performed. The volunteers were instructed to perform the breath holds in a consistent manner with end-expiration chest positions.

Imaging protocol

All CMR was performed on a GE Optima 450w 1.5 T MR system using a 32-channel cardiac phased-array coil. The coronary artery imaging protocol consisted of 4 steps: (1) Localization: MR-Echo, the stock realtime sequence, was used to find and bookmark the short-axis 2-chamber view, and the long-axis 2-chamber through the left ventricle; (2) Cine CMR gating window calibration: the bookmarked views were used to prescribe a 4-chamber slice for a cine acquisition, from which the diastasis imaging window is determined; (3) MR Septal Scout gating window calibration: from the 4-chamber cine view, a slice is prescribed along the ventricular septum for fast, projection imaging. From this Septal Scout data, the timing of diastasis is also determined; and, (4) High-resolution MRA acquisition: a 4-cm slab is prescribed obliquely from above the aortic valve to the right lateral atrioventricular (AV) groove for 3-dimensional (3D) SSFP imaging. The prescription is intended to cover: the left and right coronary ostia; the entire right coronary artery up to the posterior-lateral branch; the left main (LM), proximal left anterior descending (LAD) and left circumflex (LCx) coronary arteries; and, the associated branches including the proximal conus and sino-atrial (SA) nodal arteries. The latter 3 steps are detailed below.

Cardiac gating calibration using cine CMR

To determine the optimal data acquisition window relative to the R-peak of the ECG, a long-axis 4-chamber cine was acquired using a breath-held SSFP sequence with an in-plane resolution of 1.4×1.8 mm and 5-mm slice thickness (FOV: 35 cm; TR/TE/flip angle: 3.9 ms/1.7 ms/45°; retrospective gating: 30 phases/cardiac cycle; LPS: 16). The cine MR images were cropped by a rectangle that encompassed the 4 chambers of the heart across all frames to reduce the amount of stationary background tissue. The images were exported to MATLAB® and processed using a custom script. Frame-to-frame correlation coefficients (CC) were calculated [8]. The CC function was spline-interpolated and the inflection points (second-derivative nulls) between the E and A wave peaks were used to define the start and end times of the diastasis window (W_{cine}) as determined by cine-CMR. This method of using inflection points is intended to capture the points of approach toward and departure from a diastasis period that is presumed to (1) exist; and (2) be stationary according to the cine-CMR images. In our experience, compared to threshold methods, this approach is more robust against minor motion variations observed within diastasis.

Cardiac gating calibration using the MR Septal Scout

The Septal Scout is a high-temporal-resolution motion monitoring sequence for the ventricular septum. In particular, it observes the expansion and compression of the basal interventricular septum (IVS) along the long axis of the heart, which has been found to correlate with global epicardial motion [9]. The high temporal resolution is achieved by foregoing one dimension of spatial encoding. It is similar to a respiratory navigator for the diaphragm except rather than being interleaved with an imaging sequence, it is currently implemented as a pre-scan for calibrating ECG gating.

The Septal Scout is a modified SSFP sequence with phase encodes turned off. It acquires a one-dimensional (1D) projection of the prescribed septal Scout Plane (5 to 10 mm thick) every TR, which may be as short as 3 ms (see Figure 1a). In our experience, a 10-ms TR provides an ample data frame rate and is chosen to permit relatively fast data processing. The rest of the imaging parameters are as follows: flip angle = 55°; FOV = 31 cm; spatial resolution along the scout = 0.8 mm.

Successive Septal Scout projections are appended along a time axis, much like in M-mode ultrasound (see Figure 1c). An ROI spanning a depth ± 2.5 mm is selected to coincide with the location of the basal septum. This ROI height is set arbitrarily to be small enough for the ROI to be considered rigid, and large enough to allow for spatial signal averaging. The signals along the depth dimension (spatial axis) within the ROI are averaged to improve the signal-to-noise ratio (SNR). Along the time axis, the ROI spans at least one cardiac cycle to provide at least one estimate of diastasis timing. This produces, for the basal septum, an intensity plot over time.

To estimate tissue motion, we apply the gradient optical flow method [10] to the intensity plot. This method calculates pixel intensity variations over time to determine object motion at a location. In our case, this is feasible for tracking septal motion because the septum comprises of non-uniform pixel intensities as seen in Figure 1b. Also, this method may be simplified in our application because to identify the timing of diastasis, we only require displacement and velocity indices on a relative rather than an absolute scale. Hence, the ROI intensity plot is treated as a pseudo-displacement function of tissues moving across the basal septum ROI. The pseudo-velocity function is obtained by taking the temporal derivative of the pseudo-displacement plot, which reveals the characteristic E and A waves that border the diastasis period (see Figure 1d). Similar to the processing of the cine-CC function, inflection points between the E and A waves are considered to be the start and end times of the diastasis period.

The Septal Scout acquisition is triggered from the R-peak of the ECG and lasts 5 seconds. Currently, the scout is performed at the beginning and end of a practice 20-second breath hold. In over half of the subjects, heart rate was observed to increase during the course of a 20-second breath hold by 5 to 10 bpm. The intersection of diastases across all heartbeats observed produces the multi-heartbeat diastasis window (W_{sep}) as determined by the Septal Scout. The two Septal Scout acquisitions at the beginning and end of a breath hold allow us to find a cardiac rest period that is robust across the expected heart rate variation. This is not feasible for the cine acquisition, which needs to acquire data for the full duration of the breath hold.

Comparison with tissue doppler echocardiography

It has been shown that tissue Doppler echocardiography (TDE) of the IVS was able to identify accurate coronary artery diastasis windows [9]. The first six subjects in this study formed a subcohort for comparing the Septal Scout to the TDE technique with respect to the timing estimation of diastasis windows. TDE of the IVS was performed by an experienced ultrasound technologist in this subcohort using a Philips iE33 system with a phased array transducer operating at 3.5 MHz. The IVS was imaged in an apical 4-chamber view at 150 fps; velocity was resolved at ± 15 cm/s near the basal septum. Diastasis window estimates were determined from the IVS velocity plots using a custom MATLAB® script. For each velocity plot, similar to the Septal Scout method, the inflection points between the E and A waves were determined to be the start and end of the associated diastasis period, respectively.

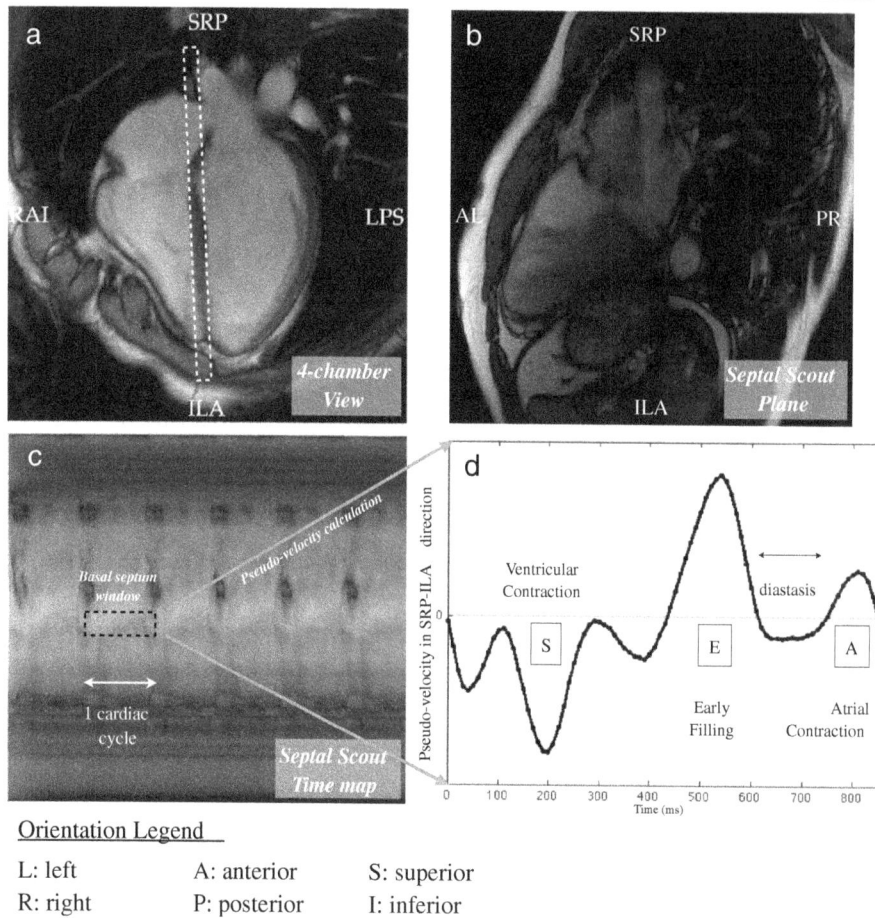

Orientation Legend

L: left   A: anterior   S: superior

R: right   P: posterior   I: inferior

Figure 1 An illustration of the Septal Scout method. The Septal Scout monitors long-axis motion of the septum using projection imaging of a slice along the ventricular septum. **(a)** The 4-chamber long-axis view from which the Septal Scout is prescribed is shown. The dashed white rectangle shows the graphical prescription of the Scout Plane, which is perpendicular to the 4-chamber view and runs along the ventricular septum. **(b)** An image of the Scout Plane is shown here for illustration. The Septal Scout does not acquire this image, rather, it acquires much more quickly projections (in the AL-PR direction) of this image plane. **(c)** Successive Septal Scouts are displayed as vertical line images and appended along a horizontal time axis. An ROI (dotted black box) is chosen at a depth near the basal septum spanning one cardiac cycle. The image intensities in this ROI are processed using optical gradients to form a pseudo-velocity graph. **(d)** The pseudo-velocity graph is shown. The diastasis period is visible as a plateau region in between the early filling (E-wave) and atrial contraction (A-wave) cardiac phases.

MRCA acquisition

Each volunteer was imaged twice with 3D SSFP, once with the cine-calibrated imaging window, and once with the septal-motion-calibrated window. The parameters for the acquisition were: 3D fat-suppressed SSFP; TR = 3.9 ms; TE = 1.9 ms; flip angle = 55°; FOV = 35 × 35 × 4 cm; resolution = 1.5 × 1.5 × 2.0 mm; slice oversampling = none. The sequence employed a Cartesian trajectory, with an $\alpha/2$ pre-pulse and 20 dummy cycles to obtain steady state. The number of TRs per heart beat, and thus also the total scan time, varied with the gating window used.

Qualitative image comparison

Subjective assessment of image quality was performed by two experienced observers, who were blinded to each other's results and to the technique with which each dataset was acquired. A 5-point Likert scale was used: 0 = not visible; 1 = artery visible with significant blurring of edges; 2 = artery visible with moderate blurring of edges; 3 = artery visible with mild blurring of edges; and, 4 = artery visible with sharply defined edges. Both observers graded, for each 3D dataset, the large vessel segments: proximal RCA, mid RCA, LM, proximal LAD, and prox LCx; and the small vessel segments: 1st acute marginal branch, 1st obtuse marginal branch, 1st diagonal branch, conus artery, and SA nodal artery. The scores were averaged within each vessel size category.

Quantitative image comparison

To compare the image quality of the two gating calibration methods, we measured the SNR, and vessel sharpness. The SNR was determined by taking the mean signal intensity measured in a region-of-interest (ROI) in the aortic root blood pool and dividing it by the standard deviation of a noise ROI measured outside the patient. The same ROIs were used between the cine-calibrated and Septal-Scout-calibrated scans. Vessel sharpness was determined by full width half maximum (FWHM) measurements that are made using a custom MATLAB® script. For each coronary artery segment, 3 cross-sectional views at 1 mm increments along the vessel were selected. For each view, the inside of the vessel is selected by a user via a mouse click. The centroid is automatically identified as the centre, and 12 radial edge profiles separated by 30° are generated. The FWHMs are calculated and averaged across the radial profiles. In this case, the FWHM serve as both a metric of vessel boundary sharpness, and an estimate of vessel diameter.

Statistical analysis

Pearson's correlation coefficient and Bland-Altman analysis were used to compare the start and end times of the diastasis windows as estimated by the Septal Scout and tissue Doppler techniques. General statistics are reported as mean ± standard deviation.

The Wilcoxon signed-ranks test was used to test for differences in all the qualitative as well as quantitative metrics between the Septal Scout and cine-CMR methods for gating window identification. This test is also used to evaluate whether the inter-observer scores are significantly different. All comparisons from the signed-ranks tests are presented as the median [IQR], where IQR is the interquartile range representing the difference between the third and first quartile marks. A

two-tailed test with P-values ≤ 0.05 was interpreted to indicate statistical significance.

Results

Comparison of the Septal Scout with tissue Doppler echocardiography

In the sub-cohort component of this study comparing the Septal Scout to TDE of the IVS, high agreement was observed in the estimation of the start and end times of the diastasis window. The correlation coefficients of the two techniques for both the start and end times were greater than 0.98 ($p < 0.001$). Figure 2 shows the corresponding Bland-Altman plots. We modified the Bland–Altman technique to plot, on the independent axis, the TDE timing data instead of the mean between the two compared data sets. The purpose of this was to reflect the fact that the TDE timing data is in this case the reference.

Angiography image quality

MRCA was successfully performed in all subjects. The identified start and end times of the cardiac gating windows by the Septal Scout and cine-CMR techniques are summarized in Table 1; the corresponding Bland-Altman plots are shown in Figure 3. A small amount of heart rate variability (HRV) of typically less than 10 bpm was observed in each subject during the breath holds. In all of the subjects except one, the heart rate was monotonically increasing over the course of the breath hold; the exceptional case experienced a monotonic decrease.

Vessel segments were sharper when imaged during the Septal Scout gating windows for both the large and small

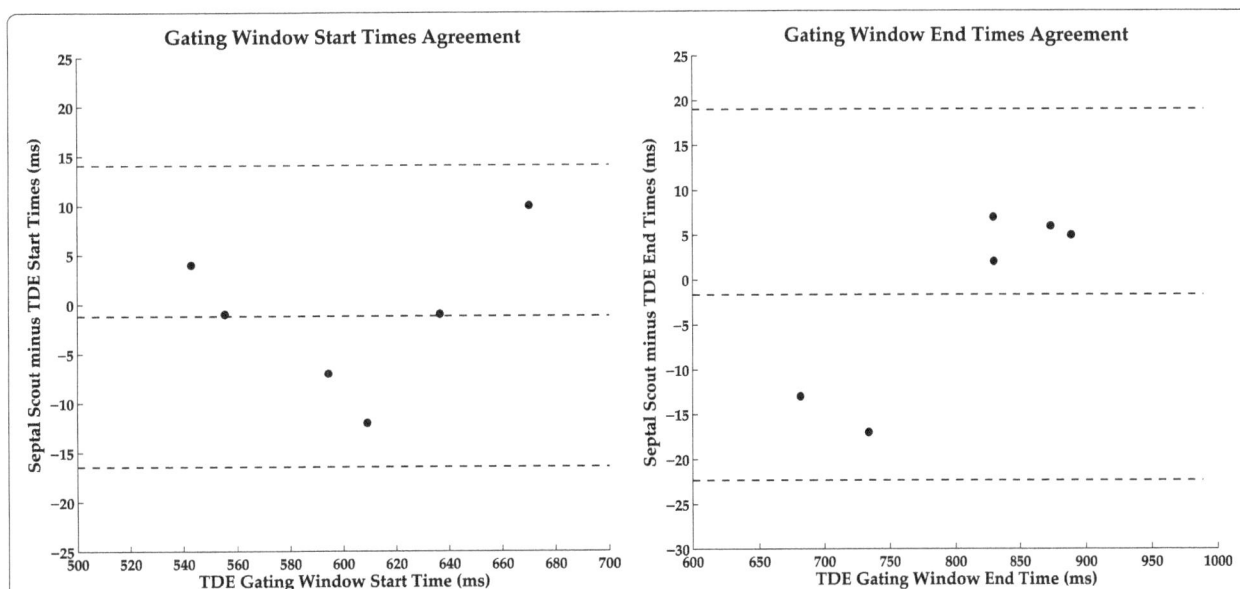

Figure 2 Comparison of the Septal Scout with tissue Doppler. Bland-Altman plots showing high agreement of the start and end times (relative to the R-peak on the ECG) of gating windows determined by the TDE and MRI Septal Scout methods.

Table 1 Septal Scout vs Cine-CMR gating windows

Subject #	Heart rate (BPM)	Gating window start time* (ms)		Gating window end time* (ms)		Gating window duration (ms)	
		Septal scout	Cine-CMR	Septal scout	Cine-CMR	Septal scout	Cine-CMR
1	56 - 62	621	602	780	825	159	223
2	68 - 75	545	580	640	662	95	82
3	61 - 67	591	571	690	710	99	139
4	55 - 60	672	649	816	850	144	201
5	53 - 59	675	652	832	853	157	201
6	52 - 62	650	676	810	846	160	170
7	59 - 63	584	575	721	777	137	202
8	55 - 50	604	582	797	757	193	175
9	68 - 72	615	644	733	771	118	127

*Start and end times are relative to the R-peak on the ECG.

diameter groups (see Figure 4). The large vessel segments were consistently measured to have a smaller FWHM in the Septal Scout group than the cine-CMR group, with a significant difference ($p = 0.03$) between the median widths of 3.6 [0.7] mm versus 4.1 [0.6] mm, respectively. The small vessel segments were also measured to have a significantly ($p = 0.03$) smaller FWHM in the Septal Scout group than in the cine-CMR group, with median widths of 2.1 [0.2] mm versus 2.4 [0.2] mm, respectively.

Subjective assessment of vessel sharpness also showed an improvement for the Septal Scout-gated scans. Large vessel segments from the Septal Scout group obtained higher sharpness scores from both Observer 1 (2.8 [0.9] vs. 1.9 [1.2], $p = 0.008$; see Figure 5) and Observer 2 (3.3 [0.9] vs. 2.5 [1.0], $p = 0.008$; see Figure 6). Similarly, small vessel segments from the Septal Scout group obtained higher sharpness scores from Observer 1 (2.4 [0.8] vs.

1.7 [0.8], $p = 0.016$; see Figure 5) and Observer 2 (3.0 [1.1] vs. 2.0 [1.0], $p = 0.016$; see Figure 6). The difference between the scores of two observers were not statistically significant (Large vessels: 2.6 [1.2] vs. 3.1 [1.1], $p = 0.10$; small vessels: 2.3 [0.7] vs. 2.4 [1.0], $p = 0.49$). Sample images and the corresponding gating windows are shown in Figures 7, 8, and 9.

There were no significant differences in SNR between the MRCA images acquired with the Septal Scout and cine-CMR techniques (23.5 [12.3] vs. 25.0 [6.6], $p = 0.18$).

Discussion

In this study, we have successfully applied the MR Septal Scout technique to find more accurate cardiac gating windows than those obtained by cine-CMR. The use of gating windows determined by the Septal Scout led to a significant increase in vessel sharpness in MRCA images.

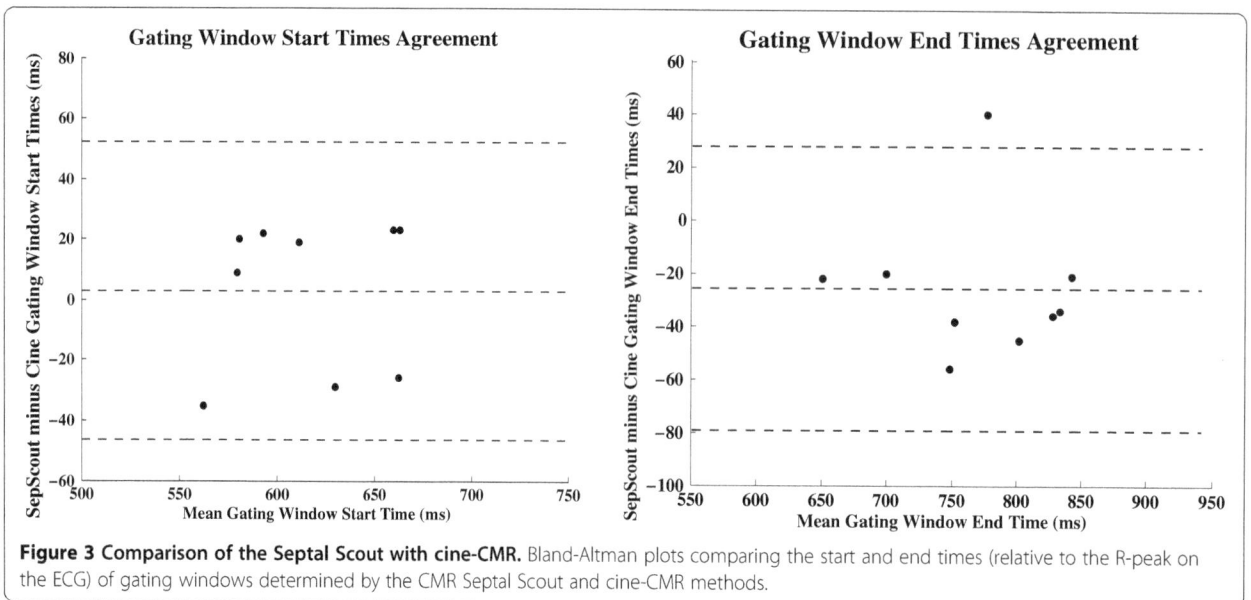

Figure 3 Comparison of the Septal Scout with cine-CMR. Bland-Altman plots comparing the start and end times (relative to the R-peak on the ECG) of gating windows determined by the CMR Septal Scout and cine-CMR methods.

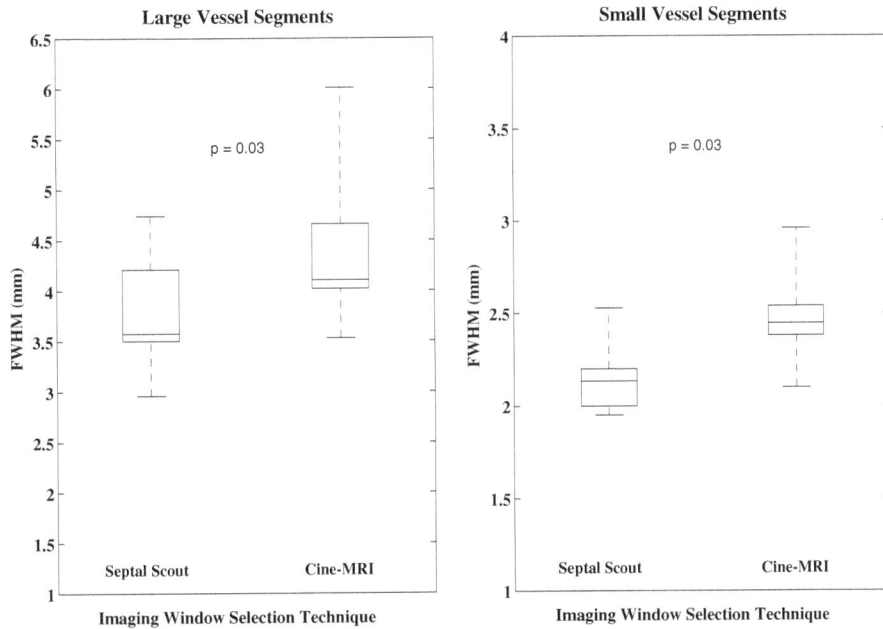

Figure 4 Full width half maximum measurements of vessel segments. Box plots of the FWHM measurements of the large and small vessel segments groups comparing the Septal Scout to the cine-CMR technique for selecting the timing parameters of imaging windows.

The principle behind the Septal Scout is to trade off extraneous spatial data, specifically a dimension of spatial encoding, for faster sampling of a targeted component of cardiac motion, specifically, the 1D long-axis motion of the basal ventricular septum. While the comparison of the Septal Scout to the cine-CMR technique is affected by other factors such as (1) imaging tissues in the Septal Scout plane which is perpendicular to the 4-chamber plane, and (2) acquiring 1D vs 2D data, it is believed that the superior temporal resolution of the Septal Scout is the most important factor for its improved performance.

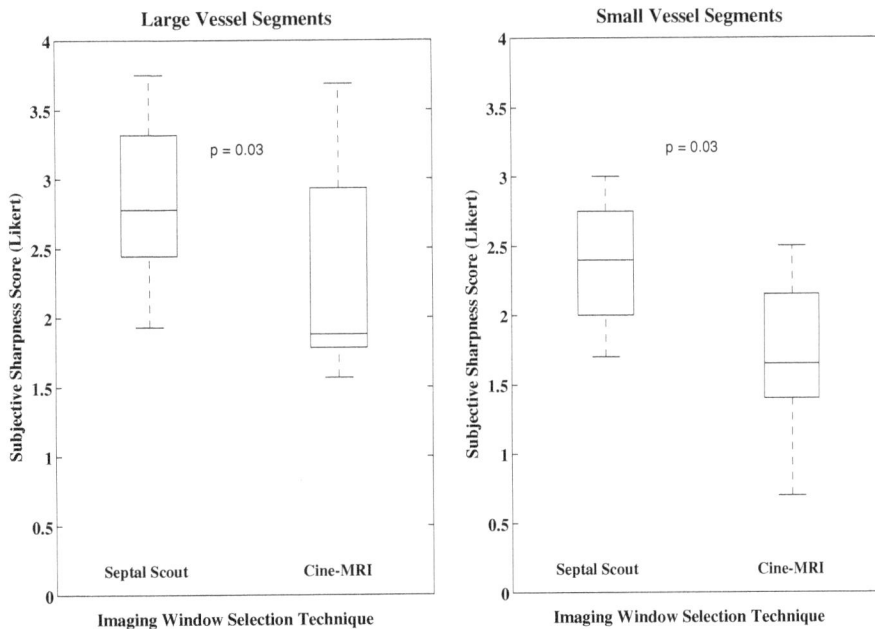

Figure 5 Observer #1 sharpness scores. Box plots of the Observer #1 sharpness scores of the large and small vessel segments groups comparing the Septal Scout to the cine-CMR technique.

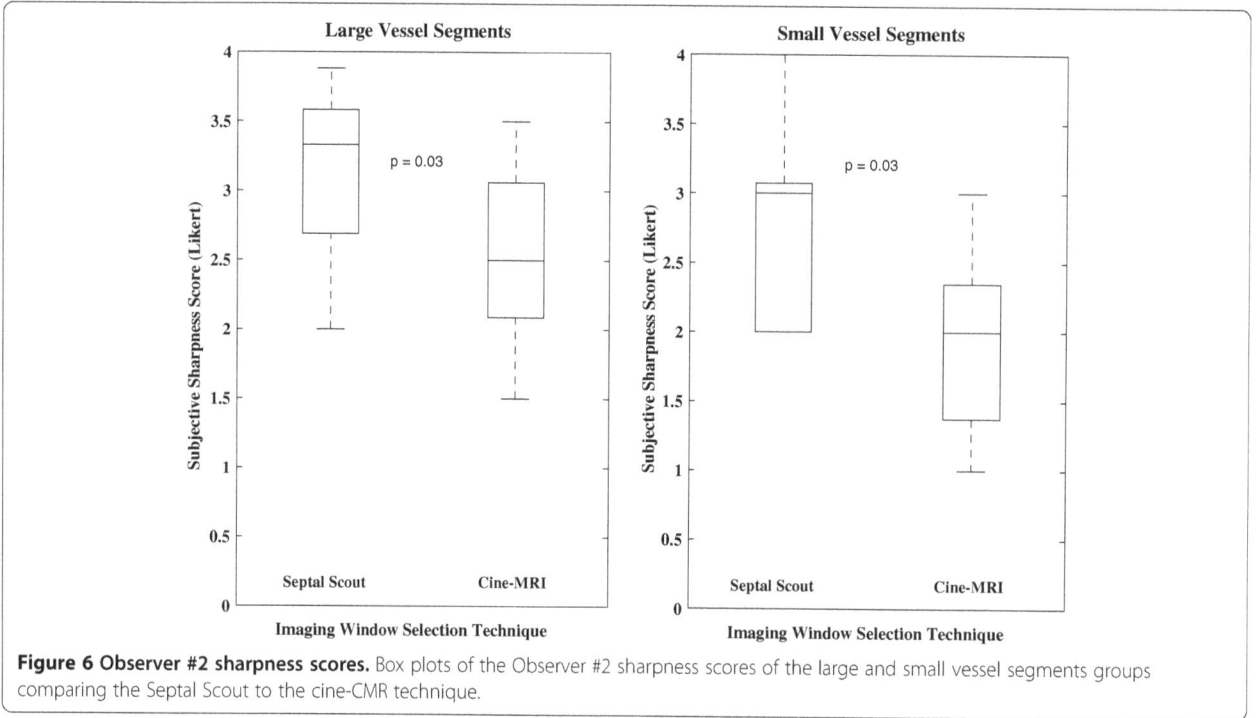

Figure 6 Observer #2 sharpness scores. Box plots of the Observer #2 sharpness scores of the large and small vessel segments groups comparing the Septal Scout to the cine-CMR technique.

In the subcohort comparison between the Septal Scout and TDE methods, the timing differences of the estimated diastasis periods sometimes reached as high as 15–20 ms. Since the Bland-Altman plots (see Figure 2) reveal no biases, this may reflect inherent variability within the methods.

The Septal Scout technique was superior to the cine-CMR technique in terms of being able to adapt to the

HRV that was observed during a breath hold. For cine-CMR, modest HRV may cause incorrect data binning, which in turn may cause motion blurring. In contrast, the Septal Scout essentially freezes cardiac motion within its 10-ms frames. The superior acquisition speed permits the identification of the diastasis window on a per heart-beat basis, and provides a set of gating windows over multiple heartbeats that varies with heart rate. This ability to

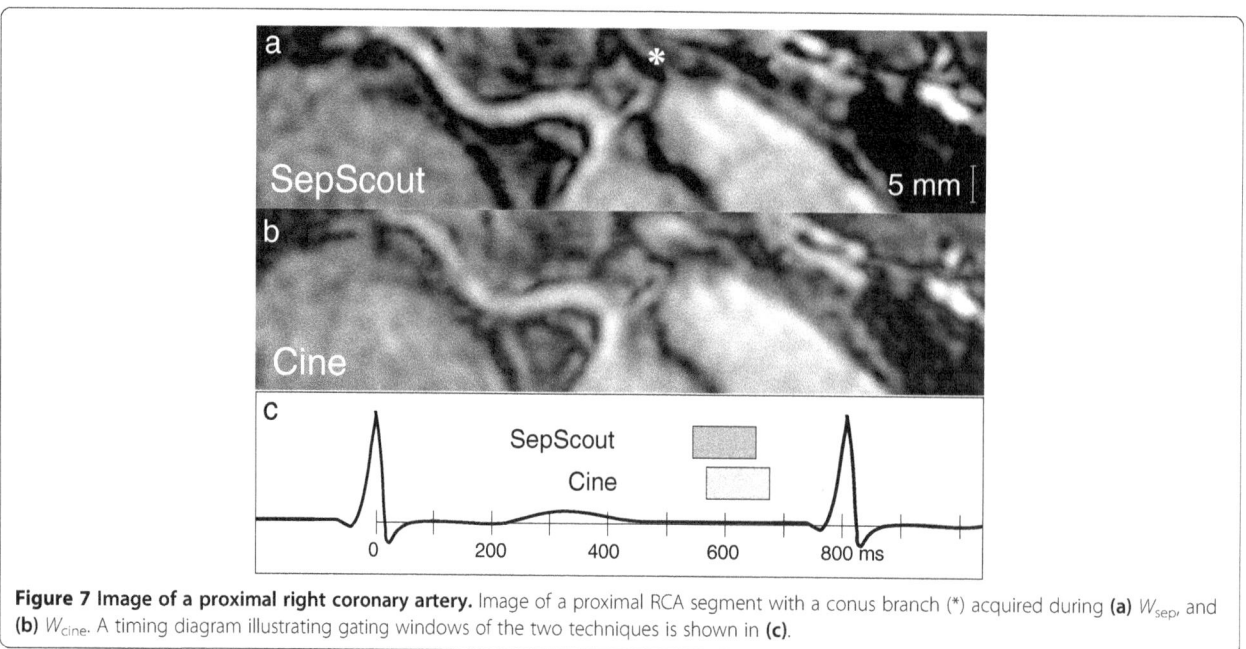

Figure 7 Image of a proximal right coronary artery. Image of a proximal RCA segment with a conus branch (*) acquired during **(a)** W_{sep}, and **(b)** W_{cine}. A timing diagram illustrating gating windows of the two techniques is shown in **(c)**.

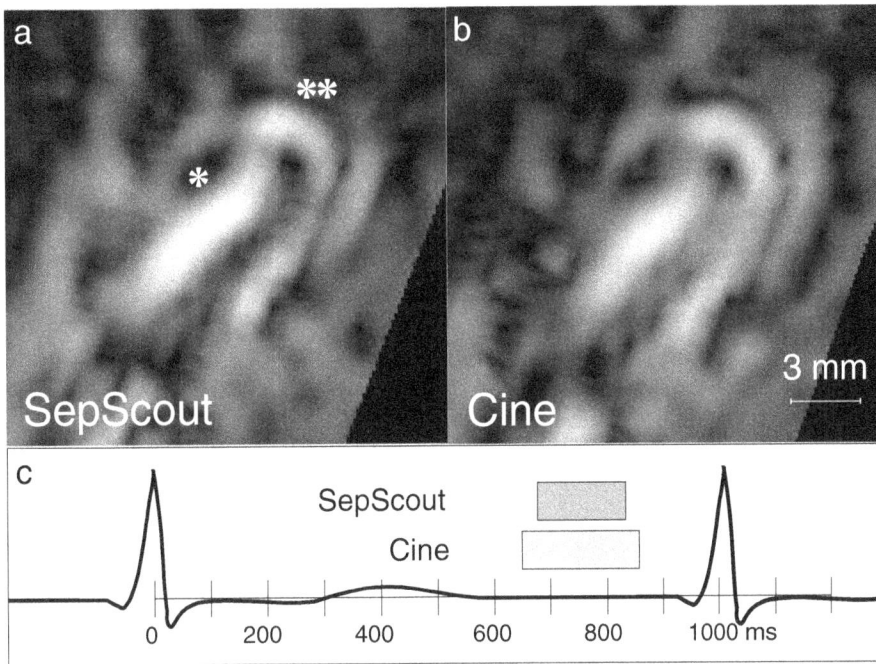

Figure 8 Image of a conus artery. Image of a conus artery (**) branching off of the proximal RCA (*) acquired during **(a)** W_{sep}, and **(b)** W_{cine}. A timing diagram illustrating gating windows of the two techniques is shown in **(c)**.

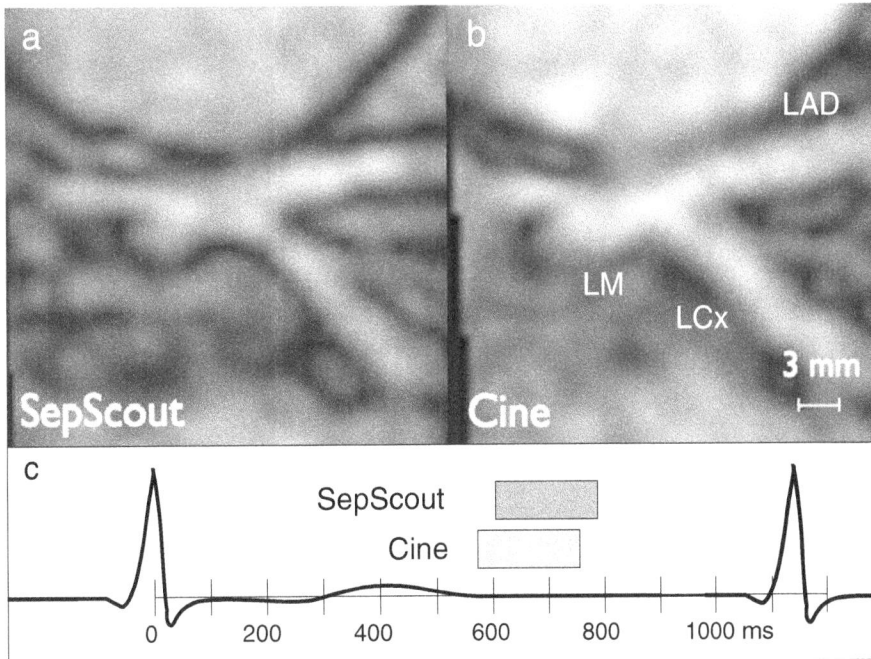

Figure 9 Image of a left main artery bifurcation. Image of a left main artery bifurcation acquired during **(a)** W_{sep}, and **(b)** W_{cine}. A timing diagram illustrating gating windows of the two techniques is shown in **(c)**.

determine a gating window that is robust across an observed range of HRV during a breath hold is believed to have contributed to the ability of the Septal Scout method to obtain sharper MRCA images in this study.

As a result of the slice excitation, the Scout Plane extends beyond the beating septum to include many unwanted static signal sources such as from the chest and back. The Septal Scout acquisition may alternatively be obtained by the use of 2D RF excitation pulses to further isolate the ventricular septum. For example, a 2D spiral RF pulse [11,12] may be used to excite a cylinder of tissue along the septal wall on the 4-chamber long-axis plane. Note that 2D RF pulses typically require longer durations. This alternative implementation must therefore consider the trade-off between the duration of the excitation pulse, the quality of the excitation profile, and the resultant TR. Generally, sharper excitation profiles require longer excitation pulses. A TR equal to or less than 10 ms should be maintained to provide sufficient temporal resolution for motion tracking. The design specifics of this alternative excitation method are left for future investigation.

The use of a 10-ms TR for the Septal Scout may introduce susceptibility-related artifacts that otherwise may be avoided with a shorter TR. In this study, however, this did not appear to have affected the ability of the Septal Scout to monitor the displacement of the basal septum and identify periods of quiescence. This is likely because the basal septum is a small ROI in a well-shimmed area.

The FWHM assessment of vessel profiles required the reformatting of vessel segments into a cross-sectional orientation. Theoretically, the asymmetric intrinsic resolution of the MRA data (1.5×1.5 mm^2 in-slice; 2 mm through slice) may affect the FWHM comparison if the actual vessel orientations were significantly different between the cine-guided vs. the septal scout-guided acquisitions. For example, if one method produced a gating window during which a vessel segment is oriented much more perpendicular to the slice orientation of the 3D image acquisition, the vessel cross-sections would appear sharper due to the higher in-slice resolution. We did not, however, observe this effect. The intrinsic resolution was near isotropic. And, this effect should not have systematically favoured one method of the study in particular.

The Septal Scout, in general, is sensitive to placement. There are two main types of septal localization errors: vertical and horizontal. Prescribed from a 4-chamber long-axis cine, vertical localization is achieved by aligning the Scout Plane such that it contains the septal wall throughout the cardiac cycle. Missing the septum at any time will result in the loss of the signal of interest. This type of error should be avoided. The prescription of the

4-chamber long-axis plane is the horizontal localization. Deviation by the 4-chamber cine from the horizontal plane of the heart is, however, not a significant concern. This is because the long-axis septal motion will still be the dominant component of motion observed on the Septal Scout. Assuming a good placement, respiratory and general patient motion may still introduce septal localization errors. Currently, this method relies on the use of breath holds to suppress respiratory motion. Like previous authors, this was found to work well for breath holds near or under 20 seconds [13].

In this study, a gradient optical flow calculation [10] was used to determine septal motion from the Septal Scout data. A correlation-based alternative was considered during experimental design using preliminary data. In this approach, a line ROI from a Septal Scout projection was tracked using maximum correlation to a new position in the subsequent projection. The ROI is updated at the new position, and tracked in the subsequent projection, and so on. In our initial experience, the correlation approach was inferior to the optical flow approach because the line ROIs have very few data points to statistically overcome image noise.

In CMR, navigators are 1D signals that monitor the displacement of an edge structure such as the diaphragm during tidal breathing [14]. Navigators are typically performed continuously (on their own and interleaved with imaging) and processed in realtime in conjunction with ECG gating to provide triggers for starting and stopping image data acquisition depending on the navigator position and cardiac phase. The Septal Scout may potentially be adapted into a Septal Navigator. The Septal Navigator function would be a realtime cardiac motion signature; it also may be compatible with a respiratory navigator. In an integrated gating system, the ECG R-peak may be used to trigger contrast preparation and the Septal Navigator may be used to trigger the start and end of imaging per heartbeat. A possible limitation may arise from the Septal Navigator interfering with the image acquisition during diastasis. The Scout Plane excitation may saturate signal sources in coplanar segments of coronary arteries, making them unavailable for imaging. 2D RF pulse excitations may be a solution being less intrusive than a slice excitation. Another issue is that the Septal Navigator may not maintain steady state magnetization, and may require a switch to low-flip-angle spoiled gradient recall methods instead of SSFP. These potential considerations are left for future investigations.

Direct cardiac motion monitoring is a shared concept between the Septal Scout and the anterior left ventricular (LV) wall navigator presented in the past by Stuber et al. [15]. A major distinguishing feature, however, is the location of the Septal Scout versus that of the LV navigator. Different epicardial regions have been known to have different diastasis timings [4,5,16]. The Septal Scout is more suitable for whole-heart angiography; basal septal diastasis is an accurate surrogate for ventricular diastasis [9]. To our knowledge, there has not been work presented on the CMR monitoring of septal motion for determining cardiac gating windows.

The performance of the Septal Scout in the presence of cardiac pathology has yet to be tested. In general, septal wall defects will likely change the relationship between septal and ventricular diastasis. One particularly problematic condition is known as the Septal Bounce, which is a paradoxical bouncing motion of the IVS initially toward and subsequently away from the LV during the beginning of diastole [17]. This condition is typically observed in constrictive cardiomyopathy, and is visible on a 4-chamber long-axis cine CMR. Septal Bounce may cause vertical plane localization errors in the Septal Scout technique. The behaviour of the Septal Scout in the presence of various septal defects should be an investigative component in future patient studies. It is important to know if and when septal diastasis is no longer an accurate surrogate for ventricular diastasis.

In our future work, we intend to explore the use of the Septal Scout to determine the onset of ventricular systole, which is currently detected by the R-peak of the ECG. This provides the benefit of not having to maintain an ECG signal to perform cardiac-gated MR imaging. Currently, the ECG signal may arbitrarily deteriorate due to loosened connections at the chest electrodes; also, R-peak detection may fail due to significant T-wave amplification [18], which may sometimes be a problem even with the use of the vector cardiogram.

Conclusions

In this chapter, the MR Septal Scout was shown in a healthy volunteer study to be effective at determining accurate cardiac gating windows. Specifically, this new technique is consistently more accurate than the cine-CMR method, the current clinical standard. The improvement in cardiac gating accuracy provided by the Septal Scout lead to sharper coronary MRA images. Furthermore, the Septal Scout was shown to provide diastasis windows that are in close agreement with those provided by TDE measurements of septal motion.

Abbreviations

1D: One-dimensional; 2D: Two-dimensional; 3D: Three-dimensional; AV: Atrioventricular; CAD: Coronary artery disease; CC: Correlation coefficient; CMR: Cardiovascular magnetic resonance; CMR-CGS: Cardiovascular magnetic resonance based cardiac gating system; ECG: Electrocardiogram; FOV: Field of view; FWHM: Full width half maximum; HRV: Heart rate variability; IQR: Inter-quartile range; IVS: Interventricular septum; LAD: Left anterior descending (artery); LCx: Left circumflex (artery); LM: Left main (artery); LV: Left ventricle; MR: Magnetic resonance; MRA: Magnetic resonance angiography; RCA: Right coronary artery; RF: Radio-frequency; ROI: Region of interest; SNR: Signal to noise ratio; SSFP: Steady state free precession;

TDE: Tissue Doppler echocardiography; TE: Echo time; TR: Repetition time; LPS: Lines per segment.

Competing interests

This work was supported in part by GE Healthcare. The authors declare that there are no other competing interests.

Authors' contributions

GL and GAW contributed in the design of the study and drafted the manuscript. GL coordinated the study and performed the statistical analysis. All authors contributed in discussions and approved the final manuscript.

Acknowledgements

I would like to thank Dr. Anna Zavodni, MD, and Dr. Laura Jimenez Juan, MD, for their work in reviewing images; Rhonda Walcarius, MRT (R) (MR), BSc, for CMR operations; and, Xiu-ling Qi, PhD, for ultrasound operations. This study was supported by funding from the Canadian Institutes of Health Research, and GE Healthcare.

References

1. Stathopoulos I, Jimenez M, Panagopoulos G. The decline in PCI complication rate: 2003–2006 versus 1999–2002. Hellenic J Cardiol. 2009; 50:379–87.
2. Ammann P, La Rocca HB. Procedural complications following diagnostic coronary angiography are related to the operator's experience and the catheter size - Ammann - 2003 - Catheterization and Cardiovascular Interventions - Wiley Online Library. Cathet Cardiovasc Interv. 2003; 59:13–8.
3. Kaufmann PA, Knuuti J. Ionizing radiation risks of cardiac imaging: estimates of the immeasurable. Eur Heart J. 2011; 32:269–71.
4. Johnson K, Patel S, Whigham A, Hakim A, Pettigrew R, Oshinski J. Three? Dimensional, time? Resolved motion of the coronary arteries. J Cardiovasc Magn Reson. 2004; 6:663–73.
5. Shechter G, Resar JR, McVeigh ER. Displacement and velocity of the coronary arteries: cardiac and respiratory motion. IEEE Trans Med Imaging. 2006; 25:369–75.
6. Wang Y, Vidan E, Bergman GW. Cardiac motion of coronary arteries: variability in the rest period and implications for coronary MR Angiography1. Radiology. 1999; 213:751–8.
7. Shechter G, Resar JR, Mcveigh ER. Rest period duration of the coronary arteries: Implications for magnetic resonance coronary angiography. Med Phys. 2005; 32:255.
8. Jahnke C, Paetsch I, Nehrke K, Schnackenburg B, Bornstedt A, Gebker R, Fleck E, Nagel E. A new approach for rapid assessment of the cardiac rest period for coronary MRA. J Cardiovasc Magn Reson. 2005; 7:395–9.
9. Liu GKC, Qi X-L, Robert N, Dick AJ, Wright GA. Ultrasound-guided identification of cardiac imaging windows. Med Phys. 2012; 39:3009–18.
10. Beauchemin SS, Barron JL. The computation of optical flow. ACM Comput Surv. 1995; 27:433–66.
11. Hardy CJ, Cline HE. Broadband nuclear magnetic resonance pulses with two-dimensional spatial selectivity. J Appl Phys. 1989; 66:1513.
12. Pauly J, Nishimura D, Macovski A. A k-space analysis of small-tip-angle excitation. J Magn Reson (1969). 1989; 81:43–56.
13. Jahnke C, Paetsch I, Achenbach S, Schnackenburg B. Coronary MR imaging: breath-hold capability and patterns, coronary artery rest periods, and β-blocker Use. Radiology. 2006; 239:71–8.
14. Bernstein MA, King KF, Zhou XJ. Handbook of MRI Pulse Sequences. Massachusetts, USA: Elsevier Academic Press; 2004.
15. Stuber M, Botnar R, Danias P, Kissinger K. Submillimeter three-dimensional coronary MR angiography with real-time navigator correction: comparison of navigator locations. Radiology. 1999; 212:579–87.

2

Evaluation of a comprehensive cardiovascular magnetic resonance protocol in young adults late after the arterial switch operation for *d*-transposition of the great arteries

Daniel Tobler[1,2], Manish Motwani[3], Rachel M Wald[1,4], Susan L Roche[1], Flavia Verocai[4], Robert M Iwanochko[4], John P Greenwood[3], Erwin N Oechslin[1] and Andrew M Crean[1,4]*

Abstract

Background: In adults with prior arterial switch operation (ASO) for *d*-transposition of the great arteries, the need for routine coronary artery assessment and evaluation for silent myocardial ischemia is not well defined. In this observational study we aimed to determine the value of a comprehensive cardiovascular magnetic resonance (CMR) protocol for the detection of coronary problems in adults with prior ASO for *d*-transposition of the great arteries.

Methods: Adult ASO patients (≥18 years of age) were recruited consecutively. Patients underwent a comprehensive stress perfusion CMR protocol that included measurement of biventricular systolic function, myocardial scar burden, coronary ostial assessment and myocardial perfusion during vasodilator stress by perfusion CMR. Single photon emission computed tomography (SPECT) was performed on the same day as a confirmatory second imaging modality. Stress studies were visually assessed for perfusion defects (qualitative analysis). Additionally, myocardial blood flow was quantitatively analysed from mid-ventricular perfusion CMR images. In unclear cases, CT coronary angiography or conventional angiography was done.

Results: Twenty-seven adult ASO patients (mean age 23 years, 85% male, 67% with a usual coronary pattern; none with a prior coronary artery complication) were included in the study. CMR stress perfusion was normal in all 27 patients with no evidence of inducible perfusion defects. In 24 cases the coronary ostia could conclusively be demonstrated to be normal. There was disagreement between CMR and SPECT for visually-assessed perfusion defects in 54% of patients with most disagreement due to false positive SPECT.

Conclusions: Adult ASO survivors in this study had no CMR evidence of myocardial ischemia, scar or coronary ostial abnormality. Compared to SPECT, CMR provides additional valuable information about the coronary artery anatomy. The data shows that the asymptomatic and clinically stable adult ASO patient has a low pre-test probability for inducible ischemia. In this situation it is likely that routine evaluation with stress CMR is unnecessary.

Keywords: Transposition of the great vessels, Cardiovascular magnetic resonance, Nuclear cardiology, Ischemia

* Correspondence: andrew.crean@uhn.ca
[1]Toronto Congenital Centre for Adults, Peter Munk Cardiac Centre, University Health Network, Toronto General Hospital, 585 University Avenue, 5 N-525, Toronto, ON M5G 2N2, Canada
[4]Department of Medical Imaging, Toronto General Hospital, Toronto, Canada
Full list of author information is available at the end of the article

Background

Good long-term outcome in adults after the arterial switch operation (ASO) has been reported [1]. In historical cohorts, there were intermittent cases after ASO of ostial coronary stenosis and ischemic symptoms occurring as a result of coronary distortion at the re-implantation site [2]. In those early cohorts, cardiovascular events have been reported in up to 7% of childhood ASO survivors, most of these occurred early after the operation [3]. In the current era, late coronary complications are rare in both, children and adults [4]. Nevertheless, evaluation of inducible ischemia in asymptomatic adult ASO patients is controversial. Non-invasive testing for myocardial ischemia, usually performed by stress echocardiography or nuclear imaging techniques, has shown insufficient sensitivity [3].

Cardiovascular Magnetic Resonance (CMR) has emerged as the reference standard for non-invasive imaging of patients with many forms of congenital heart disease [5]. Because children and adults with congenital heart disease often need serial imaging, CMR is the ideal modality to screen and to follow these complex patients due to its lack of ionizing radiation [6]. Furthermore, the recently published CE-MARC trial has established the high diagnostic accuracy of stress CMR in coronary heart disease [7]. Therefore, the objective of this study was to determine the value of a comprehensive CMR protocol in the detection of coronary problems in an adult ASO population.

Methods

Patients

After institutional research ethics board approval, adult ASO survivors (≥18 years) were recruited consecutively during routine clinic visits and studied between March 2009 and July 2013. Patients with a permanent pacemaker were excluded from the study. All patients gave informed written consent.

Patients underwent a comprehensive CMR protocol including rest and stress perfusion, Late Gadolinium Enhancement (LGE), CINE functional analysis and coronary CMR for the detection of occult coronary lesions. Additionally, SPECT imaging was done on the same day as a confirmatory second imaging modality. Figure 1 details the combined single stress - dual perfusion SPECT/CMR protocol.

Cardiovascular magnetic resonance

All patients underwent CMR on a 1.5 T scanner (Siemens Avanto, Siemens Medical Systems, Erlangen, Germany). After standard localizer sequences, steady state free precession (SSFP) images were acquired in the axial and short axis planes providing full ventricular coverage (6 mm slice thickness, 2 mm interslice gap, TR 35-50 ms, reconstructed to 25 frames per cardiac cycle). LGE images were acquired 10 minutes after the injection of a total dose of 0.2 mmol/kg of gadodiamide using a standard segmented inversion recovery gradient echo sequence at slice locations matched to the short axis SSFP images. Whole heart CMR angiography was performed as an axial block acquired in 1 mm thick partitions using a free-breathing navigated 3D SSFP sequence (end-diastolic trigger, in-plane resolution of 1.0-1.5 × 1.0-1.5 mm, gate and drift on, central acquisition window ±2.5 mm). Additional high resolution SSFP cine imaging targeted to the coronary ostia was used in selected cases (1.0 × 1.0 × 2.5-3.0 mm voxel size, TR 50-70 ms).

CMR post processing

Short axis SSFP stacks were manually contoured at end-systole and end-diastole using offline post processing

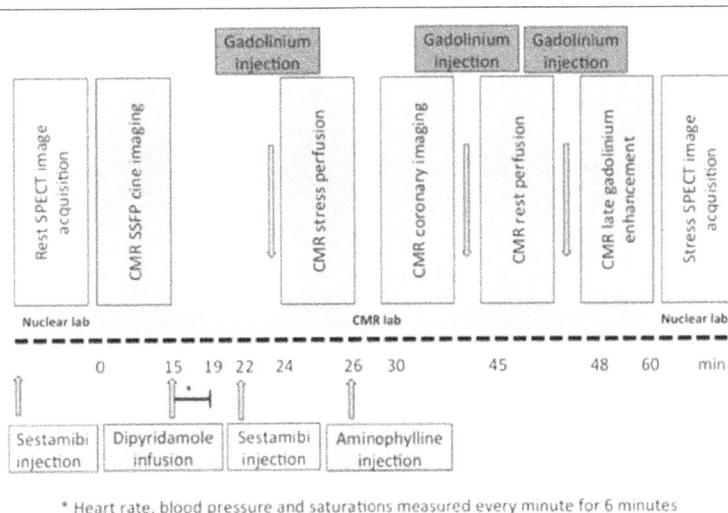

Figure 1 Schematic demonstrating the timeline of the integrated CMR/SPECT assessment of myocardial function, perfusion, scar and coronary anatomy.

software (cmr42, Circle Cardiovascular Imaging, Calgary, Canada) and volumes and ejection fraction calculated using Simpson's rule of discs. Endo- and epicardial contours of the short axis turboflash LGE image stack were traced and percentage of enhanced myocardium was defined as that exceeding a signal intensity of 5SD from a region of interest placed in remote normal myocardium. Whole heart coronary CMR volumes were examined at native resolution and plane of acquisition as well as following centre-line reformat and creation of orthogonal maximum intensity projection views (Vitrea workstation, Vital Images, Minneapolis, USA).

Myocardial blood flow estimation by CMR

Perfusion images were processed offline using previously validated in-house software (PMI 0.4; written in IDL 6.4 (ITT Visual Information Systems, Boulder, CO) [8]. Following manual rigid motion-correction, a circular region of interest was drawn in the basal left ventricular cavity to derive the arterial input function. A myocardial circular region of interest excluding any dark-rim artifact was drawn for the entire myocardium in the mid-ventricular slice. Signal intensity–time data were converted to concentration-time data by subtracting the baseline signal, and myocardial blood flow was estimated at stress and rest using constrained deconvolution with a delayed Fermi-model applied to the first pass [9-11]. Myocardial perfusion reserve was calculated as stress myocardial blood flow divided by rest myocardial blood flow.

Technetium[99m] Sestamibi™ image acquisition and analysis

Images were acquired on a Philips Forte (Philips Medical Systems, Netherlands) fitted with a high resolution VXHR collimator. Prior to SPECT image acquisition, a 30 second left anterior oblique image was acquired with the counts derived from the most count-dense pixel used to determine the time per frame for the SPECT image. Data were acquired in roving field of view step and shoot mode with 3 degree angular steps. Attenuation-corrected data were reconstructed iteratively and subsequently re-binned to create 8 cardiac phases for function and volume assessments. Summed stress, rest and difference scores (SSS, SRS, SDS) were calculated from segmental defect size using a commercially available package (QPS, Cedars-Sinai, Los Angeles, USA).

Combined single stress – dual perfusion protocol

Patients were instructed to withhold all caffeinated products for 24 hours prior to stress imaging. Prior to CMR, patients underwent rest perfusion imaging in the nuclear laboratory following injection of 300Mbq of technetium[99m] methoxyisobutylisonitrile (Sestamibi™). Four hours later the patient was transferred to the CMR suite where vasodilator stress was performed in the magnet with a 4 minute

infusion of dipyridamole at a total dose of 0.56 mg/kg. At 6 minutes from the start of infusion (maximal hyperemia) the patient was given a bolus of 650Mbq intravenous Sestamibi™ followed by a saline flush. The i.v line was then

Table 1 Patient characteristics

	Early repair* n = 24	Late repair n = 3
Age at enrolment (years)	21 ± 3	24 ± 8
Male, n (%)	21 (88)	2 (66)
Age at surgery (days)	6 ± 5	397 ± 592
Era of ASO surgery	1986 - 1991	1979 - 1985
Cardiac anatomy		
TGA with IVS	14	-
TGA with VSD	10	2
Taussig-Bing	-	1
Additional lesions		
Atrial septal defect	2	1
Coarctation	2	1
Subvalvular aortic stenosis	-	1
Subvalvular pulmonary stenosis	-	1
Coronary pattern		
1LCx2R (usual)	17	1
2RLCx (single ostium)	2	2
1L2RCx (CX from RCA)	4	
1Cx2RL (LAD from RCA)	1	
Bypass time, min	141 ± 99	203 ± 25
Cross clamp time, min	99 ± 22	55 ± 39
Additional repair		
Takeuchi repair	1	-
RV-PA conduit	-	1
Subclavian flap repair of coarctation	1	1
End-to-end repair of coarctation	1	-
Indication for exam		
Chest pain	5	2
Coronary surveillance	19	1
Prior ischemia testing as a child[†]		
Yes	13	1
No	9	2
Unknown	2	-
Type of prior ischemia testing		
Treadmill	1	
Thallium	8	
Technetium	7	
Coronary angiography	3	

IVS = Interventricular septum; RV-PA = Right ventricular to pulmonary artery; TGA = Transpostion of the great arteries; VSD = Ventricular septal defect.
*Early repair defined as occurring within the first 30 days of life.
†Median number = 1 (range 1–3).

reconnected to the power injection and a bolus of 0.05 mmol/kg gadodiamide injected at 5 ml/sec followed by a saline flush of 25 ml at 5 ml/sec. An saturation recovery gradient echo sequence was used to acquire 3 short axis slices (base, mid ventricle and apex) every heart beat (8 mm slice thickness, in plane resolution $1.5\text{-}1.8 \times 1.5 \times 1.8$ mm, 80 cardiac phases). Once the stress portion was complete, dipyridamole was reversed in every case with a slow intravenous bolus of aminophylline 2 mg/kg up to a maximum dose of 200 mg, until complete relief of symptoms or return to baseline heart rate. After a minimum period of 20 minutes the rest perfusion CMR study was acquired with the same anatomic and technical parameters. At the end of the examination the patient was transferred to the nuclear laboratory where SPECT perfusion images pertaining to the in-magnet episode of stress were obtained. Time between in-magnet injection of Sestamibi™ during stress and SPECT image acquisition in the nuclear laboratory was set at 60 minutes.

Statistical methods

Statistical analysis was performed using SPSS software version 20 (IBM SPSS 20, 2011) Descriptive statistics of continuous data are presented as mean ± standard deviation. Changes from baseline to hyperemic flow were compared by the paired Student's t test.

Table 2 Comparison of patient characteristics between the studied cohort and the entire cohort of ASO patients under active care

	STUDY COHORT	TORONTO COHORT	p-value
	n = 27	n = 65	
Age at enrolment (years)	21 ± 3*	24 ± 8	NS
Male, n (%)	23 (85)	40 (62)	0.03
Age at surgery (days)	6 ± 5*	6 ± 5	NS
Era of ASO surgery	1979 - 1991	1979 - 1991	
Cardiac anatomy			
TGA with IVS	14	36	NS
TGA with VSD	12	27	
Taussig-Bing	1	2	
Coronary pattern			
1LCx2R (usual)	18	42	NS
2RLCx (single ostium)	4	5	
1L2RCx (CX from RCA)	4	13	
1Cx2RL (LAD from RCA)	1	3	
Bypass time, min	141 ± 99*	150 ± 54	NS
Cross clamp time, min	99 ± 22*	93 ± 21	NS

ASO = arterial switch operation, Cx = circumflex artery; IVS = intact ventricular septum; LAD = left coronary artery; RCA = right coronary artery; TGA = transposition of the great arteries; VSD = ventricular septum defect.
*Patients with early repair only.

Results

Patient population

Of 65 adult ASO patients under active care in our center at the time of inclusion, 33 patients were approached consecutively and 28 agreed to participate. One patient was claustrophobic at the time of the CMR examination and no useful data were obtained. The CMR results are therefore based on 27 patients in total. Basic demographic data are provided in Table 1. Historically, at the Hospital for Sick Children in Toronto, ASOs were performed only in complex patients (with ventricular septal defect) until 1986. After 1986, the strategy changed and also simple TGA (with intact ventricular septum) were operated with the Jatene procedure. In our cohort, 2

Table 3 CMR (n = 27) and SPECT (n = 25) findings*

	Stress CMR	Coronary ostia	LGE	SPECT
Patient 1	N	N	No	A – SDS 3
Patient 2	N	N	No	N
Patient 3	N	N	No	N
Patient 4	N	N	No	N
Patient 5	N	N	No	N
Patient 6	N	N	No	A – SDS 2
Patient 7	N	N	Yes	A – SDS 2
Patient 8	N	N	No	E – SDS 0
Patient 9	N	N	No	N
Patient 10	N	N	No	N
Patient 11	N	A	Yes	N
Patient 12	N	A	No	N
Patient 13	N	N	No	E – SDS 0
Patient 14	N	N	No	Declined
Patient 15	N	N	No	A – SDS 3
Patient 16	N	N	No	N
Patient 17	N	N	No	A – SDS 2
Patient 18	N	N	No	A – SDS 2
Patient 19	N	N	No	N
Patient 22[§]	N	A	No	A – SDS 4
Patient 23	N	N	No	N
Patient 25	N	N	Yes	A – SDS 0
Patient 26	N	N	No	E – SDS 0
Patient 27	N	N	No	E – SDS 0
Patient 28	N	N	No	A – SDS 5
Patient 29	N	N	No	Declined
Patient 30	N	N	No	N

*Note that patients are not all numbered consecutively.
[§]Patient 22 was scored as having an abnormal proximal right coronary artery on CMR, however SPECT perfusion defect was in the LAD territory with normal left main ostium and no LGE on CMR (see text).
N = normal; A = abnormal; E = equivocal; LGE = late gadolinium enhancement; SDS = summed difference score; N/A = not available.

patients with late repair had complex TGA and one patient had Taussig Bing anatomy (DORV with subpulmonary ventricular septal defect and TGA). In all of these 3 patients, a pulmonary artery banding was performed as palliation prior to ASO. Of study patients, 23 (85%) were male (compared to 62% in the entire cohort under active care, p = 0.03). Otherwise, patients studied by CMR did not differ in basic demographic details compared to ASO patients under active care (Table 2) [1].

CMR studies

The imaging protocol was completed successfully in all participants. Mean left ventricular and right ventricular ejection fraction were 55 ± 5% and 51 ± 7%, respectively and mean left and right end-diastolic volume assessment indexed to body surface area were 105 ± 22 ml/m^2 and 113 ± 23 ml/m^2, respectively.

Stress perfusion was visually normal in all participants with no evidence of inducible perfusion defects (Table 3) despite appropriate physiologic and symptomatic response to dipyridamole (mean rise in rate-pressure product from 8296 bpm*mmHg to 12389 bpm*mmHg, p < 0.01). Whole heart coronary MR angiography was successfully completed in 18 patients (67%) – in the remaining 9 cases, coronary ostial evaluation was instead performed with high resolution SSFP cine imaging due to either poor navigator efficiency with the whole heart sequence and/or constraints on available scan time. LGE images were acquired in all 27 patients but were abnormal in only 3 (Table 3) where very small volumes of enhancement were apparent (Figure 2). The ostia were seen and evaluated as normal in 24 cases, abnormal in 2 cases and nondiagnostic in one case (Table 3).

Cases in which a coronary abnormality was recorded on CMR

In the first of the abnormal cases (Patient 12) the left main coronary artery could not be identified (Figure 3) – however it later transpired that the patient had previously been documented to have a single coronary system arising from the right coronary ostium.

The second case was a patient with possible compression of the right coronary artery on CMR but negative CMR perfusion study (Patient 22). A small SPECT defect was recorded in the LAD territory and was therefore not congruent with the potential right coronary artery anomaly. Subsequent multiplanar reformats of the whole heart data set demonstrated tortuosity rather than obstruction (Figure 4). The patient remains asymptomatic and has declined further investigation by either CT coronary angiography or conventional catheterization.

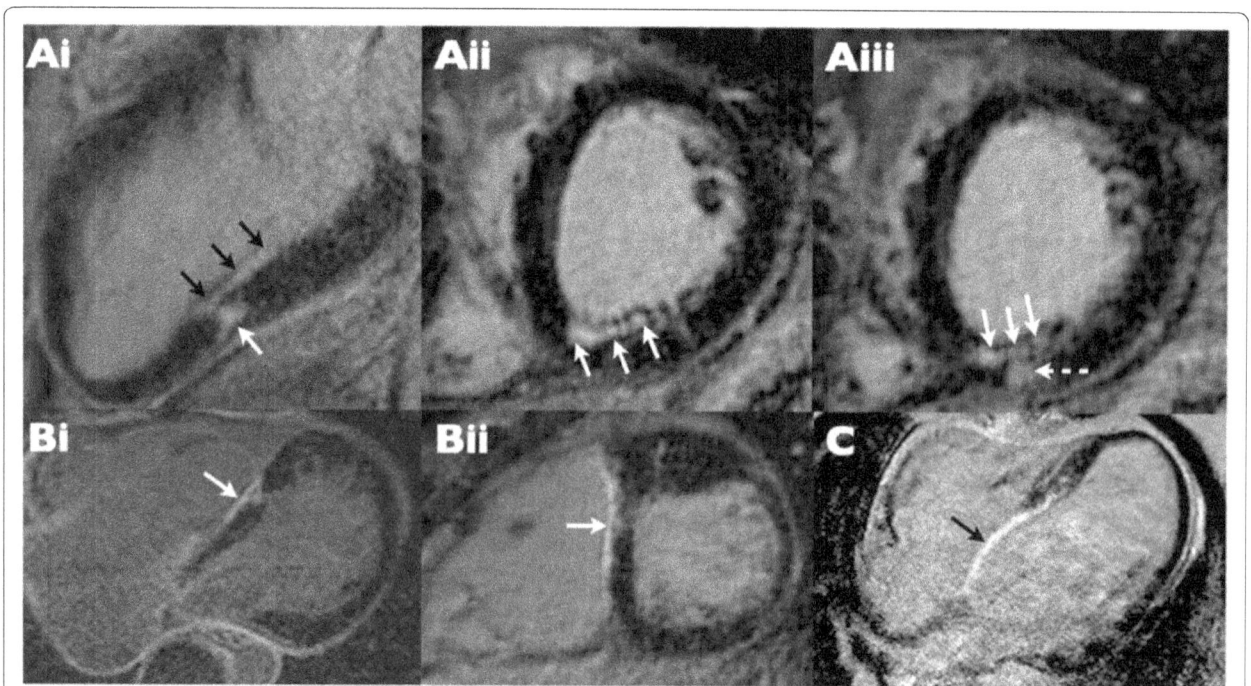

Figure 2 Real and 'pseudo-real' late gadolinium enhancement (LGE) in 3 patients with positive LGE studies. (Ai-iii) Genuine LGE is evident in the mid inferior wall in the 2-chamber view **(Ai)** with both linear (black arrows) and more focal (white arrow) enhancement. Confirmation of these findings is provided by short axis cross cuts through this region, which also show subendocardial (white arrows) and midwall nodular (dotted arrow) myocardial scar. **(Bi-ii)** "Pseudo" LGE (white arrow) is present at the site of ventricular septal defect (VSD) repair shown in 4-chamber **(i)** and short axis **(ii)** views. **(C)** "Pseudo" LGE (black arrow) evident in a large surgical patch placed for VSD repair.

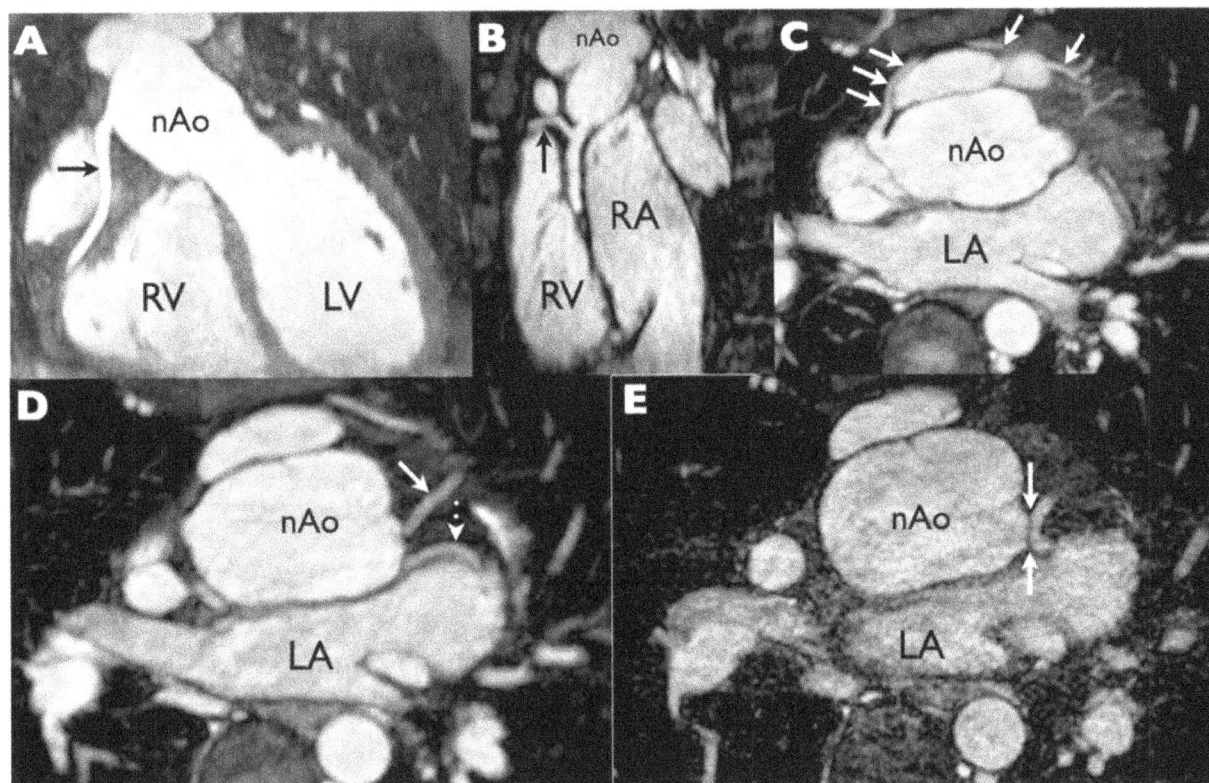

Figure 3 Whole heart coronary magnetic resonance angiography (MRA) at 1×1×1 mm resolution with multiplanar maximum intensity projection reformats to demonstrate the coronary arteries. (A) The right coronary artery (RCA) is seen to have a normal origin and course. **(B)** Excellent image quality is evident from the depiction of a small RCA marginal branch (arrow). **(C)** A large conal branch (arrows) takes a pre-pulmonic course and anastomoses with the left coronary system at the apex. **(D, E)** The left anterior descending (**D** solid arrow) and left circumflex (**D** dotted arrow) coronary arteries are shown in their proximal portions. Although the bifurcation of these vessels is clearly depicted, note that the left main coronary artery is not visible and that there is a'gap' between the aortic root and the LAD/Cx bifurcation even on ultrahigh resolution (0.5 × 0.5 × 0.5 mm) MRA (**E** arrows). This was misinterpreted as an occlusion of the left main segment as the diagnosis of single coronary artery had not been recognized. RV = right ventricle; LV = left ventricle; nAo = neo-aorta; RA = right atrium; LA = left atrium.

In the third case (Patient 11), the ostia were unevaluable due to the presence of bilateral pulmonary artery stents (Figure 5); visual and quantitative CMR perfusion and SPECT were all normal and the subsequent coronary CT was unremarkable.

In one additional case (Patient 4), stress CMR perfusion and whole heart coronary angiography were read as normal but - because of ongoing complaints of chest pain and a SPECT study read as mildly abnormal (SDS 2) - went on to conventional angiography, which confirmed undistorted coronary ostia and normal distal vessels (Figure 6).

Quantitative stress perfusion CMR

There was a significant increase in absolute myocardial blood flow from the resting to vasodilated state (1.39 ± 032 ml/min/g at rest increasing to 3.21 ± 0.62 ml/min/g with stress, p < 0.0001). Nine patients had resting myocardial blood flow greater than 1.5 ml/min/g. Mean myocardial perfusion reserve for the cohort was 2.44 ± 0.77.

Technetium 99 m Sestamibi™ perfusion studies

Twenty-five patients underwent rest-stress SPECT of whom 22/25 underwent the single stress dual perfusion (SSDP) protocol (Table 3). The remaining 3 patients returned for resting SPECT on another day. Two patients declined SPECT examination - one of whom subsequently underwent (normal) CT coronary angiography (Patient 14). Twelve patients were reported as having a normal SPECT scan (entirely normal in 10 cases (40%); probably normal in 2 cases (8%)). Four patients (16%) were reported as equivocal, and 9 (36%) were reported as abnormal. For these latter 13 patients the reported defects were relatively small with a mean summed stress score of 2.65 ± 3.55, mean summed rest score of 1.81 ± 3.36 and a mean summed difference score of 1.1 ± 1.61. One patient with an abnormal SPECT scan (SDS 0) subsequently had normal computed tomographic coronary angiography (Patient 25). Median effective dose was 11 mSv (range 9-14 mSv).

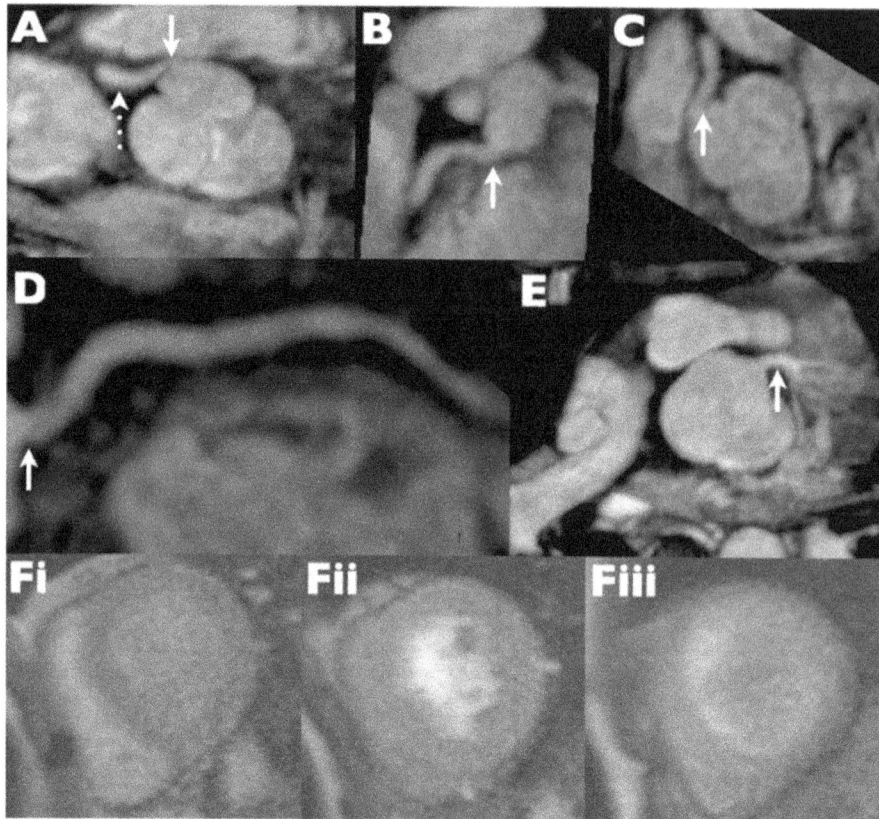

Figure 4 Evaluation of a "kinked" right coronary artery. (A) Straight axial image from a whole heart magnetic resonance angiogram demonstrates an apparent "kink" at the right coronary artery origin. **(B-D)** Subsequent multiplanar and centre line reformats however demonstrate that the ostium is in reality unobstructed. **(E)** The left coronary origin is also unobstructed. **(Fi-iii)** Stress perfusion magnetic resonance frames at basal, mid and apical left ventricular level show no evidence of any inducible perfusion defect. Quantitative perfusion measured in the right coronary territory was normal (not shown).

Discordant CMR-SPECT studies

There was complete agreement between CMR and SPECT for the absence of visually assessed perfusion defects in 11 out of 24 (46%) paired comparisons and disagreement in 13 studies (54%). Disagreements were generally minor – in 5 out of 13 mismatches the SPECT SDS was zero, indicating that the defect seen at SPECT was not due to the presence of inducible ischemia, implicating either scar or artifact as the cause.

In the remaining 8 cases of disagreement the SDS scores were 2 in four patients, SDS 3 in two patients, SDS 4 in one patient and SDS 5 in the final case (Figure 7). In 6 out of these 8 cases CMR demonstrated normal coronary ostia, perfusion and absent LGE suggesting that the SPECT defects were artifactual. In the two other cases, a small amount of LGE was present in one case (patient 7); in the other case (patient 22), proximal RCA kinking was called, with a small SPECT perfusion defect in the LAD territory that was felt to be artifactual in view of the normal ostial left main appearances and absence of LGE in the anterolateral wall (Figure 4).

Discussion

In this observational study of stable adult patients with prior ASO, none had evidence of stress -induced perfusion deficit by CMR, neither visually nor with fully quantitative measurement of blood flow. We further demonstrated a low incidence of overt focal myocardial fibrosis, which principally related to enhancement in the region of prior ventricular septal defect repair rather the intrinsic myocardial injury. Similarly, we were able to visualize the coronary ostia with a high degree of success (24/27 cases) and in no case did coronary CMR show potential proximal luminal obstruction when images were analysed with centre-line reformatting. Importantly, in the one case where there was significant clinical concern regarding ischemic chest pain there was no evidence of perfusion abnormality, myocardial scar or coronary distortion by CMR - corresponding to subsequent normal invasive coronary angiography.

We have demonstrated the feasibility of using CMR with dynamic stress perfusion, ventricular function, coronary artery and scar imaging to provide comprehensive

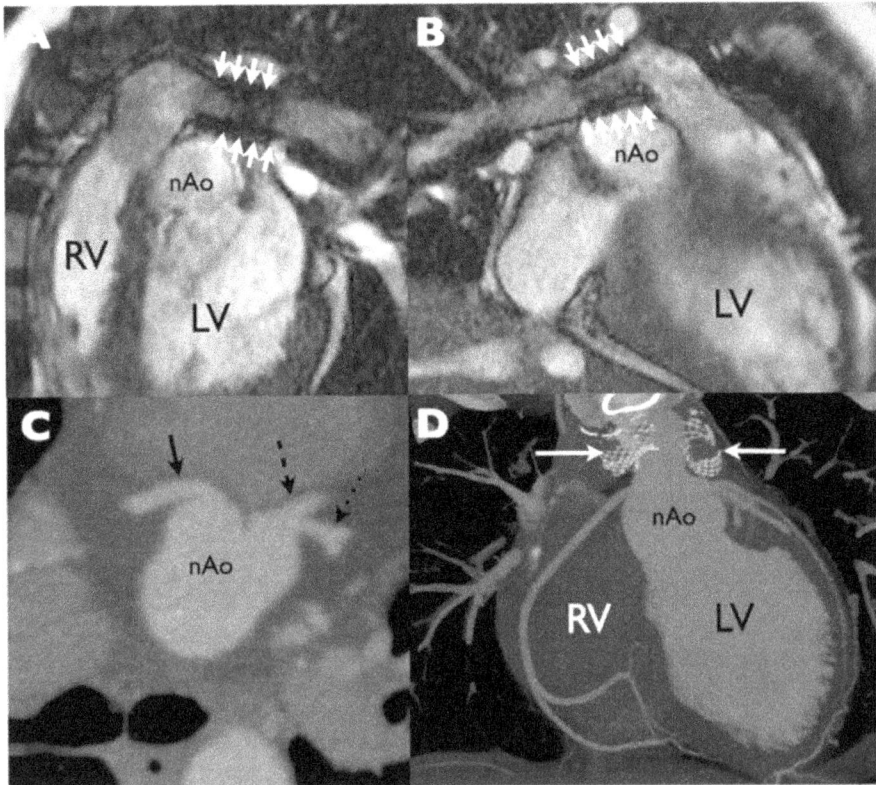

Figure 5 Bilateral pulmonary artery stents obscuring coronary origins at CMR. (A, B) Metallic artifact from bilateral pulmonary artery (PA) stents (arrows) on steady state free precession cine imaging obscures the coronary arteries as they emerge from the neo-aortic root. **(C)** Multiplanar reformat from low dose cardiac gated computed tomography reveals normal origins of the right coronary artery (solid arrow), left anterior descending (dashed arrow) and circumflex (dotted arrow) coronary arteries. **(D)** Lack of effect of bilateral PA stents (arrows) on visibility of the coronary arteries at cardiac CT is apparent on this coronal reformat. RV = right ventricle; LV = left ventricle; nAo = neo aorta.

assessment. Since the standard of care at our institution (and at the Labatt Family Heart Centre at SickKids, Toronto) has historically involved the use of radio-isotopes (SPECT), our study also includes data from this method. Our cohort underwent both stress SPECT and CMR examinations under identical physiologic conditions since a single episode of stress with the long-acting vasodilator dipyridamole allowed sequential delivery of both Sestamibi™ and gadolinium tracers while the patient remained on the magnet table. The relatively long half-life of technetium made it possible to then acquire the stress SPECT images back in the nuclear laboratory once the remainder of the CMR study was complete.

Coronary complications in adults after the arterial switch procedure

In the current era, coronary complications including coronary-related deaths late after ASO are rare events in both children and adults [4]. In historical cohorts, however, these complications have been described by several series and case reports [12-15] associated with coronary distribution as an independent risk factor [15]. The major problem with those historical surgical series was the common use of the single ostium technique for coronary transfer, which was shown to have a high rate of coronary occlusion and therefore has now been abandoned. Although a single right coronary artery was an independent risk factor for cardiovascular events in one study [15], in the current era coronary anatomy no longer determines outcome [4]. Recent work seems to confirm a genuinely low rate of significant coronary complications - at least in early adult life [1,15,16]. In these series, none of the adults suffered acute coronary syndrome during follow-up.

The vast majority of our cohort had had the ASO in the current era (after 1986). In line with the low prevalence of late coronary complication, our data confirm the absence of significant proximal coronary abnormality following reimplantation. We also demonstrate a re-assuringly low prevalence of scar despite prior cardiopulmonary bypass. Perfusion was uniformly normal on a qualitative basis but we did detect a mild increase in resting flow in some patients – a finding of unknown significance, which replicates that of earlier PET data

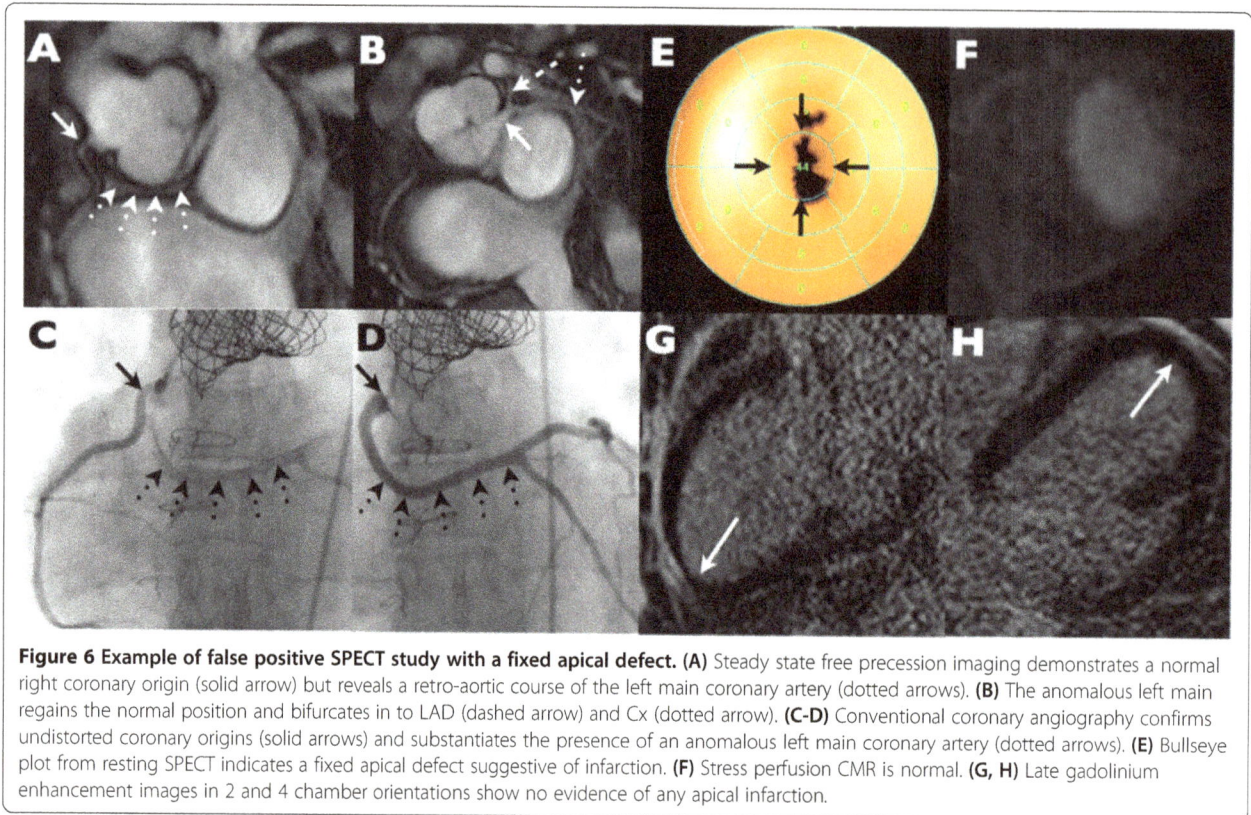

Figure 6 Example of false positive SPECT study with a fixed apical defect. (A) Steady state free precession imaging demonstrates a normal right coronary origin (solid arrow) but reveals a retro-aortic course of the left main coronary artery (dotted arrows). **(B)** The anomalous left main regains the normal position and bifurcates in to LAD (dashed arrow) and Cx (dotted arrow). **(C-D)** Conventional coronary angiography confirms undistorted coronary origins (solid arrows) and substantiates the presence of an anomalous left main coronary artery (dotted arrows). **(E)** Bullseye plot from resting SPECT indicates a fixed apical defect suggestive of infarction. **(F)** Stress perfusion CMR is normal. **(G, H)** Late gadolinium enhancement images in 2 and 4 chamber orientations show no evidence of any apical infarction.

[17]. As such, measured coronary flow reserve for the group was towards the lower end of the accepted normal range for CMR perfusion.

Assessment for silent myocardial ischemia after the arterial switch procedure

Historically, nuclear perfusion techniques were commonly employed in the follow-up of children and adults following ASO surgery in our center. However they may not be ideal in this population. Firstly, they expose radio-sensitive young adults to a significant dose of ionizing radiation. Secondly, many post-operative patients have left bundle branch block, creating perfusion defects in the absence of obstructive disease or myocardial scar. Thirdly, patients who underwent cardiopulmonary bypass as neonates may have sustained myocardial damage as a result of inadequate myocardial protection creating perfusion defects that are not linked to the longer-term patency of the translocated coronary arteries [18,19]. Resting perfusion abnormalities are very common in this population and show little correlation to symptoms or exercise-induced ECG abnormalities [20].

Stress perfusion CMR has been extensively validated in the adult ischemic heart disease population [21]. It has been shown to be superior to SPECT [7] and to have comparable diagnostic accuracy to both PET [22] and fractional flow reserve [23]. By comparison, the literature

on use of stress CMR in congenital heart disease populations is sparse [24,25]. The study by Manso et al. [26] employed stress perfusion CMR to look at survivors of the ASO procedure in a younger age group (median age of 14 years). In keeping with our results, they found no evidence of visible perfusion abnormality but did not seek to quantitatively assess absolute myocardial blood flow. Manso et al. also failed to find late gadolinium enhancement in the myocardium - providing further indirect support for our contention that perfusion defects seen on SPECT but unmatched by scar on late gadolinium enhancement imaging are most likely related to artifact.

Although ostial obstrucion has been described as the main reason for late onset myocardial infarction, other mechanism leading to myocardial ischemia may be discussed in the setting of prior ASO. After the Lecompte maneuvre, compression of the coronary arteries by the pulmonary arteries may occur and in this case, exercise could induce ischemia [14]. In this scenario, pharmacological stress testing may not trigger the underlying mechanism for ischemia and perfusion CMR may have insufficient sensitivity.

Clinical outlook

Although our data are reassuring, the ASO has only been in widespread use since the 1980s and so the ultimate fate of the coronary arteries after ASO remains

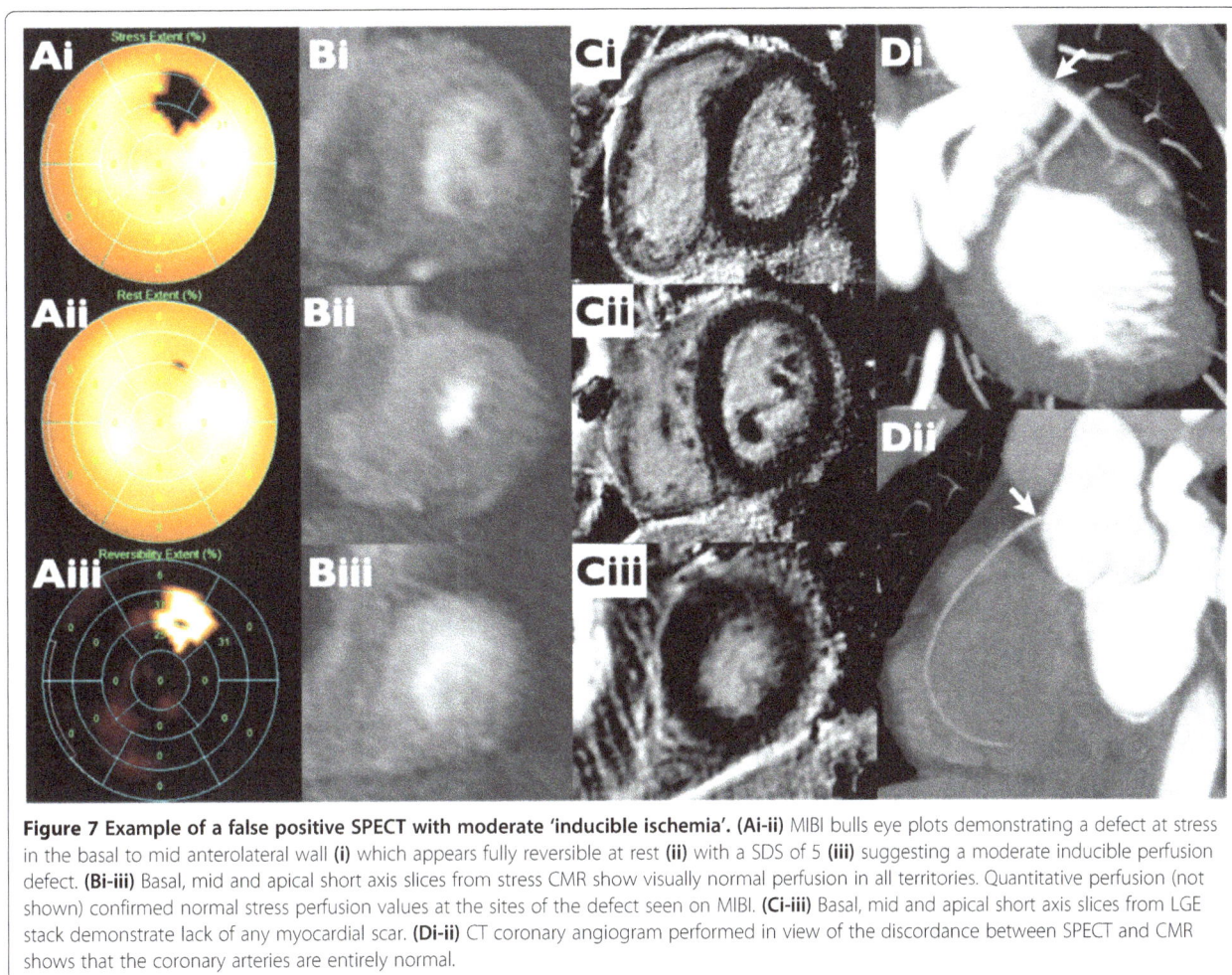

Figure 7 Example of a false positive SPECT with moderate 'inducible ischemia'. (Ai-ii) MIBI bulls eye plots demonstrating a defect at stress in the basal to mid anterolateral wall **(i)** which appears fully reversible at rest **(ii)** with a SDS of 5 **(iii)** suggesting a moderate inducible perfusion defect. **(Bi-iii)** Basal, mid and apical short axis slices from stress CMR show visually normal perfusion in all territories. Quantitative perfusion (not shown) confirmed normal stress perfusion values at the sites of the defect seen on MIBI. **(Ci-iii)** Basal, mid and apical short axis slices from LGE stack demonstrate lack of any myocardial scar. **(Di-ii)** CT coronary angiogram performed in view of the discordance between SPECT and CMR shows that the coronary arteries are entirely normal.

uncertain. At the current time there is no single accepted surveillance protocol for this patient group [22,27,28]. Notwithstanding the facts that patients with coronary denervation following ASO may not experience typical symptoms of angina, and the finding of a high prevalence of coronary atheroscleriosis by IVUS examination in a historical cohort of children with prior ASO [29], our data do not support routine and serial imaging screening for silent myocardial ischemia in asymptomatic adults after ASO. Nevertheless, we emphasize that a comprehensive evaluation by CMR - without perfusion protocol - is recommended as a baseline assessment in these patients when they present in adulthood in order to assess: coronary anatomy and the pulmonary artery tree; to rule out ostial obstruction; to evaluate for unexpected prior myocardial injury; and to determine biventricular function and volumes. In specific cases where coronary obstruction is present, or compression of the coronary artery by the pulmonary artery is suggested, then we recommend further functional ischemic testing, either with perfusion CMR in the first or with exercise SPECT in the latter scenario.

Study limitations

This was a single center study from a relatively narrow surgical era later on in the operative experience for the arterial switch procedure with a limited number of patients. Nonetheless our results are congruent with the lack of published adverse outcomes in adult ASO patients and suggest that coronary anatomical concerns may have been over-stated in an asymptomatic adult population. Almost all of the patients in our cohort underwent imaging for surveillance rather than symptomatic chest pain or breathlessness and therefore we lack confirmation of coronary normality by coronary artery catheterization in most patients. However stress perfusion CMR has been shown to have a very high degree of diagnostic accuracy compared to PET, IVUS or quantitative coronary angiography and has previously been shown to be superior to SPECT in the context of ischemic heart disease [7]. Although myocardial flow reserve obtained by quantitative perfusion CMR was comparable to prior published data, these values should be interpreted with caution as data from a healthy control group is lacking. None of our patients have had any adverse coronary events since recruitment into the study over a median follow up period of 24 months. However we accept that we cannot exclude a potential for accelerated atherosclerosis at a later time point in the natural history of operated *d*-transposition of the great arteries.

Conclusions

Adult ASO survivors in this study had no CMR evidence of myocardial ischemia, scar or coronary ostial abnormality. Compared to SPECT, CMR provides additional valuable information about the coronary artery anatomy. The data show that the asymptomatic and clinically stable adult ASO patient has a low pre-test probability for inducible ischemia. In this situation, it is likely that routine evaluation with stress CMR is unnecessary.

Abbreviations
ASO: Arterial switch operation; CMR: Cardiovascular magnetic resonance; CT: Computed tomography; LGE: Late gadolinium enhancement; PET: Positron emission tomography; SDS: Summed difference scores; SPECT: Single-photon emission computed tomography; SRS: Summed rest scores; SSS: Summed stress scores.

Competing interests
The authors declare that they have no competing interests.

Authors' contributions
The individual contributions of the authors to the current manuscript were as follows: DT: Conception and design of the study, analysis and interpretation of the data, drafting and revising of the manuscript. MM: Analysing quantitative perfusion CMR data, revising the manuscript critically for important intellectual content. RMW: Analyzing CMR data, revising the manuscript critically for important intellectual content. SLR: Revising the manuscript critically for important intellectual content. FV: Acquring SPECT data, revising the manuscript critically for important intellectual content. RMI: Acquiring SPECT data, revising the manuscript critically for important intellectual content. JPG: Analysing quantitative perfusion CMR data, revising the manuscript critically for important intellectual content. ENO: Revising the manuscript critically for important intellectual content. AMC: Conception and design of the study, analyzing CMR data, revising the manuscript critically for important intellectual content, final approval of the manuscript submitted. All authors read and approved the final manuscript.

Acknowledgements
The authors wish to acknowledge Mr. S Soubron of the Department of Medical Physics, University of Leeds for initial validation of the quantitative perfusion package used in this paper.

Author details
[1]Toronto Congenital Centre for Adults, Peter Munk Cardiac Centre, University Health Network, Toronto General Hospital, 585 University Avenue, 5 N-525, Toronto, ON M5G 2N2, Canada. [2]Department of Cardiology, University Hospital Basel, Basel, Switzerland. [3]Multidisciplinary Cardiovascular Research Centre, Leeds Institute of Genetics, Health and Therapeutics, University of Leeds, Leeds, UK. [4]Department of Medical Imaging, Toronto General Hospital, Toronto, Canada.

References
1. Tobler D, Williams WG, Jegatheeswaran A, Van Arsdell GS, McCrindle BW, Greutmann M, Oechslin EN, Silversides CK. Cardiac outcomes in young adult survivors of the arterial switch operation for transposition of the great arteries. *J Am Coll Cardiol*. 2010; 56:58–64.
2. Bonhoeffer P, Bonnet D, Piéchaud JF, Stümper O, Aggoun Y, Villain E, Kachaner J, Sidi D. Coronary artery obstruction after the arterial switch operation for transposition of the great arteries in newborns. *J Am Coll Cardiol*. 1997; 29:202–06.
3. Legendre A, Losay J, Touchot-Koné A, Serraf A, Belli E, Piot JD, Lambert V, Capderou A, Planche C. Coronary events after arterial switch operation for transposition of the great arteries. *Circulation*. 2003; 108(Suppl 1):II186–90.
4. Brown JW, Park HJ, Turrentine MW. Arterial switch operation: factors impacting survival in the current era. *Ann Thorac Surg*. 2001; 71:1978–84.
5. Kilner PJ, Geva T, Kaemmerer H, Trindade PT, Schwitter J, Webb GD. Recommendations for cardiovascular magnetic resonance in adults with congenital heart disease from the respective working groups of the European Society of Cardiology. *Eur Heart J*. 2010; 31:794–805.
6. Hoffmann A, Bremerich J. The danger of radiation exposure in the young. *Heart*. 2010; 96:251–52.
7. Greenwood JP, Maredia N, Younger JF, Brown JM, Nixon J, Everett CC, Bijsterveld P, Ridgway JP, Radjenovic A, Dickinson CJ, Ball SG, Plein S. Cardiovascular magnetic resonance and single-photon emission computed tomography for diagnosis of coronary heart disease (CE-MARC): a prospective trial. *Lancet*. 2012; 379:453–60.
8. Huber A, Sourbron S, Klauss V, Schaefer J, Bauner KU, Schweyer M, Reiser M, Rummeny E, Rieber J. Magnetic resonance perfusion of the myocardium: semiquantitative and quantitative evaluation in comparison with coronary angiography and fractional flow reserve. *Invest Radiol*. 2012; 47:332–38.
9. Costa MA, Shoemaker S, Futamatsu H, Klassen C, Angiolillo DJ, Nguyen M, Siuciak A, Gilmore P, Zenni MM, Guzman L, Bass TA, Wilke N. Quantitative magnetic resonance perfusion imaging detects anatomic and physiologic coronary artery disease as measured by coronary angiography and fractional flow reserve. *J Am Coll Cardiol*. 2007; 50:514–22.
10. Jerosch-Herold M, Wilke N, Stillman AE. Magnetic resonance quantification of the myocardial perfusion reserve with a Fermi function model for constrained deconvolution. *Med Phys*. 1998; 25:73–84.
11. Motwani M, Fairbairn TA, Larghat A, Mather AN, Biglands JD, Radjenovic A, Greenwood JP, Plein S. Systolic versus diastolic acquisition in myocardial perfusion MR imaging. *Radiology*. 2012; 262:816–23.
12. Hutter PA, Kreb DL, Mantel SF, Hitchcock JF, Meijboom EJ, Bennink GBWE. Twenty-five years' experience with the arterial switch operation. *J Thorac Cardiovasc Surg*. 2002; 124:790–97.
13. Losay J, Touchot A, Serraf A, Litvinova A, Lambert V, Piot JD, Lacour-Gayet F, Capderou A, Planche C. Late outcome after arterial switch operation for transposition of the great arteries. *Circulation*. 2001; 104:I121–26.
14. Gatlin S, Kalynych A, Sallee D, Campbell R. Detection of a coronary artery anomaly after a sudden cardiac arrest in a 17 Year-old with D-transposition of the great arteries status post arterial switch operation: a case report. *Congenit Heart Dis*. 2011; 6:384–88.
15. Khairy P, Clair M, Fernandes SM, Blume ED, Powell AJ, Newburger JW, Landzberg MJ, Mayer JE Jr. Cardiovascular outcomes after the arterial switch operation for d-transposition of the great arteries. *Circulation*. 2013; 127:331–39.
16. Kempny A, Wustmann K, Borgia F, Dimopoulos K, Uebing A, Li W, Chen SS, Piorkowski A, Radley-Smith R, Yacoub MH, Gatzoulis MA, Shore DF, Swan L, Diller GP. Outcome in adult patients after arterial switch operation for transposition of the great arteries. *Int J Cardiol*. 2013; 167:2588–93.
17. Hauser M, Bengel FM, Kühn A, Sauer U, Zylla S, Braun SL, Nekolla SG, Oberhoffer R, Lange R, Schwaiger M, Hess J. Myocardial blood flow and flow reserve after coronary reimplantation in patients after arterial switch and ross operation. *Circulation*. 2001; 103:1875–80.
18. Vogel M, Smallhorn JF, Gilday D, Benson LN, Ash J, Williams WG, Freedom RM. Assessment of myocardial perfusion in patients after the arterial switch operation. *J Nucl Med: Offic Publ Soc Nucl Med*. 1991; 32:237–41.
19. Hayes AM, Baker EJ, Kakadeker A, Parsons JM, Martin RP, Radley-Smith R, Qureshi SA, Yacoub M, Maisey MN, Tynan M. Influence of anatomic correction for transposition of the great arteries on myocardial perfusion: radionuclide imaging with technetium-99m 2-methoxy isobutyl isonitrile. *J Am Coll Cardiol*. 1994; 24:769–77.
20. Weindling SN, Wernovsky G, Colan SD, Parker JA, Boutin C, Mone SM, Costello J, Castaneda AR, Treves ST. Myocardial perfusion, function and exercise tolerance after the arterial switch operation. *J Am Coll Cardiol*. 1994; 23:424–33.
21. Hamon M, Fau G, Nee G, Ehtisham J, Morello R, Hamon M. Meta-analysis of the diagnostic performance of stress perfusion cardiovascular magnetic resonance for detection of coronary artery disease. *J Cardiovasc Magn Reson: Offic J Soc Cardiovasc Magn Reson*. 2010; 12:29.

Evaluation of a comprehensive cardiovascular magnetic resonance protocol in young adults late after...

23

22. Schwitter J, Nanz D, Kneifel S, Bertschinger K, Buchi M, Knusel PR, Marincek B, Luscher TF, von Schulthess GK. Assessment of myocardial perfusion in coronary artery disease by magnetic resonance: a comparison with positron emission tomography and coronary angiography. *Circulation.* 2001; **103**:2230–35.

23. Watkins S, McGeoch R, Lyne J, Steedman T, Good R, McLaughlin MJ, Cunningham T, Bezlyak V, Ford I, Dargie HJ, Oldroyd KG. Validation of magnetic resonance myocardial perfusion imaging with fractional flow reserve for the detection of significant coronary heart disease. *Circulation.* 2009; **120**:2207–13.

24. Buechel ER, Balmer C, Bauersfeld U, Kellenberger CJ, Schwitter J. Feasibility of perfusion cardiovascular magnetic resonance in paediatric patients. *J Cardiovasc Magn Reson: Offic J Soc Cardiovasc Magn Reson.* 2009; **11**:51.

25. Deva DP, Torres FS, Wald RM, Roche SL, Jimenez-Juan L, Oechslin EN, Crean AM. The value of stress perfusion cardiovascular magnetic resonance imaging for patients referred from the adult congenital heart disease clinic: 5-year experience at the Toronto General Hospital. *Cardiol Young.* 2014; **24**:822–30.

26. Manso B, Castellote A, Dos L, Casaldaliga J. Myocardial perfusion magnetic resonance imaging for detecting coronary function anomalies in asymptomatic paediatric patients with a previous arterial switch operation for the transposition of great arteries. *Cardiol Young.* 2010; **20**:410–17.

27. Warnes CA, Williams RG, Bashore TM, Child JS, Connolly HM, Dearani JA, Del Nido P, Fasules JW, Graham TP Jr, Hijazi ZM, Hunt SA, King ME, Landzberg MJ, Miner PD, Radford MJ, Walsh EP, Webb GD, Smith SC Jr, Jacobs AK, Adams CD, Anderson JL, Antman EM, Buller CE, Creager MA, Ettinger SM, Halperin JL, Hunt SA, Krumholz HM, Kushner FG, Lytle BW, et al. ACC/AHA 2008 Guidelines for the Management of Adults with Congenital Heart Disease: Executive Summary: a report of the American College of Cardiology/American Heart Association Task Force on Practice Guidelines (writing committee to develop guidelines for the management of adults with congenital heart disease). *Circulation.* 2008; **118**:2395–451.

28. Baumgartner H, Bonhoeffer P, De Groot NM, de Haan F, Deanfield JE, Galie N, Gatzoulis MA, Gohlke-Baerwolf C, Kaemmerer H, Kilner P, Meijboom F, Mulder BJ, Oechslin E, Oliver JM, Serraf A, Szatmari A, Thaulow E, Vouhe PR, Walma E. ESC Guidelines for the management of grown-up congenital heart disease (new version 2010). *Eur Heart J.* 2010; **31**:2915–57.

29. Pedra SRFF, Pedra CAC, Abizaid AA, Braga SLN, Staico R, Arrieta R, Costa JR, Vaz VD, Fontes VF, Sousa JER. Intracoronary ultrasound assessment late after the arterial switch operation for transposition of the great arteries. *J Am Coll Cardiol.* 2005; **45**:2061–68.

3

Downstream clinical consequences of stress cardiovascular magnetic resonance based on appropriate use criteria

Sloane McGraw[1], Omer Mirza[1], Michael A Bauml[1], Vibhav S Rangarajan[1] and Afshin Farzaneh-Far[1,2]*

Abstract

Background: Appropriate use criteria (AUC) have been developed by professional organizations as a response to the rising costs of imaging, with the goal of optimizing test-patient selection. Consequently, the AUC are now increasingly used by third-party-payers to assess reimbursement. However, these criteria were created by expert consensus and have not been systematically assessed for CMR. The aim of this study was to determine the rates of abnormal stress-CMR and subsequent downstream utilization of angiography and revascularization procedures based on the most recent AUC.

Methods: 300 consecutive patients referred for CMR-stress testing were prospectively enrolled. Two cardiologists reviewed all clinical information before the CMR-stress test and classified the test as "appropriate', "maybe appropriate" or "rarely appropriate" according to the 2013 AUC. Patients were followed for 2 months for the primary outcomes of coronary angiography and/or revascularization.

Results: 49.7% of stress CMRs were appropriate, 36.7% maybe appropriate, and 13.6% rarely appropriate. Ischemia was significantly more likely to be seen in the appropriate (18.8%) or maybe appropriate groups (21.8%) than the rarely appropriate group (4.8%) ($p = 0.030$ and $p = 0.014$ respectively). Referral for cardiac catheterization was not significantly different in the appropriate (10.1%) and maybe appropriate groups (10.0%) compared to the rarely appropriate group (2.4%) ($p = 0.119$ and $p = 0.127$ respectively). No patients undergoing catheterization in the rarely appropriate group went on to require revascularization, in contrast to 53.3% of the appropriate vs 36.4% of the maybe appropriate patients ($p = 0.391$). Presence of ischemia led to referral for cardiac catheterization in 50.0% of the appropriate group vs 33.3% of the maybe appropriate group ($p = 0.225$); in contrast to none of the rarely appropriate group.

Conclusions: The great majority of tests were classified as appropriate or maybe appropriate. Downstream cardiac catheterization rates were similar in all 3 groups. However, rarely appropriate studies never required revascularization, suggesting suboptimal resource utilization. Studies classified as maybe appropriate had similar rates of abnormal findings and led to similar rates of downstream catheterization and revascularization as those that were deemed appropriate. This suggests that consideration could be given to upgrading some of the common maybe appropriate indications to the appropriate category.

* Correspondence: afshin@uic.edu
[1]Section of Cardiology, Department of Medicine, University of Illinois at Chicago, 840 South Wood St. M/C 715, Suite 920 S, Chicago, IL 60612, USA
[2]Division of Cardiology, Department of Medicine, Duke University Medical Center, Durham, NC, USA

Background

As a response to fiscal pressures and with the goal of optimizing test-patient selection, appropriate use criteria (AUC) have been developed by several professional organizations - including the American College of Cardiology, the Society for Cardiovascular Magnetic Resonance, the American Society of Nuclear Cardiology and the American Society of Echocardiography [1–5]. Consequently, the AUC are now increasingly used by payers to assess the suitability of reimbursement for imaging procedures. Moreover, recent approval of the "Protecting Access to Medicare Act" (PAMA) by the United States Congress has very significant implications for the application of AUC to CMR reimbursement [6,7]. It states that starting in 2017 - in order to be paid by Medicare for advanced imaging - certification must be provided that the ordering physicians consulted the AUC. The claim to Medicare must specify whether the requested imaging adheres to the AUC. The act also states that criteria must be developed by national medical societies or provider-led entities and should be evidence based, to the extent possible. By November 2015, the Centers for Medicare and Medicaid Services (CMS) must select the specific AUC to be used. Finally, in 2020 CMS must identify up to 5% of physicians as outliers in adherence to AUC, who may then be subject to prior authorization.

Stress CMR is increasing used in the management of patients with known or suspected coronary artery disease [8]. The initial AUC for stress CMR was recently replaced by the AUC for stable ischemic heart disease, as part of a new multimodality approach [1,5]. The AUC were developed by a panel who were asked to rate 80 clinical indications as being "appropriate", "maybe appropriate", or "rarely appropriate". However, these criteria were created by expert consensus and have never been systematically assessed or validated for CMR. In particular, there is no data regarding the impact of the AUC on downstream cardiac procedures.

The aims of this study were to determine the rates of abnormal stress CMR results and subsequent downstream utilization of angiography and revascularization procedures based on the most recent AUC.

Methods

Study population

Three hundred consecutive patients referred for CMR stress testing were prospectively enrolled in a single academic medical center. Patients were excluded if they had metallic implants incompatible with CMR, glomerular filtration rate < 30 ml/min, high degree atrio-ventricular block, severe active wheezing from asthma or severe claustrophobia. Subjects were asked to abstain from caffeine-containing products for at least 12 h prior to the test.

Clinical variables

Demographic and clinical characteristics were recorded prospectively at the time of CMR stress testing from patient interviews and the electronic medical record. Patients gave informed written consent for the protocol, which was approved by the local institutional review board.

CMR acquisition

Images were acquired on a 3 T scanner (Philips Achieva, Philips Medical Systems, Best, the Netherlands) using a six-element phased-array receiver coil as previously described [9]. Steady-state free-precession cine images were acquired in multiple short-axis and three long-axis views (repetition time, 3.0 ms; echo time, 1.5 ms; flip angle, 40°; slice thickness 6 mm).

The patient table was then partially pulled outside the scanner bore to allow direct observation of the patient and full access. A 0.4 mg bolus of regadenoson (Lexiscan, Astellas Pharma Inc) was infused under continuous electrocardiography and blood pressure monitoring. Approximately 1 min after regadenoson administration, the perfusion sequence was applied and Gadolinium contrast (0.075 mmol/kg gadoteridol, Bracco Diagnostics) followed by a saline flush (30 ml) was infused (4.5 ml/s) via an antecubital vein. On the console, the perfusion images were observed as they were acquired, with breath-holding starting from the appearance of contrast in the right ventricular cavity. Imaging was completed 10 to 15 s after the gadolinium bolus had transited the left ventricular myocardium. Perfusion images consisted of three to four short-axis slices obtained every heartbeat with a saturation-recovery, gradient-echo sequence (repetition time 2.8 ms; echo time 1.1 ms; flip angle 20°; voxel size, 2.5 × 2.5 × 8 mm). Aminophylline (100 mg IV) was administered immediately after stress perfusion imaging [9]. Rest perfusion images were acquired 15 min after stress imaging with an additional contrast bolus (0.075 mmol/kg gadoteridol) using identical sequence parameters. Five minutes after rest perfusion, late gadolinium enhancement (LGE) imaging was performed with a 2D segmented gradient echo phase-sensitive inversion-recovery sequence in the identical views as cine-CMR. Inversion delay times were typically 280 to 360 ms. Perfusion and LGE images were visually interpreted by standard methods [10]. The pattern of LGE was classified as either infarct or non-CAD type on the basis of subendocardial enhancement [11,12].

Patient classification for AUC

Two independent general cardiologists reviewed all clinical information dated before the CMR stress test. These reviewers were blinded to the results of the CMR and to the clinical course subsequent to the test. The CMR stress tests were classified as "appropriate", "maybe appropriate" or "rarely appropriate" as defined by the 2013 AUC [5]. A third blinded independent physician adjudicated any discrepancy between the interpreters.

Follow-up

After CMR, patients were prospectively followed for 2 months for the primary outcomes of coronary angiography and/or revascularization. Clinical follow-up was based on review of the electronic medical records or from telephone interviews with patients or their physicians.

Statistical analysis

Normally distributed data were expressed as mean ± SD. Continuous variables were compared by the Student's t-test or Wilcoxon rank-sum (depending on data normality). Comparisons of discrete variables were made using the chi-square test; Fisher's exact test was used when the assumptions of the chi-square test were not met. A p value of <0.05 was considered statistically significant.

Results

Patient characteristics

Table 1 summarizes the baseline patient characteristics. The mean age of the study population was 59 years. 54% of patients were female and 36% had diabetes mellitus. 32% had known coronary artery disease, including prior PCI (17%) and CABG (4%). The mean ejection fraction was 61%. Of the 300 CMRs reviewed, arbitration for AUC assignment by a third cardiologist was required for just 1 patient.

Primary outcomes

At 2 months of follow-up, the endpoint of coronary angiography occurred in 27 patients and the endpoint of revascularization occurred in 12 patients (PCI = 11, CABG = 1).

Appropriateness

Based on the 2013 AUC, 49.7% of stress CMRs were classified as appropriate, 36.7% as maybe appropriate, and 13.6% as rarely appropriate. A comparison of the baseline characteristics across AUC is given in Table 1. There were significant differences in age, prevalence of diabetes, hyperlipidemia, smoking, hypertension, and known CAD across the three groups.

The six most frequent AUC categories accounted for 179 patients (Table 2). Of patients with these common six indications approximately 69% were classified as appropriate and 31% as maybe appropriate.

Relationship of appropriateness to CMR results

Abnormal CMR stress results (defined as presence of ischemia or scar) were more common in the appropriate (29.5%) and maybe appropriate (28.2%) groups compared with the rarely appropriate (14.6%) group although the differences did not reach statistical significance ($p = 0.055$ and $p = 0.085$ respectively) (Fig. 1). Ischemia was significantly more likely to be seen in patients in the appropriate (18.8%) or maybe appropriate groups (21.8%) than the rarely appropriate group (4.8%) ($p = 0.030$ and $p = 0.014$ respectively) (Fig. 2).

Relationship of appropriateness to downstream angiography and revascularization

There was a trend towards more referral for cardiac catheterization in the appropriate (10.1%) and maybe

Table 1 Baseline Characteristics Stratified by Appropriate Use Criteria

CHARACTERISTICS	Total N = 300	Appropriate N = 149	Maybe Appropriate N = 110	Rarely Appropriate N = 41	P Value
Age (±SD)	59 (±13.6)	61 (±12.0)	61 (±13.3)	46 (±14.4)	<0.0001
Female %	54.0	49.7	55.0	66.7	0.1703
BMI (±SD)	30.8 (±5.7)	31.3 (±5.4)	30.8 (±6.1)	29.2 (±5.5)	0.1000
Diabetes %	36.2	43.6	32.4	16.7	0.0049
Hyperlipidemia %	53.6	60.4	55.9	23.8	0.0002
Current Smoking %	16.3	18.8	8.5	27.8	0.0089
Hypertension %	73.0	78.5	74.8	45.2	0.0002
Known CAD %	32.1	39.6	29.7	11.9	0.0032
Prior MI %	13.6	16.1	13.5	4.8	0.1793
Prior PCI %	16.9	22.8	14.4	2.4	0.0061
Prior CABG %	4.3	3.4	7.3	0	0.1058
LVEF (±SD)	61 (±10.9)	60.3 (±12.0)	61 (±10.7)	62 (±6.8)	0.4800

BMI, Body Mass Index; CAD, Coronary Artery Disease; LVEF, Left Ventricular Ejection Fraction; MI, myocardial infarction; PCI, Percutaneous Coronary Intervention; CABG, Coronary Artery Bypass Grafting; SD, standard deviation

Table 2 AUC categories in our study population

AUC Description	N	Classification
Follow-up testing (>90 days) for new or worsening symptoms with non-obstructive CAD on coronary angiography (invasive or noninvasive) OR normal prior stress imaging study	48	A
Symptomatic in intermediate pre-test probability of CAD with interpretable ECG AND able to exercise	32	M
Symptomatic in intermediate pre-test probability of CAD with uninterpretable ECG OR unable to exercise	27	A
Newly diagnosed systolic heart failure (resting LV function previously assessed but no prior CAD evaluation)	25	A
Evaluation for symptomatic (ischemic equivalent) post-revascularization (PCI or CABG)	24	A
Sequential or follow up testing (≤90 days) with uncertain results on prior stress imaging study (not stress CMR) where obstructive CAD remains a concern	23	M
Symptomatic in low pre-test probability of CAD with interpretable ECG AND able to exercise	20	R
Pre-operative clearance in poor or unknown functional capacity (<4 METS); intermediate risk surgery with ≥1 clinical risk factor	12	M
High pre-test probability of CAD with an interpretable ECG and able to exercise	8	A
High pre-test probability of CAD with an uninterpretable ECG and unable to exercise	6	A
Follow up testing for new or worsening symptoms with an abnormal prior stress imaging study	6	M
Follow up testing (>90 Days) in an asymptomatic or symptomatically stable patient whose last study was ≥ 2 years ago	4	M
Follow up testing (>90 Days) in an asymptomatic patient without ischemic equivalent, who has a normal prior stress imaging study or non-obstructive CAD on angiogram who is intermediate to high global CAD risk with a study ≥ 2 years ago	4	M
Follow up testing (>90 Days) in an a patient with stable symptoms, who has a normal prior stress imaging study or non-obstructive CAD on angiogram who is intermediate to high global CAD risk with a study ≥ 2 years ago	4	M
Symptomatic patients who are low pre-test probability of CAD with an uninterpretable ECG or unable to exercise	3	M
Newly diagnosed diastolic heart failure	3	A
Evaluation of arrhythmias without ischemic equivalent with frequent PVCs	3	M
Syncope without ischemic equivalent in a patient with low global CAD risk	3	R
Follow up testing (>90 Days) in an asymptomatic or symptomatically stable patient with a history of abnormal prior stress imaging study < 2 years ago	3	R
Follow up testing (>90 Days) in an asymptomatic patient with a normal prior stress imaging study OR non-obstructive CAD on angiogram	3	R
Follow up testing for new or worsening symptoms in a patient with prior obstructive CAD on invasive coronary angiography	3	M
Pre-op risk stratification in a patient with poor or unknown functional capacity (<4 METs) in a patient who is undergoing vascular surgery with ≥ 1 clinical risk factor	3	M

AUC, Appropriate Use Criteria; *A*, Appropriate; *M*, Maybe Appropriate; *R*, Rarely Appropriate; *CAD*, Coronary Artery Disease; *ECG*, Electrocardiogram; *LV*, Left Ventricular; *PCI*, Percutaneous Coronary Intervention; *CABG*, Coronary Artery Bypass Grafting; *PVC*, Premature Ventricular Beat

appropriate groups (10.0%) compared to the rarely appropriate group (2.4%), but the differences were not statistically significant ($p = 0.119$ and $p = 0.127$ respectively). However, none of the patients undergoing catheterization in the rarely appropriate group went on to require revascularization, in contrast to 53.3% of the appropriate vs 36.4% of the maybe appropriate patients ($p = 0.391$) (Fig. 3).

Relationship of abnormal CMR results with referral to downstream angiography

The finding of ischemia on CMR led to referral for cardiac catheterization in 50.0% of the appropriate group vs 33.3% of the maybe appropriate group ($p = 0.225$). In contrast none of the rarely appropriate patients with ischemia were referred for cardiac catheterization. Based on an angiographic cut-off of ≤50% major epicardial stenosis, stress-CMR had a sensitivity = 94%,

specificity = 44%, positive predictive value = 77%, and negative predictive value = 80%, in this biased referral population.

Discussion

Due to rising healthcare costs, appropriate use of cardiovascular imaging is increasingly emphasized by professional societies, third party payers and accreditation agencies [6,7,13,14]. To the best of our knowledge this is the first study to systematically and prospectively assess the downstream utilization of angiography and revascularization procedures based on the AUC for stress-CMR. We have shown that tests categorized by the AUC as rarely appropriate, infrequently demonstrate ischemia, but the rates of downstream cardiac catheterization were not significantly different to those categorized as appropriate or maybe appropriate. Importantly when patients underwent cardiac catheterization none of the rarely

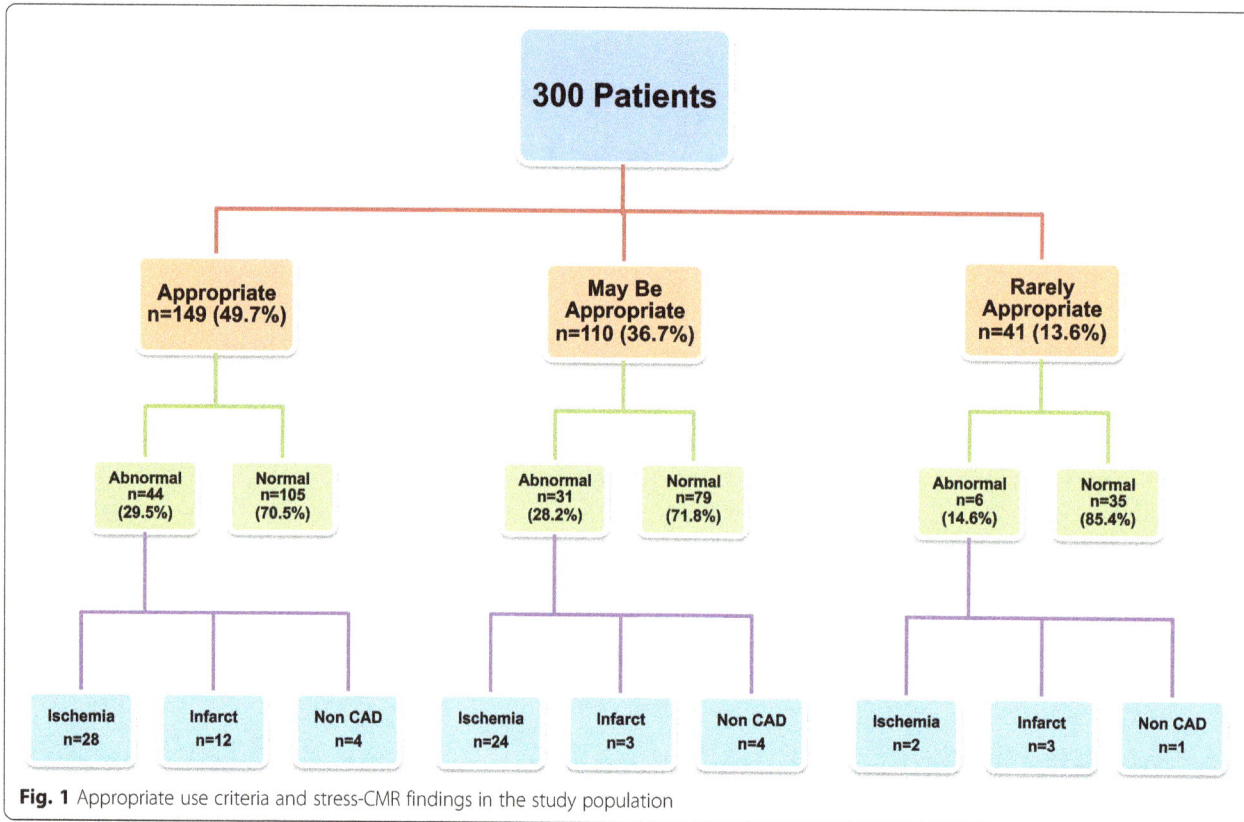

Fig. 1 Appropriate use criteria and stress-CMR findings in the study population

appropriate group went on to require subsequent revascularization. These findings appear to support the current AUC classification of rarely appropriate stress-CMR studies, since this group appears to result in suboptimal resource utilization.

In our study population, the great majority of tests ordered were deemed as appropriate or maybe appropriate. Only, approximately 14% of the stress-CMRs were categorized as rarely appropriate. This is similar to the inappropriate proportions reported for stress echocardiography

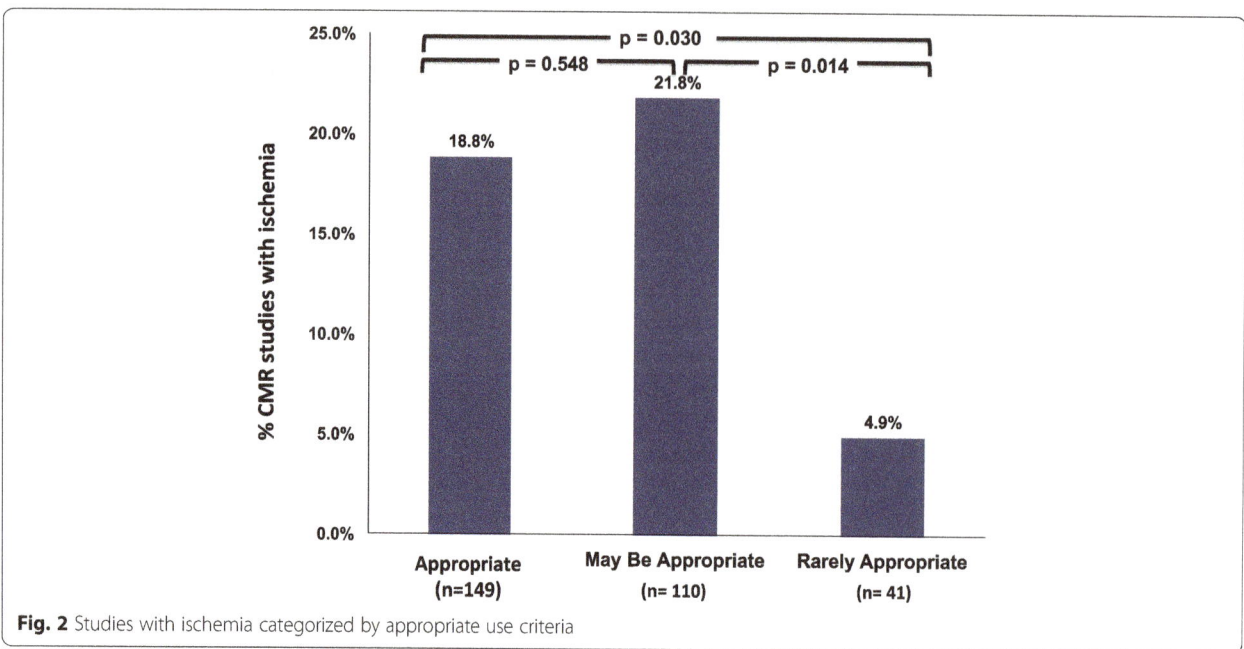

Fig. 2 Studies with ischemia categorized by appropriate use criteria

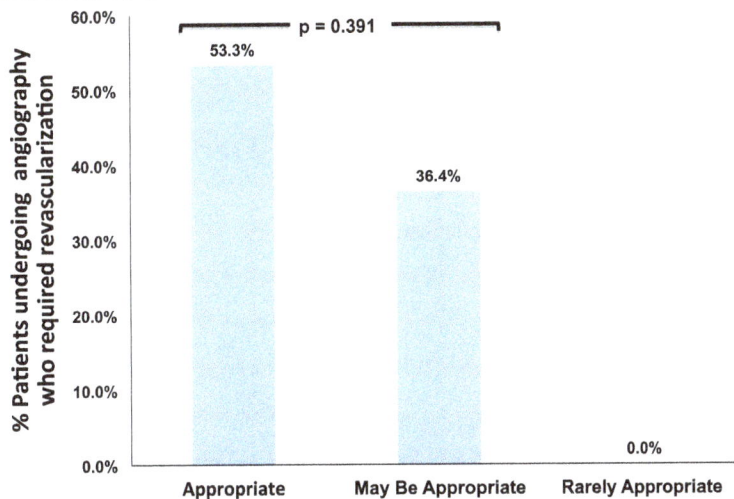

Fig. 3 Patients undergoing cardiac catheterization who required revascularization, categorized by appropriate use criteria

(9–33%) [15,16], Single Photon Emission Computed Tomography (SPECT) (7–46%) [17–19], and Positron Emission Tomography (PET) (10.2%) [20]. It is interesting to speculate whether growing pre-certification demands by third-party payers may have affected physicians test orderings patterns, but this cannot be assessed from this study.

We found that studies that were classified as maybe appropriate had similar rates of ischemia and led to similar rates of downstream catheterization and revascularization as those that were deemed appropriate. This suggests that consideration could be given to upgrading some of the common maybe appropriate indications to the appropriate category (Table 2).

It is interesting to note that even when ischemia was reported, patients were more likely to be referred for cardiac catheterization in the appropriate and maybe appropriate groups. In fact none of the patients with ischemia in the rarely appropriate group were referred for cardiac catheterization. The reasons for this are unclear but may relate to physician's assessment that invasive testing and revascularization would not significantly change outcomes or symptoms in this patient group.

In this study we have looked at the rates of abnormal stress tests and the endpoints of downstream angiography and revascularization to help assess optimal test-patient selection and imaging utilization. However, there are a number of important caveats to bear in mind. Higher rates of abnormal findings and greater use of angiography or revascularization doesn't necessarily imply better outcomes. Such validation would require performance of prospective randomized outcome trials. Ideally these studies should be part of larger initiatives to compare the effectiveness of different imaging modalities. Although, such studies will be challenging to

perform and fund, they are of critical importance in clarifying optimal imaging strategies. Another important point to emphasize is that stress testing can be very useful in patient management even when it does not lead to angiography or revascularization [21]. For example a normal study may lead to exclusion of coronary artery disease as a cause of symptoms, as well as to clinic/hospital discharge; or it may lead to 'surgical clearance' in patients referred prior to elective non-cardiac surgery. Further studies are required to more comprehensively assess these types of clinical impact and management change [22,23].

Future steps in assessing and validating AUC for stress-CMR should aim to compare the prognostic ability of the test across the various AUC categories. Such an approach was recently undertaken by Doukky et al. in a large nuclear study [19]. They demonstrated that inappropriate use of SPECT was associated with reduced prognostic value. In those patients whose scans were appropriate or uncertain, abnormal scans were of significant value in predicting major adverse cardiac events (hazard ratio 3.1–3.7) compared with normal scans. However, in those with inappropriate scans, abnormal studies did not achieve significance in predicting adverse cardiac events. Moreover, all abnormal SPECT findings were associated with increasing rates of revascularization, irrespective of the level of appropriateness.

Limitations

Our study was limited by a small sample size ($n = 300$) drawn from a single academic institution and may not be representative of the wider population. However, this may have the advantage of providing uniform scanning, interpretation and follow-up protocols. Larger studies with greater statistical power and more events (particularly revascularization) will allow a more comprehensive analysis of subgroups. The results of this study should therefore be regarded as preliminary, until larger multicenter studies are completed. As mentioned above, cardiac catheterization and revascularization are only part of the downstream clinical consequences of CMR-stress. Cost-effectiveness was not assessed in this study and clearly needs to be the subject of future studies aiming to establish the validity of the AUC.

Conclusions

The great majority of tests ordered in our population were classified as appropriate or maybe appropriate. Downstream referral for cardiac catheterization was not significantly different in the 3 groups. However, rarely appropriate studies never required revascularization, suggesting suboptimal resource utilization. Studies classified as maybe appropriate had similar rates of abnormal findings and led to similar rates of downstream catheterization and revascularization as those that were deemed appropriate. This suggests that consideration could be given to upgrading some of the common maybe appropriate indications to the appropriate category.

Competing interests
The authors declare that they have no competing interests.

Authors contributions
AF conceived the study, participated in its design and coordination, supervised imaging and drafted the manuscript. SM and OM participated in the study design and conduct, and helped to draft the manuscript. MAB and VR participated in the study coordination and supervised the performance of the studies. All authors read and approved the final manuscript.

References
1. Hendel RC, Patel MR, Kramer CM, Poon M, Hendel RC, Carr JC, et al. ACCF/ACR/SCCT/SCMR/ASNC/NASCI/SCAI/SIR 2006 appropriateness criteria for cardiac computed tomography and cardiac magnetic resonance imaging: a report of the american college of cardiology foundation quality strategic directions committee appropriateness criteria working group, american college of radiology, society of cardiovascular computed tomography, society for cardiovascular magnetic resonance, american society of nuclear cardiology, north american society for cardiac imaging, society for cardiovascular angiography and interventions, and society of interventional radiology. J Am Coll Cardiol. 2006;48(7):1475–97.
2. Hendel RC, Berman DS, Di Carli MF, Heidenreich PA, Henkin RE, Pellikka PA, et al. ACCF/ASNC/ACR/AHA/ASE/SCCT/SCMR/SNM 2009 appropriate Use criteria for cardiac radionuclide imaging: a report of the american college of cardiology foundation appropriate Use criteria task force, the american society of nuclear cardiology, the american college of radiology, the american heart association, the american society of echocardiography, the society of cardiovascular computed tomography, the society for cardiovascular magnetic resonance, and the society of nuclear medicine. J Am Coll Cardiol. 2009;53(23):2201–29.
3. American College of Cardiology Foundation Appropriate Use Criteria Task F, American Society of E, American Heart A, American Society of Nuclear C, Heart Failure Society of A, Heart Rhythm S, Society for Cardiovascular A, Interventions, Society of Critical Care M, Society of Cardiovascular Computed T et al. ACCF/ASE/AHA/ASNC/HFSA/HRS/SCAI/SCCM/SCCT/SCMR 2011 appropriate Use criteria for echocardiography. A report of the american college of cardiology foundation appropriate Use criteria task force, american society of echocardiography, american heart association, american society of nuclear cardiology, heart failure society of america, heart rhythm society, society for cardiovascular angiography and interventions, society of critical care medicine, society of cardiovascular computed tomography, and society for cardiovascular magnetic resonance endorsed by the american college of chest physicians. J Am Coll Cardiol. 2011;57(9):1126–66.
4. Taylor AJ, Cerqueira M, Hodgson JM, Mark D, Min J, O'Gara P, et al. ACCF/SCCT/ACR/AHA/ASE/ASNC/NASCI/SCAI/SCMR 2010 appropriate use criteria for cardiac computed tomography. A report of the american college of cardiology foundation appropriate Use criteria task force, the society of cardiovascular computed tomography, the american college of radiology, the american heart association, the american society of echocardiography, the american society of nuclear cardiology, the north american society for cardiovascular imaging, the society for cardiovascular angiography and interventions, and the society for cardiovascular magnetic resonance. J Am Coll Cardiol. 2010;56(22):1864–94.
5. Wolk MJ, Bailey SR, Doherty JU, Douglas PS, Hendel RC, Kramer CM, et al. ACCF/AHA/ASE/ASNC/HFSA/HRS/SCAI/SCCT/SCMR/STS 2013 multimodality appropriate use criteria for the detection and risk assessment of stable ischemic heart disease: a report of the American college of cardiology foundation appropriate use criteria task force, american heart association, american society of echocardiography, american society of nuclear cardiology, heart failure society of america, heart rhythm society, society for cardiovascular angiography and interventions, society of cardiovascular computed tomography, society for cardiovascular magnetic resonance, and society of thoracic surgeons. J Am Coll Cardiol. 2014;63(4):380–406.
6. Ferrari VA, Whitman B, Blankenship JC, Budoff MJ, Costa M, Weissman NJ, et al. Cardiovascular imaging payment and reimbursement systems: understanding the past and present in order to guide the future. J Am Coll Cardiol Img. 2014;7(3):324–32.
7. Soman P, Kelly R. Imaging at the 2014 ACC legislative conference: a debrief. J Am Coll Cardiol Img. 2015;8(1):118–20.
8. Greenwood JP, Maredia N, Younger JF, Brown JM, Nixon J, Everett CC, et al. Cardiovascular magnetic resonance and single-photon emission computed tomography for diagnosis of coronary heart disease (CE-MARC): a prospective trial. Lancet. 2012;379(9814):453–60.
9. Dandekar VK, Bauml MA, Ertel AW, Dickens C, Gonzalez RC, Farzaneh-Far A. Assessment of global myocardial perfusion reserve using cardiovascular magnetic resonance of coronary sinus flow at 3 Tesla. J Cardiovascular Magnetic Resonance Off J Soc Cardiovascular Magnetic Resonance. 2014;16(1):24.
10. Klem I, Heitner JF, Shah DJ, Sketch Jr MH, Behar V, Weinsaft J, et al. Improved detection of coronary artery disease by stress perfusion cardiovascular magnetic resonance with the use of delayed enhancement infarction imaging. J Am Coll Cardiol. 2006;47(8):1630–8.
11. Reimer KA, Jennings RB. The "wavefront phenomenon" of myocardial ischemic cell death. II. Transmural progression of necrosis within the framework of ischemic bed size (myocardium at risk) and collateral flow. Laboratory Investigation J Technical Methods Pathol. 1979;40(6):633–44.
12. McCrohon JA, Moon JC, Prasad SK, McKenna WJ, Lorenz CH, Coats AJ, et al. Differentiation of heart failure related to dilated cardiomyopathy and coronary artery disease using gadolinium-enhanced cardiovascular magnetic resonance. Circulation. 2003;108(1):54–9.
13. Hendel RC. Utilization management of cardiovascular imaging pre-certification and appropriateness. J Am Coll Cardiol Img. 2008;1(2):241–8.
14. Iglehart JK. Health insurers and medical-imaging policy–a work in progress. N Engl J Med. 2009;360(10):1030–7.
15. Bhattacharyya S, Kamperidis V, Chahal N, Shah BN, Roussin I, Li W, et al. Clinical and prognostic value of stress echocardiography appropriateness criteria for evaluation of coronary artery disease in a tertiary referral centre. Heart. 2014;100(5):370–4.
16. Willens HJ, Nelson K, Hendel RC. Appropriate use criteria for stress echocardiography: impact of updated criteria on appropriateness ratings, correlation with pre-authorization guidelines, and effect of temporal trends and an educational initiative on utilization. J Am Coll Cardiol Img. 2013;6(3):297–309.
17. Medolago G, Marcassa C, Alkraisheh A, Campini R, Ghilardi A, Giubbini R, et al. Applicability of the appropriate use criteria for SPECT myocardial perfusion imaging in Italy: preliminary results. Eur J Nucl Med Mol Imaging. 2014;41(9):1695–700.

18. Hendel RC, Cerqueira M, Douglas PS, Caruth KC, Allen JM, Jensen NC, et al. A multicenter assessment of the use of single-photon emission computed tomography myocardial perfusion imaging with appropriateness criteria. J Am Coll Cardiol. 2010;55(2):156–62.

19. Doukky R, Hayes K, Frogge N, Balakrishnan G, Dontaraju VS, Rangel MO, et al. Impact of appropriate use on the prognostic value of single-photon emission computed tomography myocardial perfusion imaging. Circulation. 2013;128(15):1634–43.

20. Winchester DE, Chauffe RJ, Meral R, Nguyen D, Ryals S, Dusaj R, Shaw L, Beyth RJ: Clinical utility of inappropriate positron emission tomography myocardial perfusion imaging: Test results and cardiovascular events. J Nuclear Cardiol Off Publication Am Soc Nuclear Cardiol 2014.

21. Armstrong W, Eagle KA. Appropriate use criteria in echocardiography: is no change the same as no benefit? JAMA Internal Med. 2013;173(17):1609–10.

22. Matulevicius SA, Rohatgi A, Das SR, Price AL, DeLuna A, Reimold SC. Appropriate use and clinical impact of transthoracic echocardiography. JAMA Internal Med. 2013;173(17):1600–7.

23. Abbasi SA, Ertel A, Shah RV, Dandekar V, Chung J, Bhat G, et al. Impact of cardiovascular magnetic resonance on management and clinical decision-making in heart failure patients. J Cardiovascular Magnetic Resonance Off J Soc Cardiovascular Magnetic Resonance. 2013;15:89.

4

A review of 3D first-pass, whole-heart, myocardial perfusion cardiovascular magnetic resonance

Merlin J. Fair[1,2]*, Peter D. Gatehouse[1,2], Edward V. R. DiBella[3] and David N. Firmin[1,2]

Abstract

A comprehensive review is undertaken of the methods available for 3D whole-heart first-pass perfusion (FPP) and their application to date, with particular focus on possible acceleration techniques. Following a summary of the parameters typically desired of 3D FPP methods, the review explains the mechanisms of key acceleration techniques and their potential use in FPP for attaining 3D acquisitions. The mechanisms include rapid sequences, non-Cartesian k-space trajectories, reduced k-space acquisitions, parallel imaging reconstructions and compressed sensing. An attempt is made to explain, rather than simply state, the varying methods with the hope that it will give an appreciation of the different components making up a 3D FPP protocol. Basic estimates demonstrating the required total acceleration factors in typical 3D FPP cases are included, providing context for the extent that each acceleration method can contribute to the required imaging speed, as well as potential limitations in present 3D FPP literature. Although many 3D FPP methods are too early in development for the type of clinical trials required to show any clear benefit over current 2D FPP methods, the review includes the small but growing quantity of clinical research work already using 3D FPP, alongside the more technical work. Broader challenges concerning FPP such as quantitative analysis are not covered, but challenges with particular impact on 3D FPP methods, particularly with regards to motion effects, are discussed along with anticipated future work in the field.

Keywords: Myocardial perfusion, 3D, Whole heart, Cardiovascular magnetic resonance

Introduction

Detection of coronary artery disease (CAD) through examination of dynamically contrast-enhanced myocardial perfusion cardiovascular magnetic resonance (CMR) is well established clinically [1, 2], following its first demonstrations in 1990 [3]. Dynamic contrast enhancement (DCE), here called first-pass perfusion (FPP), has shown high diagnostic accuracy [4] and compares favourably with other modalities as a "gate-keeper" to invasive coronary x-ray angiography [5]. Despite this, there are a multitude of desired properties in an ideal FPP protocol that CMR is currently unable to simultaneously meet with standard imaging speeds. In particular is the extension of FPP protocols from 2D non-contiguous coverage of the left ventricle (LV) to 3D whole-heart imaging, which has been hypothesised as a way of increasing the competitiveness of CMR for perfusion imaging [6]. Whilst there is debate over the clinical utility of 3D FPP when coverage is at the expense of other imaging parameters (discussed further in section *Imaging parameters for FPP*), there is interest in its potential; for example, possible increased confidence by obtaining more slices over the same cardiac regions and the slices being all at the same cardiac phase. There has therefore been a recent surge in publications on 3D FPP (see Table 1), and with it increasing application of extreme acceleration to FPP.

The purpose of this review is exploration of this wide range of current and potential techniques for achieving 3D FPP, in particular the acceleration of data acquisition. The characteristics of ideal FPP methods are reviewed first, with some reflection on the issues governing typical multi-slice 2D FPP. This follows into a justification for

* Correspondence: M.Fair@rbht.nhs.uk
[1]National Heart & Lung Institute, Imperial College London, London, UK
[2]Cardiovascular Magnetic Resonance Unit, Royal Brompton Hospital, Sydney Street, London SW3 6NP, UK
Full list of author information is available at the end of the article

Table 1 Overview of technical developments in 3D whole-heart first-pass perfusion

Lead Author	Year	Reconstruction Method	Trajectory	Other Stated Efficiencies*	US Factor (Nominal)	US Factor (True)	Resolution/mm	Acquisition Window/ms	Stress Agent	Free Breathing†	Field Strength/T
Shin [70]	2008	TSENSE	Cartesian	–	6	6	3.0 × 4.5 × 10.0	304	No	No	3
Shin [19]	2010	TSENSE	Cartesian	–	6	6	4.5 × 6.7 × 10.0[a]/ 2.8 × 4.2 × 10.0[b]	116-145[a]/254-305[b]	No	No	3
Manka [79]◊	2011	k-t SENSE	Cartesian	Partial Fourier	NS	6.3	2.3 × 2.3 × 10.0	200	Yes	No	3
Vitanis [81]	2011	k-t PCA (compartment based)	Cartesian	Elliptical Shutter (75 %); Partial Fourier (75 %)	10	5.6 - 7.5	2.3 × 2.3 × 10.0	225	Yes	No	3
DiBella [25]	2012	CS (temporal)	Radial	–	~14‡	~14‡	2.2 × 2.2 × 8.0	310	No	No	3
Manka [125] ◊	2012	k-t PCA	Cartesian	Partial Fourier	10	7	2.3 × 2.3 × 10.0	NS	Yes	No	1.5
Jogiya [126] ◊	2012	k-t PCA	Cartesian	Partial Fourier	10	7	2.3 × 2.3 × 5.0	NS	Yes	No	3
Chen [44]	2012	CS (spatio- temporal)	Radial	Partial Fourier (75 %)	~9-11‡	~9-11‡	(1.8-2.8) × (1.8-2.8) × (6.0-10.0)	300	No	No	3
Shin [39]	2013	k-t SENSE	Spiral	–	5	5	2.4 × 2.4 × 9.0¯	230	No	No	1.5
Giri [24]	2014	TWIST (GRAPPA)	Cartesian	2D Partial Fourier§ (87.5 %/87.5 %)	3	3	2.2 × 2.8 × 8.0	300-380	No	No	1.5
Motwani [56]	2014	k-t PCA	Cartesian	2D Partial Fourier (70 %/70 %)	10	7	2.3 × 2.3 × 5.0	192	Yes	No	3
Schmidt [58]	2014	k-t PCA (motion-corrected)	Cartesian	Elliptical Shutter; 3D Partial Fourier (62.5 %/75 %/75 %)	10	NS	2.3 × 2.3 × 10.0	205-225	No	Yes	3
Akçakaya [105]	2014	CS (localised constraints)	Cartesian	Elliptical Shutter (75 %)	10	10	2.3 × 2.3 × 10.0	250	No	Both	1.5
Jogiya [57]◊	2014[e]	k-t PCA	Cartesian	Elliptical Shutter; 2D Partial Fourier (75 %/75 %)	10	7	2.3 × 2.3 × 5.0	191	Yes	No	3
Jogiya [21]	2014	k-t PCA	Cartesian	Elliptical Shutter; 3D Partial Fourier (NS/75 %/75 %)	10	7	2.3 × 2.3 × 5.0	191	Yes	No	3
Wang [45]	2014[e]	CS (spatio-temporal)	Cartesian	Partial Fourier (83 %)	11	11	(2.0-2.4) × (2.0-2.4) × (4.0-6.0)	255	No	No	3
Manka [130]◊	2015[e]	k-t PCA	Cartesian	Elliptical Shutter; 2D Partial Fourier (75 %/75 %)	10	7	2.3 × 2.3 × 5.0	200	Yes	No	3

◊Clinically relevant/tested techniques – see Table 2 for details

*Zero padding typically not stated when applied, so not included in the table

†Imaging during breath-hold assumed in cases where literature did not state

‡US factor estimated from number of radial projections and number of readouts: $N_{Nyquist} = (\pi/2) * N_{readouts}$ N.b. using this definition radial trajectories require $\pi/2$ greater acceleration to be equivalent to a Cartesian acquisition time

§Only applied in cases of high HR

[a]Systolic acquisition values

[b]Diastolic acquisition values

¯Nominal spatial resolution can be affected by off-resonance errors in long spiral readouts

[e]Date of early online publication, yet to be published fully at time of print

NB The acquisition window as far as possible is the pure image data acquisition time not including saturation recovery delay pre-imaging as that is not normally motion-sensitive

Abbreviations: US undersampling; NS not stated; others as defined in text

the approximate acceleration required for translation to 3D, before a review and explanation of two main categories of acceleration methods applicable to 3D FPP. These are referred to as pulse sequence modification and sub-Nyquist reconstruction techniques, and include non-Cartesian k-space trajectories, k-space efficiencies, and multiple varieties of parallel imaging and compressed sensing. Having presented these methods concurrent with examples in 3D FPP literature, the smaller amount of clinical research is summarised. The issues arising with applying such acceleration techniques to FPP are then examined before finally discussing future considerations and requirements.

Imaging parameters for FPP

As with most medical imaging, the ideal parameters for 2D or 3D FPP are many, interdependent and often contradictory, causing a 'trade-off' in any realistic setting. They can broadly be broken down into the following areas: High spatial and temporal resolution, high signal-to-noise ratio (SNR) and coverage of the LV that supports the clinical purpose effectively. Unlike some other CMR applications, however, reliability is also critical for FPP of gadolinium-based contrast agents (GBCA) because reacquisition is impracticable.

Fine spatial resolution is required in-plane in order to adequately resolve the transmurality and extent of perfusion defects. It is also important for the problematic dark-rim artefact (DRA) [7], which frequently confounds imaging of perfusion defects. The DRA is partly caused by a Gibbs truncation effect at the sharp signal changes between the subendocardial myocardium and brighter contrast-enhanced blood-pool, and has been shown to be reduced at increased spatial resolutions [8]. For visual analysis of most defects, an isotropic in-plane resolution of 2 mm to 2.5 mm is generally deemed a sufficient balance in the trade-off against image acquisition duration and other parameters. Through-plane resolution is less important for clinical evaluation because the slice (or for 3D, 2nd phase-encoding) direction is typically along the long-axis of the heart. The impact of Gibbs artefacts in the through-plane direction has however so far undergone little investigation for 3D FPP [9]. An acquired slice-direction resolution of around 10 mm is typical in FPP, but in 3D imaging the final slice resolution is sometimes interpolated from coarser acquisitions, as will be reviewed later.

The temporal resolution of FPP imaging, i.e. imaging each slice every single cardiac cycle ("single-RR") or alternate cycles ("alternate-RR"), is another important consideration without a clear consensus and to some extent depending on the clinical application [10]. Acquiring single-RR multi-slice 2D arguably might increase diagnostic confidence in some situations. On the other hand, alternate-RR can deliver greater myocardial

coverage and with careful setup has potential to avoid imaging during phases of rapid cardiac motion [1, 11]. To date the topic of 3D FPP has entirely used single-RR, presumably due to the risk of data inconsistency if split over two cycles. This would be a more extreme version of some 3D FPP methods reviewed below in which some aspects of their raw data are potentially shared between adjoining cardiac cycles. However, some type of dual-slab alternate-RR method may have potential for reducing the toughest constraints on single-RR 3D FPP.

Myocardial SNR is of increased concern in the topic of 3D FPP due to the potential for SNR loss caused by many of the acceleration techniques presented here. The related contrast-to-noise ratio (CNR) is required to be high in distinguishing a perfusion defect from the normal tissue, especially as a defect may be only a mild limitation of blood supply. However CNR depends on many other factors such as contrast agent dose, T1 sensitivity, etc (see, for example, reference [10]).

Full coverage of the LV is often cited as a reason for investigating 3D FPP, but this is subject to the following discussion. Other perfusion modalities such as SPECT and PET, whilst providing lower resolutions, usually offer full coverage of the LV, whereas conventional CMR FPP acquires typically 3 or 4 equi-distant short-axis slices along the LV – although long-axis myocardial motion modulates their true myocardial coverage. There is some debate over the clinical utility of coverage of the whole LV [1, 12], hereafter referred to as "whole-heart" coverage, particularly when at the expense of other factors such as spatial resolution [13]. 2D FPP has already been proven a reliable method of investigating CAD, showing high accuracy in comparison to other techniques, as is reflected in multiple clinical guidelines. It has been shown that coverage with 3 or 4 short-axis slices is ample for clinical accuracy [1]. However, some potential clinical advantages of full coverage have been proposed. Most important of these is to assess the "ischaemic burden", due to its link to survival prognosis [14]. Secondly, it may improve confidence that no defects have been missed, although the coverage by 2D multi-slice has been shown sufficient as discussed. Thirdly, it may also assist in distinguishing between DRAs and true perfusion defects, as 3D may enable improved tracking of the hypointense region through-plane for discriminating between the two, in some situations employing knowledge of typical coronary territories as already used where appropriate in 2D FPP clinical work [15].

Continuous coverage (even if not whole-heart) supports the use of 3D imaging, with a potentially strong benefit that all the images in each cycle are at the same cardiac phase and respiratory phase, even if both are liable to intra-shot motion artefacts. 3D imaging acquires the raw data (k-space) with additional repeated acquisitions of phase-encoding ($N_{partitions}$) used to collect the third dimension, called slice or partition encoding. Along with providing contiguous coverage, this delivers a fundamental increase in SNR. From Edelstein et al. [16], keeping all other factors the same, it can be derived that the SNR in 3D compared to its 2D equivalent is

$$SNR_{3D} = SNR_{2D} \times \sqrt{N_{partitions}}.$$

A limitation to this equation is that it does not account for alterations in saturation caused by the slab RF excitation pulses compared to multi-slice. No direct measurement of this predicted SNR gain in 3D FPP has been performed, largely due to the modification of SNR by the acceleration methods required for 3D.

Whilst attempting to achieve the above parameters the final factor of note is in achieving reliability of the protocol. The imaging of the first-pass of GBCA makes repetition of acquisitions impracticable due to dose limits and wash out time, therefore making reliability key. Practically, a requirement for breath-hold, in support of the acceleration methods discussed later, introduces unreliability over whether the breath-hold is maintained during the key frames of contrast arrival, although the importance of this is debated. A requirement of breath-hold or gentle breathing is made more difficult by the potential impact of adenosine or other stressors on respiratory motion. The additional effect of misgating on acceleration methods is another concern for reliability.

Requirement for acceleration in 3D FPP

As has been mentioned, the above requirements cannot normally be achieved simultaneously, with spatial resolution, temporal resolution, LV coverage, reliability and SNR being traded off against each other. To gain an understanding of the shortfall of a basic imaging sequence in achieving all these properties, timings of a 3D fast low flip-angle spoiled gradient-echo (FLASH) sequence were calculated to illustrate potential optimal acquisition times (see Appendix). Despite using a sequence based on timing minimisation rather than image quality, this gives an acquisition time of around 2.8 s to acquire data of the whole-heart with the proposed parameters; this illustrates the scale of the challenge because FPP imaging requires at least alternate-cycle imaging of GBCA distribution, so the usual "segmented" methods for accumulating resolution over multiple cardiac cycles cannot be applied.

Whilst the above timings already prevent a temporal resolution of one (or two) cardiac cycles, the cardiac motion itself further limits the acquisition "window" for FPP to either the mid-diastolic or end-systolic pause (Fig. 1). Although some formulations exist for predicting these pause times based on the R-R interval, generally in CMR it is best practice to measure them using cine imaging [17]. For 3D FPP, the end-systolic period has a benefit of the heart being contracted along its long-axis, therefore requiring a smaller 3D partition-direction

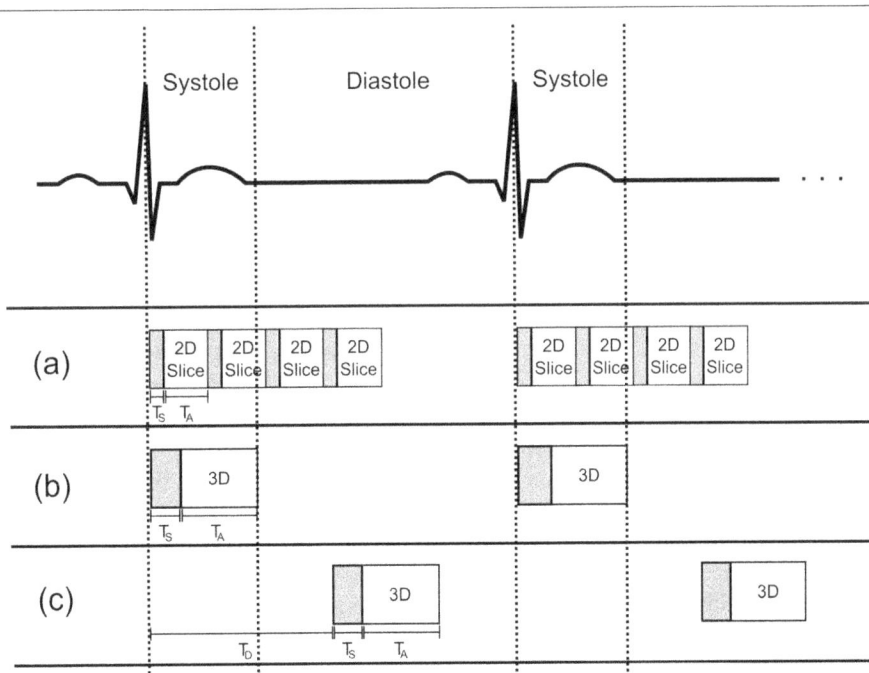

Fig. 1 Acquisition timings. Whilst conventional 2D multi-slice FPP is acquired throughout the cycle, typically starting in early systole (a), there are two popular options in 3D FPP. The 3D acquisition can be placed either in mid-systole (b) or mid-diastole (c), although the durations of these periods of minimal motion can be problematic (see text). Trigger delay (TD), saturation time (TS) and acquisition time (TA) are labelled for each in the first cardiac cycle

field-of-view (FOV) which directly reduces the imaging time needed per image. In this phase the myocardium is also transmurally thicker, which has been shown to give greater visualisation of perfusion defects [18]. End-systolic imaging in healthy subjects has been shown in 3D FPP to produce image quality comparable to diastole [19]. The systolic pause is however very short, so a large number of 3D FPP acquisitions to date are acquired in the diastolic pause. During physiological or pharmaco-logical stress both pauses become shorter, particularly at mid-diastole, and so potential acquisition windows are shortened further. Whilst 3D FPP work has a wide range of stated acquisition windows (Table 1), here an ideal time of less than 150 ms for the readout time is used in our estimates. With diastasis durations of ≤100 ms associated with HRs of ≥75 bpm [20], even 150 ms is a compromise towards the longer acquisi-tion windows currently being reported in 3D FPP literature.

The potential utility of 3D FPP has driven a surge in improvement of current acceleration techniques, as well as development of entirely novel processes. Acceleration factors of this magnitude are unlikely to be achieved dir-ectly through one method alone. Acceleration methods to date have used a combination of two broad areas: **pulse sequence modification (Section Pulse sequence modification)** and **sub-Nyquist sampling reconstruc-tion techniques (Section Acceleration through sub-Nyquist reconstruction).** This review will focus on the current and potential schemes used in these two areas to attain 3D FPP, along with the difficulties arising from their application and discussion on what the future may hold for this rapidly growing field.

Pulse sequence modification

Many of the acceleration methods described here can be applied to various CMR pulse sequence types. After a brief recap of the sequences used in FPP, an examination of the potential acceleration techniques will be presented.

Basic sequence types

Spoiled gradient-echo (SGRE) sequences at low flip-angles are widely used in FPP to produce a steady-state of longitudinal magnetisation, where "spoiling" scram-bles or dephases transverse magnetisation to become effectively zero before each RF pulse. Also known as Fast Low Angle Shot (FLASH), these sequences typically further increase the spoiling effectiveness through RF spoiling methods. For SGRE, the choice of flip-angle and the linked impact of B1-inhomogeneity are important in optimising scarce SNR, as reviewed later (Section Alternative k-space coverage).

The transverse magnetisation can effectively be recycled instead of discarded, in the sequence known generically as balanced steady-state free precession (bSSFP, or here as SSFP) [21] which can deliver higher SNR than SGRE as a higher flip-angle can be used. In theory SSFP is a good candidate for FPP; however, increased blood-myocardium contrast in SSFP imaging causes greater artefacts from ringing [22, 23]. The increased flip-angle of SSFP runs into specific absorption rate (SAR) limits, particularly at 3 T, sometimes enforcing a slowdown of the sequence. As well, there is increased unreliability of SSFP at 3 T due to off-resonance effects, whereas SGRE is more robust in regards to both SAR and off-resonance. Despite this, recent work has applied SSFP to 3D FPP at 3 T, investi-gating use of dual-source parallel transmit capabilities [21]. The application of this technique resulted in SSFP acquired 3D FPP datasets of similar quality to equi-valent 3D SGRE datasets, with predicted increased SNR and CNR; however, increased artefacts (including DRAs) were still present.

An extension to SSFP specifically for FPP, called Steady-State First-Pass Perfusion (SSFPP), applies the inherent sqrt(T2/T1) weighting of SSFP in the setting of short native myocardial T2 to deliver myocardial T1-weighting by continuous imaging without saturation pulses [24]. This was presented in 2D FPP as well as showing initial 3D experience. Earlier work used the SGRE steady-state to eliminate saturation pulses [25] with continuous ungated acquisition, before data with similar cardiac phase are identified and reconstructed. Focus was on good SNR and CNR in the myocardium, ig-noring effects in the blood pool including inflow artefacts from unsaturated blood, making this implementation of most benefit to non-quantitative FPP. However, for 3D FPP, the acquisition window per 3D image requires further acceleration before this approach may become more realistic.

Almost all 3D FPP work has been based on gated SGRE sequences and the focus of this review will continue with their optimisation.

Alternative k-space coverage

As with 2D encoding, coverage of k-space in 3D need not necessarily be Cartesian, and two such approaches can accelerate imaging.

Echo-planar Imaging (EPI) is geometrically closest to typical Cartesian k-space coverage (Fig. 2a) [23]. The premise is to collect multiple 'lines' of raw data by a series of gradient echoes after each RF pulse, allowing acceleration by omitting RF excitations. Due mainly to the limited echo-train length (ETL) achievable as a con-sequence of cardiac motion and main-field inhomogene-ities around the heart, hybrid EPI (h-EPI) is generally used in FPP [26] with limited applicability of true single-shot EPI [27, 28]. The compromise for h-EPI is made between increasing the ETL – which reduces total image

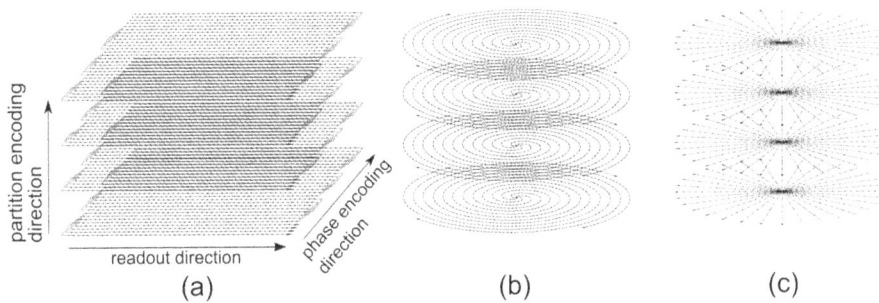

Fig. 2 Non-Cartesian trajectories. Examples of three potential alternate trajectories discussed in the text. EPI (**a**) demonstrated with an ETL of 4, a spiral trajectory (**b**) with 4 interleaves and a radial projection design (**c**). Partition encoding direction in (**b**) and (**c**) is the same as for (**a**)

time – and the corresponding increased unreliability [26, 29] which also increases with main field strength. Despite this, h-EPI in 2D FPP typically uses an ETL of around 4 at 1.5 T (no current examples at 3 T), corresponding to acceleration factors of approximately 2 compared to the FLASH timings calculated earlier (see Appendix). Early examples of 2D FPP with extended LV coverage used h-EPI [26, 30, 31] but so far 3D EPI imaging has largely been limited to non-cardiac work.

Other trajectories in k-space gain their efficiency through altering the geometry of their coverage to collect more data after each RF excitation. Spiral imaging [32, 33] collects data while spiralling outward from the central raw data through k-space (Fig. 2b), replacing the conventional phase-encode and frequency-encode gradients. Again, as with EPI, the multi-shot variants are most commonly used for FPP, due to the relatively large amount of data required and off-resonance effects with long spiral readout durations [34]. Careful choice of readout duration, flip-angle strategy and other characteristics of a spiral sequence have been shown to compensate for spiral related artefacts in FPP to produce high quality images [35]. Extension of spiral sequences to 3D can in theory provide spherical or elliptical coverage [36]. Far more common however is 3D by a stack of spiral planes with Fourier encoding in the third direction, giving a cylindrical distribution. The acceleration achieved with a stack of spiral design for the purpose discussed here is estimated to be similar to that of h-EPI (see Appendix). The spirals can be produced as uniform density, with a constant sampling interval in the radial direction of k-space, or with variable density which utilises greater sampling density radially in the central region of k-space than is used further out. These variable-density spirals have been shown to improve image quality in 2D FPP [37]. Variable density in the radial direction results in either oversampling the centre of k-space to reduce aliasing artefacts [38] or to have undersampled edges combined with a Nyquist sampled centre, suitable for combination with parallel imaging (discussed later). A 'dual-density' approach, with uniform

fully-sampled centre and uniform undersampled edges of the spirals, was applied by Shin et al. [39] in conjunction with advanced parallel imaging techniques to achieve 3D whole-heart FPP. This gave in-plane resolution of 2.4 mm × 2.4 mm, and compared favourably with the image quality and dynamics of 2D Cartesian acquisitions, with an acquisition time of 230 ms but was performed only at rest.

Sampling with projections (Fig. 2c) through the centre of k-space ('projection acquisition' or 'diametrical sampling') is now often named 'radial' imaging. For Nyquist sampling at the edges of the acquired k-space, radial trajectories massively oversample the centre, leading to high motion robustness. Even when the edges of raw data are undersampled, the full or oversampled centres naturally support parallel imaging and other acceleration techniques. Radial trajectories in themselves are fundamentally somewhat slower than the conventional phase-encoded approach, but they allow acceleration techniques to be applied efficiently. Likely due to its lower comparative efficiency, radial imaging has seen less application to 2D FPP, with its limited applications drawing on its suitability to specific purposes (e.g. multiple samples through the centre of k-space to calculate the arterial input function [40] and its inherent motion robustness for free-breathing [41]). Radial sampling does however lend itself to combination with compressed sensing methods [42] and as greater numbers of motion sensitive compressed sensing methods emerge it may be applied more to 3D FPP [43] (more discussion in Sections Compressed sensing and Motion correction & free-breathing 3D FPP). Recently, radial trajectories have been used for 3D whole-heart FPP sequences [25, 44, 45], combined with compressed sensing. In all cases, a stack of the 2D radial trajectories formed a 3D cylinder, as for the spiral examples. True 3D radial trajectories are also possible [46], with techniques such as Vastly undersampled Isotropic Projection Reconstruction (VIPR) [47] utilising the greater tolerance to undersampling, but these are less common in cardiac work. As with 2D radial, these trajectories are suited to compressed sensing and similar reconstruction techniques [48], however, the small number of projections achievable in 3D FPP and relaxed requirement for isotropic resolution make them less desirable.

Amalgamation of the benefits of the above trajectories can be achieved, for example by adding a spiral twist to the ends of radial projections, known as TWIsting Radial Lines (TWIRL) [49] or using a Cartesian grid acquisition for each projection angle, named Periodically Rotated Overlapping ParallEL Lines with Enhanced Reconstruction (PROPELLER) [50]. These have not been applied to even 2D FPP, but are possible considerations for the highly optimised sequences required for 3D FPP.

Other k-space efficiencies

To achieve the acceleration required for 3D FPP, further reductions in raw data coverage are often applied in conjunction with the other methods discussed, although they are compatible with only some non-Cartesian methods (see Section Alternative k-space coverage). These k-space "efficiencies" or 'tricks' include methods such as partial Fourier, elliptical shutters, zero padding and zonal-imaging (see Fig. 3) and are described in this section. Many of the details of these techniques can be found in textbooks, such as [51] or [52].

Partial Fourier imaging (Fig. 3a) is also sometimes known as partial averaging (fractional NEX) or partial echo when applied along phase-encode and frequency-encode directions respectively. If fully implemented, partial Fourier uses the "conjugate symmetry" [51] of k-space under certain conditions to reconstruct omitted regions. In reality, phase variations across the image FOV, caused by various factors, break the mathematical conditions supporting this method. In practice therefore, correction can use a low-resolution phase image estimated by raw data collection extending slightly into the omitted half [53–55]. A simpler alternative is more often performed, which is not true partial Fourier reconstruction, simply zero-filling the portions of k-space omitted by the truncated acquisition, for input to the reconstruction by Fourier

transformation. However, this usually requires a higher proportion of acquired k-space for acceptable accuracy, and wider Gibbs ringing artefacts are typically provoked by the sudden truncation of sampling nearer central k-space. This process is effectively a filter and consequently reduces spatial resolution. Zero-filling does however allow truncated acquisition to be applied in multiple directions simultaneously (unlike conjugate synthesis), giving greater acceleration. Cartesian examples of 3D whole-heart FPP have used this principle of zero-filled "partial Fourier" extensively, in 2 [56, 57] and all 3 [58] dimensions simultaneously.

Another type of zero-filling or "zero-padding" in raw data operates by "pads" of extra zero-valued lines added symmetrically to both edges of k-space (Fig. 3b) before applying the Fourier transform. This synthetically reduces the pixel size of the reconstructed image, without the added time of acquiring extra data. This is virtually equivalent to post-reconstruction interpolation of pixels, but differs regarding consistency of the Gibbs artefact [59]. This is prominently used in the partition direction in 3D imaging due to the significant extension in time needed to increase the acquired data in this direction, but can be applied in any or all directions. Artefacts such as Gibbs ringing are common with this technique, as previously mentioned, with the sharp cut-off in k-space manifesting as ringing artefacts at strong edges in the image. Some filtering can be applied to reduce this ringing at the cost of loss of resolution. Zero-padding is not always explicitly stated in literature, but with Gibbs ringing a particular issue in DRAs with FPP, care needs to be taken with these techniques.

Another possible efficiency gain, again by omitting regions of k-space, is to exclude the acquisition of the corner regions of k-space (Fig. 3c). This has various names but will here be referred to as an elliptical shutter, due to the typical shape of the acquired k-space afterwards. Due to the small genuine signal amplitude in outer regions compared with the uniformity of noise,

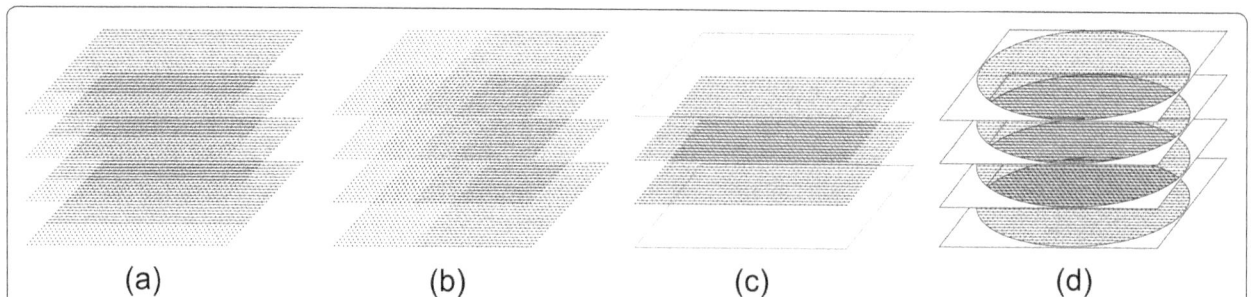

| (a) | (b) | (c) | (d) |

Fig. 3 K-space efficiencies. Three k-space acquisition modifications demonstrated for a 3D Cartesian sequence. Representations of partial Fourier in the phase-encoding (**a**) and readout (partial-echo) (**b**) directions are shown, with dashed lines denoting data points that are not acquired but later calculated (see text). Zero padding (**c**) has lines of 'data' filled with zeros added either side of the acquired data before reconstruction, artificially increasing resolution. An elliptical shutter (**d**) does not acquire the corner regions of k-space, as they are deemed less critical. Each of these methods can be applied in any encoding direction and those chosen here are simply illustrative

removal of the corners of k-space can improve the SNR. Furthermore, with an apodisation filter to reduce Gibbs ringing typically applied in a radial or elliptical fashion for isotropic resolution, the corners of k-space, even if acquired, are typically filtered to zero before reconstruction. Some efficiency can therefore be gained by omitting acquisition of these corners in the first place. However, combination with other efficiencies makes the effects of this process more complex, with the corners of k-space impacting the resolution when applying zero-padding [60]. The combination of an elliptical shutter and 3-dimensional partial Fourier mentioned in the previous paragraph, on top of other acceleration methods (see Section Parallel imaging using joint spatiotemporal redundancy), has resulted in a 3D FPP protocol acquiring just 5 % of the total k-space region [58]. These three types of "zero-filling" k-space efficiency are widely used to further accelerate 3D FPP in addition to the "headline" methods of many papers.

Inner-volume [61], zoomed or zonal-imaging reduces acquisition times by exciting only the required phase-encode FOV, therefore reducing the number of acquired data lines. This can be done by spin-echo, as previously demonstrated in 2D FPP EPI [29, 62], and by two-dimensional spatially selective pulses [63] without spin-echo limitations. The biggest drawback of this latter approach is the complexity and extended duration of zone-selection, which is much slower than ordinary slice-excitation. The scanning efficiency gained by zonal-imaging is therefore highly dependent on the application. For 2D FPP, the phase-encode FOV is typically already minimised to the smallest dimension of the patient's thorax in the typical short-axis plane, even permitting phase-encode wraparound if it does not reach the LV myocardium. This, combined with the requirement for rapid repetition of RF excitations, limits zone-selective imaging in 3D FPP, based on simple estimates balancing 2D-selective RF pulse duration, ETL, SNR and phase-encode FOV reduction.

Acceleration through sub-Nyquist reconstruction

The second broad area of acceleration techniques mentioned at the start of this review is sub-Nyquist reconstruction techniques. As with some of the methods discussed above (Section Other k-space efficiencies), they gain efficiency by sampling fewer points in k-space. However, rather than reducing the extent of k-space coverage, these methods accelerate through undersampling, defined as increasing the spacing between k-space samples to an extent that would typically cause intolerable FOV aliasing (wraparound) artefacts [64]. Each version differs in the way undersampling is performed, and also critically the method used to compensate for missing data and reconstruct an image without FOV aliasing.

These methods can achieve high acceleration factors and are an essential component in 3D FPP.

Early work using parallel imaging

One of the biggest breakthroughs in MRI, certainly with regards to imaging acceleration, was the invention and improvement of parallel imaging (PI) methods. The basic premise is to achieve acceleration by utilising spatial redundancy in multiple receiver coils [64, 65] and several varieties are standard on commercial scanners. The ability to perform accurate reconstruction with PI acceleration opened the door to the first attempts at whole-heart FPP. With only relatively low acceleration factors achievable due to the SNR losses accompanying PI, the first adaptations to whole heart coverage used multiple timeframes of FPP series data in calculating coil sensitivity (so called temporal PI techniques) to maximise acceleration.

Köstler et al. used auto-SENSE in 2003 to first demonstrate whole-heart coverage every cardiac cycle, with a contiguous stack of 2D slices [66]. Despite achieving full coverage, only an undersampling acceleration factor of 2 was applied and therefore spatial resolution was coarser than the ideal values considered earlier. Kellman et al. [31] extended the use of h-EPI with TSENSE [67] to produce improved quality in extended coverage FPP, potentially whole-heart, but again limited by the parallel imaging performance to an acceleration factor of 2.

These first two works moved towards whole-heart FPP whilst utilising 2D imaging; the step from 2D to 3D requires greater acceleration. 3D trajectories do, however, allow PI to be split across the two phase-encoded directions [68]. PI performed in this way is more efficient than the same acceleration across just one direction, as increases in the g-factor dependent part of SNR loss can be lower (strongly dependent on coil design). Application of SENSE with an undersampling factor of 6 (3x2, phase-encoded and partition-encoded directions respectively) first demonstrated the feasibility of 3D whole-heart FPP [69]. A more detailed comparison with multi-slice 2D FPP was later made with similar methods but utilising the greater SNR of higher field strengths, and additionally demonstrated the benefit of 3D imaging in estimating defect size [70].

Parallel imaging using joint spatiotemporal redundancy

The feasibility of true 3D whole-heart FPP with good SNR, spatial and temporal resolution improved with the introduction of new PI methods. These take advantage of the similarity of large portions of the images during FPP, and/or the generally gradual changes in image contrast that occur, known technically as using joint spatiotemporal redundancy in dynamically acquired datasets [71]. These techniques are collectively referred to here as k-t PI techniques, due to the temporally (t) varying k-space (k) sampling pattern used in these methods. An extension to the original PI and temporal PI techniques to make simultaneous use of spatial and temporal redundancy, the roots of k-t PI methods can be traced back to the UNFOLD reconstruction algorithm [72]. Redundancy in CMR datasets across time (i.e. across the temporal dimension) can be translated mathematically as a narrower point spread function (PSF) of the series of images when transformed into representation of the different temporal frequencies in the series. This is known as the x-f domain, where x represents all of the spatial dimensions (as with an image in x-y) and f corresponds to frequency, obtained through a Fourier transform across the image in the time series (Fig. 4). This means, with appropriate sampling patterns and small enough acceleration factors, the leakage of PSF energy due to aliasing can be filtered from the true object signal (Fig. 5), which is then Fourier-transformed back to make unaliased images. The process, in effect applying a temporal filter, does not directly cause SNR degradation of gradual changes in image contrast, and therein lies its potential. However, this also ties into a limitation; that more sudden or dynamic real changes in image contrast can lose SNR locally [73], for example if a GBCA bolus remains very compact on arrival in the myocardium.

Whilst UNFOLD and its predecessors uncovered a powerful concept of capitalising on the combined redundancies in spatial and temporal dimensions, its application in cardiac work is mostly limited to acceleration factors of 2 [74] due to the dynamic region being restricted to only 50 % of the FOV. This produces a spreading of the PSF that would overlap at higher acceleration rates and therefore cannot be separated through a simple filter. This minimisation of the dynamic region therefore has a built-in assumption of perfect breath-hold, although a method of easing this constraint to improve applicability to free-breathing FPP has been presented [75].

Alone this would not support the acceleration required for 3D FPP. Extension to the concept is made through modelling of the expected signal correlations in x-f space using low-resolution unaliased data, known as "training data". This allows accurate separation of the signal in this space, even for the multiple overlaps resulting from high acceleration factors and dynamic contrast (Fig. 6). This and its enhancement to incorporate parallel imaging are known as k-t BLAST and k-t SENSE respectively [76]. Nominal undersampling factors (undersampling factor, excluding collection of training data) of 5 were demonstrated with k-t SENSE in 2D FPP by Plein et al. [8], with the recouped time used to increase resolution. Vitanis et al. [77] used SENSE to acquire higher resolution training data, which supported a higher undersampling factor (nominal 8, true 5.8) for k-t SENSE

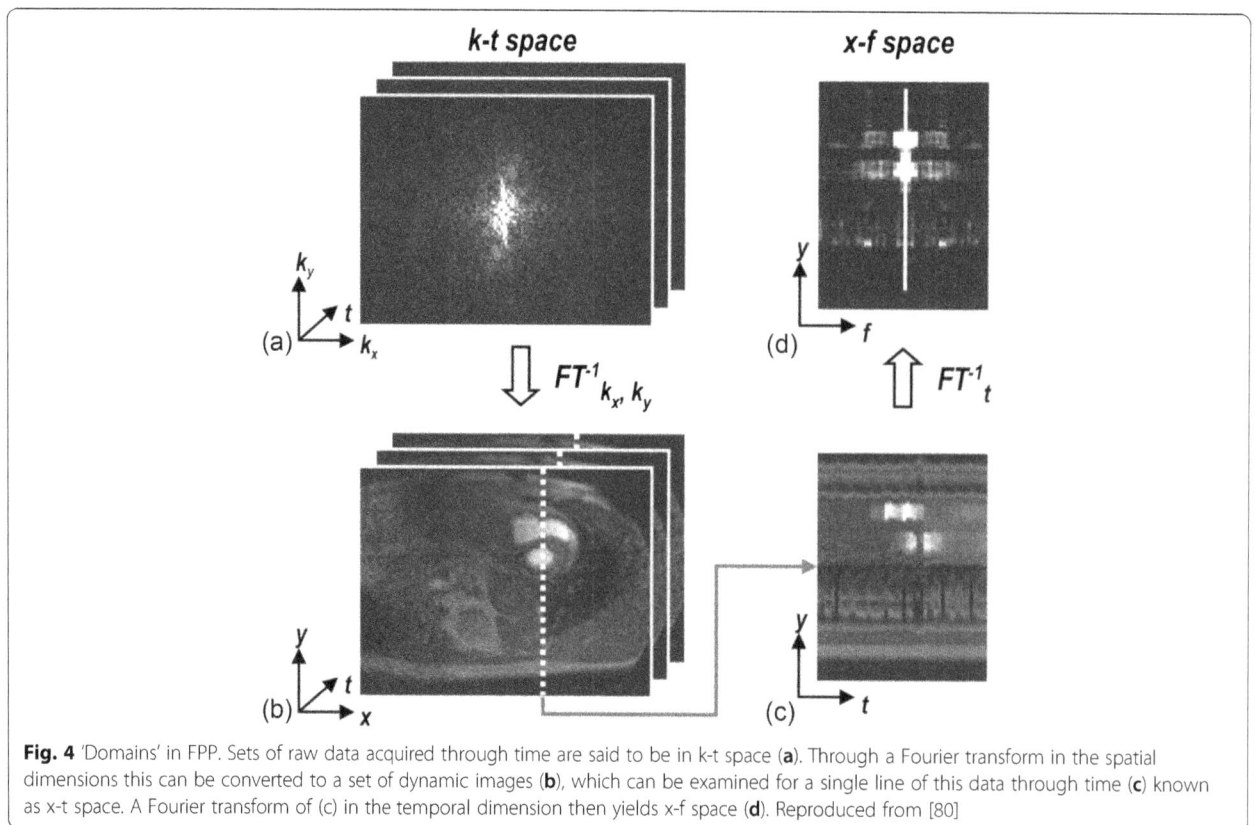

Fig. 4 'Domains' in FPP. Sets of raw data acquired through time are said to be in k-t space (**a**). Through a Fourier transform in the spatial dimensions this can be converted to a set of dynamic images (**b**), which can be examined for a single line of this data through time (**c**) known as x-t space. A Fourier transform of (c) in the temporal dimension then yields x-f space (**d**). Reproduced from [80]

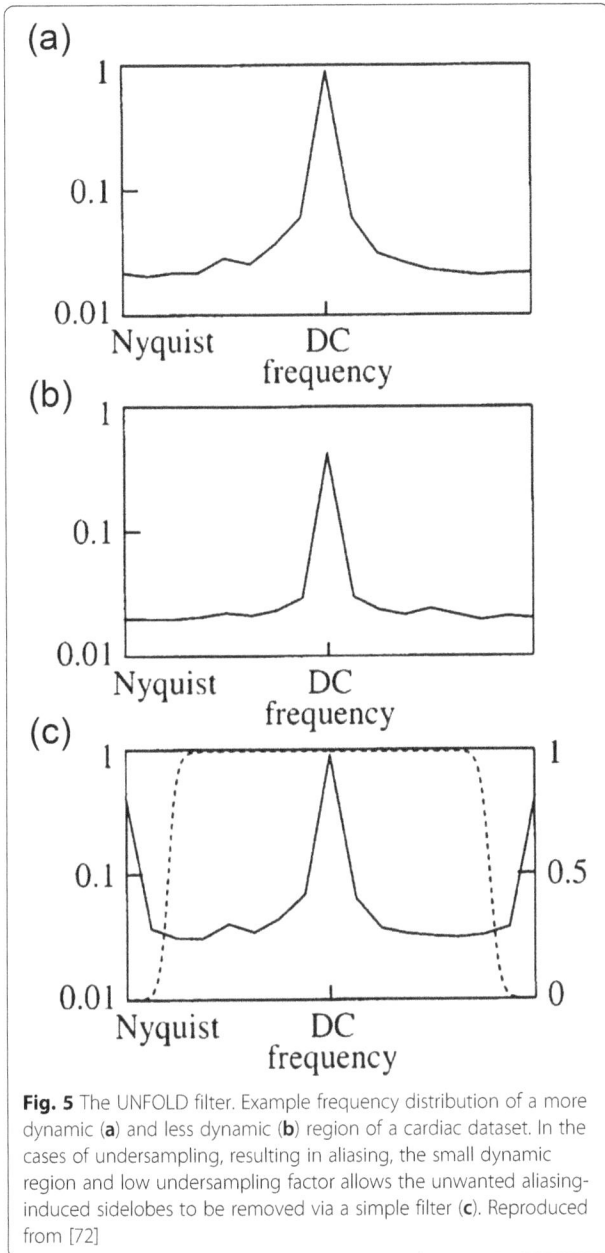

Fig. 5 The UNFOLD filter. Example frequency distribution of a more dynamic (**a**) and less dynamic (**b**) region of a cardiac dataset. In the cases of undersampling, resulting in aliasing, the small dynamic region and low undersampling factor allows the unwanted aliasing-induced sidelobes to be removed via a simple filter (**c**). Reproduced from [72]

accelerated 2D FPP. In theory training data can be collected either through a prescan or integrated into the undersampled data itself each cardiac cycle, although this latter case is by far the most popular. Due to the importance of the training data's resolution on unwanted temporal filtering effects, an auto-calibrated approach with training data derived from a TSENSE acquisition has also recently been proposed [78] and could be applicable to FPP. k-t BLAST and k-t SENSE have limits in application to FPP due to motion and contrast sensitivity limiting reliability of reconstruction accuracy [8]. As stated earlier, respiratory motion in FPP causes a further spreading of the signal in the x-f domain, beyond the limited spread due to

changing image contrast, and therefore such motion reduces the ability of the reconstruction algorithm to correct the aliased data. Despite this, Manka et al. [79] successfully applied k-t SENSE in 3D FPP with a true undersampling factor of 6.3x to a fast Cartesian sequence (including other k-space efficiencies, see Section Other K-space efficiencies), achieving an acquisition window of 200 ms and good spatial and temporal resolution. It has also been applied, using a lower total acceleration, in conjunction with a stack-of-spirals sequence design at similar resolution, though with a longer acquisition window of >300 ms [39].

Transformation of a time-series of images into the x-f domain is the essential component of each of these techniques. Many of the latest techniques aim to accelerate dynamic datasets such as FPP by extending this concept further, with additional or different transformations into mathematical domains that have properties better suiting the reconstruction of the specific dataset type. The method known as k-t PCA is a prime example of this extension and is currently the sub-Nyquist undersampling technique most commonly implemented in 3D FPP literature (see Table 1). As an extension to k-t BLAST (or k-t SENSE), k-t PCA improves the adaptive filter (described above) for removing aliasing while leaving FPP changes unfiltered, by applying principal component analysis (PCA) to the training data used for calculating that filter. This is effectively transforming the images into a new domain of temporal "basis function" components (x-PC) rather than the less suitable temporal pure frequencies as in x-f [80]. The advantage of this principal component domain is that it is more sparse, even in the cases of non-periodic motion such as respiration or misgating. Due to this, the majority of the FPP information is contained within a few principal components, allowing the rest to be discarded. This allows overlapping image space signals to be more easily separated before being converted back into images. Whilst producing large improvements in its ability to cope with greater motion and contrast changes than k-t SENSE, some artefacts and temporal resolution loss can remain in these situations, particularly at higher acceleration factors [73, 81].

Vitanis et al. [81] was the first work to examine the techniques for developing 3D whole-heart FPP with use of k-t PI methods, seen in Fig. 7, by a modified k-t PCA technique designed to support the higher acceleration factors demanded for 3D FPP at higher resolutions. A compartment-based model system was added to k-t PCA using automatic identification of compartments of interest (e.g. LV myocardium, LV blood pool, etc). By using an initial higher-resolution reconstruction process, voxels contaminated by partial volume effects in the low resolution training data could be excluded. This is thought to

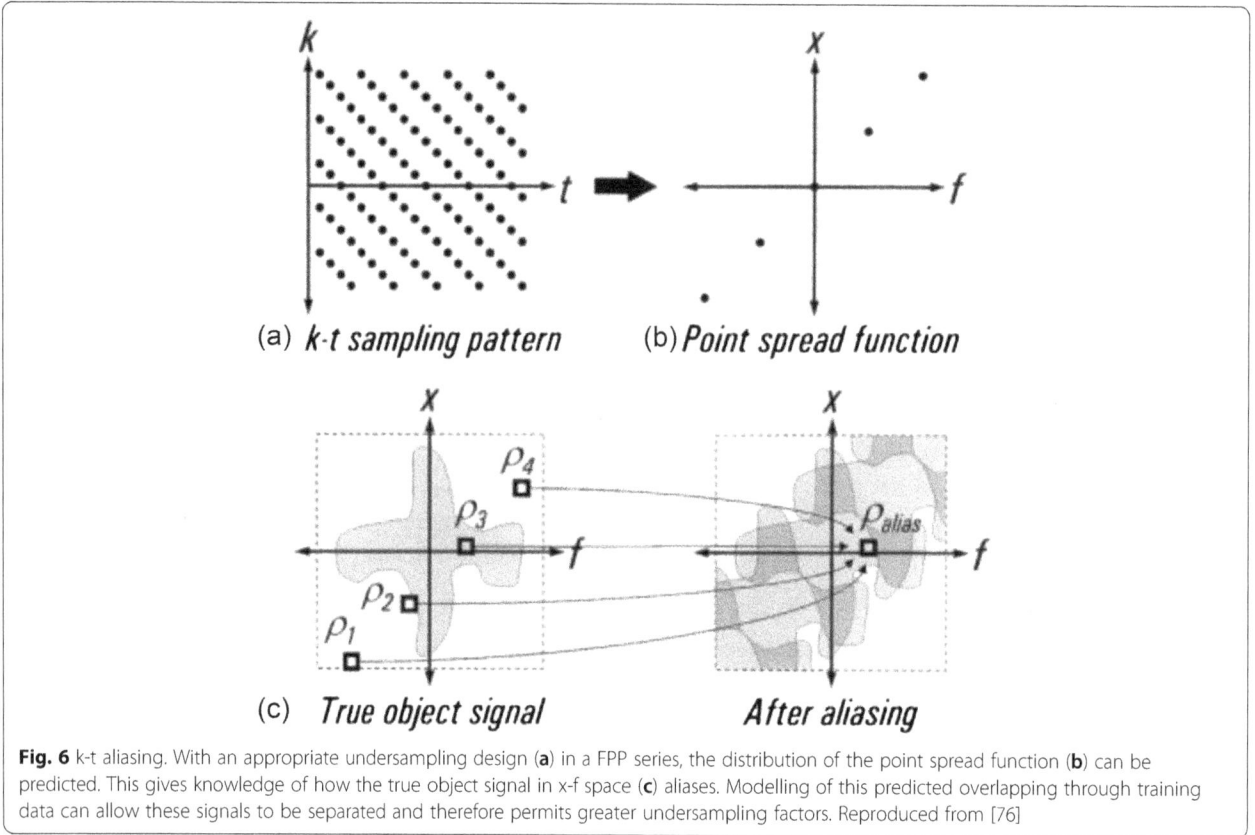

Fig. 6 k-t aliasing. With an appropriate undersampling design (**a**) in a FPP series, the distribution of the point spread function (**b**) can be predicted. This gives knowledge of how the true object signal in x-f space (**c**) aliases. Modelling of this predicted overlapping through training data can allow these signals to be separated and therefore permits greater undersampling factors. Reproduced from [76]

compensate for a large proportion of the errors in the calculation of the temporal basis functions in conventional k-t PCA. Application of this method allowed temporal and spatial resolution to be maintained (1 RR and 2.3 × 2.3 × 10.0 mm respectively) during whole-heart coverage through use of 10x nominal (5.6-7.5x true) undersampling factor, combined with additional k-space efficiencies. Work from the same group later employed non-rigid motion correction as part of an iterative version of k-t PCA so as to improve 3D FPP reconstruction in the presence

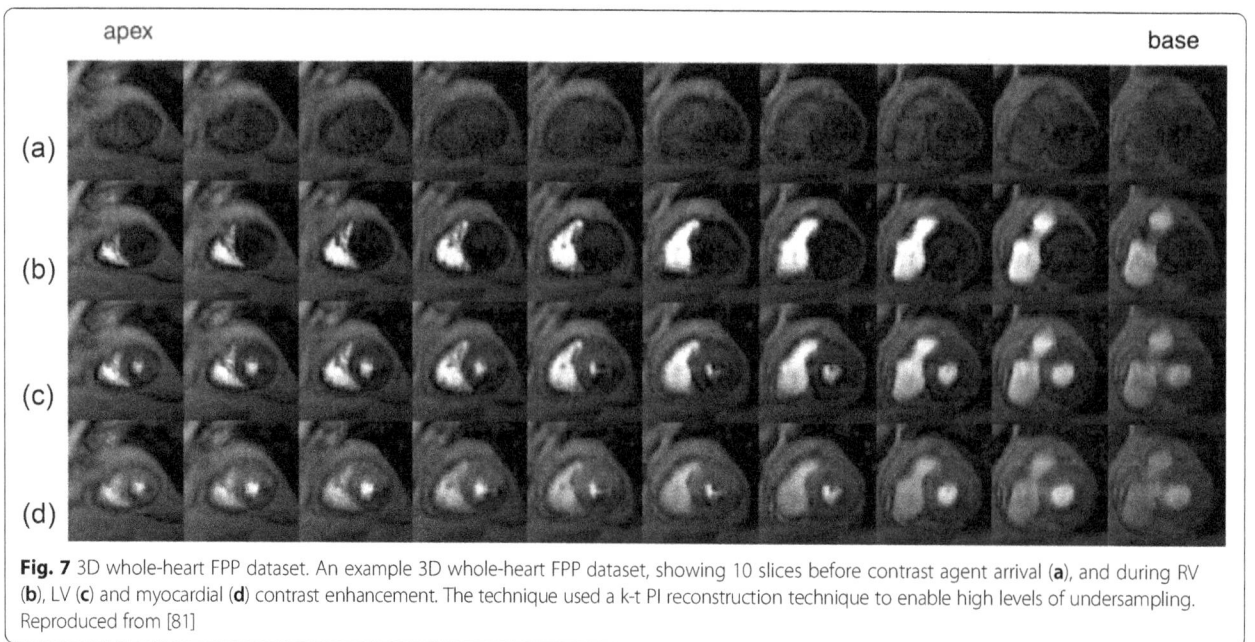

Fig. 7 3D whole-heart FPP dataset. An example 3D whole-heart FPP dataset, showing 10 slices before contrast agent arrival (**a**), and during RV (**b**), LV (**c**) and myocardial (**d**) contrast enhancement. The technique used a k-t PI reconstruction technique to enable high levels of undersampling. Reproduced from [81]

of more severe motion, particularly in the case of failed breath-hold/free-breathing [58]. Motion correction increases robustness of the reconstruction scheme to free-breathing or breath-hold failure through frame-to-frame warping of the x-PC training data to match a specified 'reference' shape, selected at one phase of the respiratory cycle. Similar acceleration factors and imaging parameters were achieved with this approach, with reported improvement of image quality.

Other parallel imaging methods

There has been a proliferation in new parallel imaging techniques, based both on spatial and spatiotemporal redundancy, with extensions to the previously described work as well as more unique implementations. While most could in theory be applied to 3D FPP, this review omits much of the parallel imaging work that has not yet been so applied.

CMR reconstruction is fundamentally a "linear" process. The term linear, in situations such as this, simply refers to an output that is proportional to an input, for example, with a tissue of twice the brightness in an image corresponding during scanning to twice the strength of its supporting components of the raw data (k-space) values. PI is also fundamentally a linear process as, using coil response profiles, it solves a set of linear equations. Recent parallel imaging has focussed on exploiting all available data in the most efficient manner. "Self consistency" is one such approach; optimising together ("joint estimation") the reconstruction of the image and estimation of the coil calibration data, called SPIRiT [82]. When it comes to finding a solution to these types of joint estimation scenarios, the system of equations to be solved no longer linearly connects the raw data to the output images. One way to solve this is "non-linear inversion" (NLINV), repeated inside an iterative search for the best-fit solution [83]. Such a non-linear scheme with an added variational penalty (described in Section Compressed sensing) has demonstrated high quality reconstructions in real time imaging of the heart, with an acceleration factor of approximately 10 [84]. Non-linear reconstructions may allow greater reconstruction accuracy for FPP at higher acceleration factors, making it a potential candidate for 3D FPP reconstruction.

Parallel imaging for non-Cartesian trajectories such as radial and spiral can be challenging, as discussed next. The SENSE category of methods, which operate by correcting phase-encode wrap-around in images, are more difficult to apply because the effects of undersampling do not give FOV wrap-around artefacts like Cartesian undersampling. Methods to solve this exist [85], but are not as simple to implement (see Section Computational efficiency). The GRAPPA category, where unsampled raw data is calculated from nearby samples in the raw data, depends on the accurate estimate of the "weighting factors" from sampled to unsampled points; for trajectories over the raw data such as radial and spiral sampling, the estimation of the GRAPPA weights is complicated due to non-equidistant spacing between k-space points. Alternative strategies for calculation of the GRAPPA weights have been proposed to rectify this difficulty for GRAPPA [86–88]. Recently 'through-time' calibration techniques for radial GRAPPA [89] and spiral GRAPPA [90] have been developed, which calculate the weights using multiple fully-sampled prescans. Through-time radial GRAPPA has been used for breath-held 2D FPP achieving whole-heart coverage with 15 slices [91] as well as in 3D for non-FPP applications [92].

Time-resolved angiography With Interleaved Stochastic Trajectories (TWIST), which builds on 'keyhole' techniques that update sections of k-space at different rates, alters the 2D phase-encode pattern. The outer portions of the raw data are collected in a pseudo-random pattern that, combined with multiple timeframes, manipulates the undersampling pattern enabling reconstruction via parallel imaging. Originally designed for angiography, it was adapted in SSFPP [24] and used with GRAPPA, as part of a 3D FPP protocol.

Close analogies can be drawn between some of the qualities exploited with these later techniques, namely nonlinear reconstruction and "random" undersampling patterns, and those used in the final main technique to be discussed – compressed sensing.

Compressed sensing

This section introduces compressed sensing (CS), followed by the applications of CS to 2D and 3D FPP.

The mathematical framework of CS [93] is relatively recent and was almost immediately considered for CMR due to the inherent suitability of aspects of CMR data. CS utilises the implicit 'sparsity' in MR images, either in the image itself or in a suitable mathematical representation (i.e. in a transform domain via a 'sparsifying transform') of the image, to reconstruct accelerated acquisitions. The term sparsity is simply used to describe a matrix, e.g. of image pixels or raw data points, that are predominately zero valued. Such sparseness may exist after a transform due to redundancy in a single image or over a series of related images. Using this property, CS allows accurate reconstruction of undersampled data, with the proviso that the sampling pattern is 'random' and that an appropriate non-linear reconstruction is used [94]. Compression of images using sparsifying transforms is well known [95] and compressed sensing attempts to implement the same concept from the reverse direction; if images can be compressed accurately, then it may be possible to scan faster by acquiring less data in the first place.

44

Handbook of Angiography

The ability to sample a reduced number of random positions in k-space is essential to realise this idea, with such *random* subsampling in k-space resulting in *incoherent* (i.e. noise-like) aliasing artefacts in images. One way to consider this is that strong signals rising above a predetermined threshold can be selected, and the expected interference pattern arising from these signals can be calculated. This interference signal can then be subtracted from the original and the process repeated on the subtracted data, with lowering thresholds, until the true sparse signals have been separated from the aliased signals [42]. In this simplistic version of CS, the process effectively 'denoises' the incoherent artefacts created by the random undersampling. In practice, reconstruction of this randomly undersampled data is performed via the solution to an appropriate constrained optimization problem [42].

In MRI, random sampling is limited to phase-encoded direction(s) but can also vary during a series of images, such as during FPP. CS techniques have accelerated 2D FPP [96] for increased resolution or LV coverage, as with k-t PI. CS has an advantage that it does not require training data which can reduce the overall acceleration. Similar temporal characteristics in the reconstructions are seen at lower acceleration factors between CS and k-t PI methods, with the most basic variants of both struggling beyond a critical value of ~5 in human FPP [97]. The increased error for higher accelerations is particularly prominent for CS, limited by insufficient sparsity that is typically achieved in FPP by transformations into other domains, as in k-t PI methods. The x-f domain was popular for early CS work, e.g. k-t SPARSE [98] and k-t FOCUSS [99]. However, in FPP, due to the changing image contrast, a wider range of temporal frequencies causes weaker sparsity in this domain, and therefore other domains have been proposed [100].

With potentially high CS acceleration factors under the ideal conditions of good breath-holding and ECG-triggering, work has gone into modifying the standard CS processes to correct for respiratory motion. A technique utilising the Sparsity and Low-Rank properties of the dynamic datasets termed k-t SLR [100] has shown promise in 2D free-breathing FPP in comparison to other CS reconstructions [101], using a transform that provides greater sparsity even in free breathing (Fig. 8). Usman et al. [102] presented free-breathing 2D FPP with more direct motion compensation, improving on methods that adjust for affine deformations (e.g. [99]), integrating a general motion correction technique directly into the CS algorithm. Block LOw-rank Sparsity with Motion-

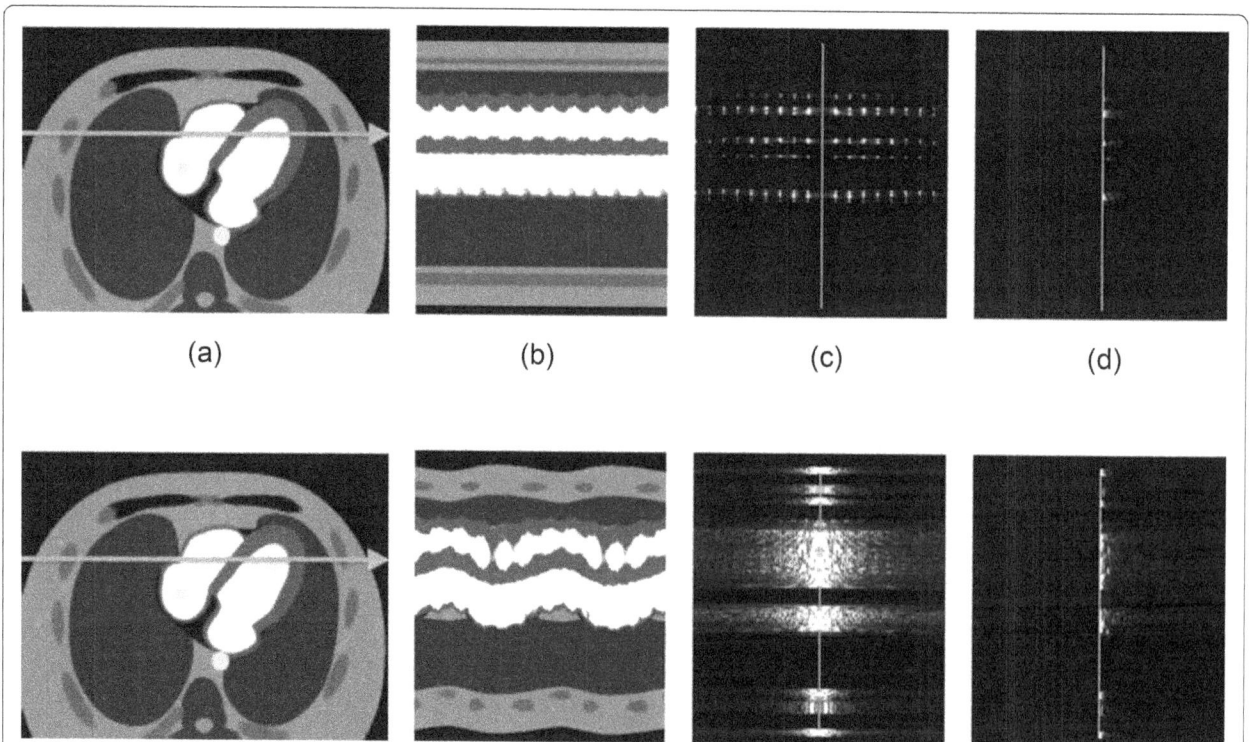

Fig. 8 Breath-held and free-breathing sparsity in different domains. The image (**a**), x-t (**b**), x-f (**c**), and x-KLT (**d**) domains of simulated breath-held (top) and free-breathing (bottom) datasets. The x-f domain (**c**) is seen to be far more sparse when the patient is breath-holding than when the patient is allowed to breathe. (**d**) shows the potential for alternate domains to increase sparsity, with improvements in both cases, but of particular importance in the case of free-breathing. KLT stands for Karhunen-Loève transform and is not discussed further - more information can be found in the references in the text. Reproduced from [100]

guidance (BLOSM) [103] is another method for motion correction in CS, designed specifically for FPP, combining similar properties of the above methods, dividing the image into regions that can be tracked over time. This was compared with the previously mentioned CS algorithms in 2D FPP under prominent respiratory motion, as well as recent preliminary work in quantitative 3D FPP [104].

Compressed sensing is particularly suited to 3D data (in the case of 3D FPP, a dynamic series of 3D images - "4D" data). The extra dimension(s) and spatial coverage allow greater compressibility of the data. Despite this theoretical advantage, the issues of respiratory motion/misgating mentioned earlier have resulted in limited application of CS to 3D FPP. 3D FPP sequences using CS [25, 44, 45] used temporal and spatiotemporal constrained reconstruction methods from 2D FPP [43]. The first [25] used this reconstruction with ungated imaging (Section Basic sequence types), whilst in [44] it was combined with a more typical radial FPP protocol to achieve good quality images in cases of optimised flip angle. [45] applied a similar reconstruction technique but to a Cartesian SGRE sequence, investigating the effect of trajectory ordering strategy due to imperfect slab excitation profiles (Section Reliability and accuracy).

Recently, a CS algorithm using localised spatiotemporal constraints allowed free-breathing 3D FPP with CS to be demonstrated [105]. Whilst a compartment-based method for k-t PI [81] broke the reconstruction process into compartments of interest, here compartments in the PCA-based sparsifying functions were broken down into smaller patches, allowing overlaps to improve quality, to similarly compensate for differing physiological characteristics during the FPP series. In addition only a subset of the images in the FPP series are considered when, in effect, reconstructing each image - this was hypothesised to suit free-breathing but has the restriction that only moderate motion is expected over a few consecutive frames. This enabled acceleration to an acquisition window of 250 ms at resolution (2.3 × 2.3 × 10.0)mm^3 and FOV of (340 × 340 × 80)mm^3 during free-breathing, that compared promisingly against other 3D FPP techniques [105], although was not tested at stress.

Combining parallel imaging with compressed sensing is an intuitive subsequent step and various methods have been proposed [106, 107], as well as CS extensions to joint estimation parallel imaging techniques [84] (see Section Other parallel imaging methods). Otazo et al. [96] applied a combined parallel imaging and CS reconstruction for 2D FPP, and later showed preliminary work in free-breathing, building the motion directly into the sparsity constraints [108]. It seems likely that more reconstruction strategies combining the two will be seen, potentially including 3D FPP.

Motion challenges

The problems arising from motion in CMR acquisition are well known [109] and FPP is no exception in requiring compensation for cardiac and respiratory induced motion. The necessity for acquiring the data during a quiescent period of the cardiac cycle and the implications of this on the allowed acquisition window were described earlier (Section Requirement for acceleration in 3D FPP). The motion susceptibility of many of the proposed sub-Nyquist reconstruction schemes (Section Acceleration through sub-Nyquist reconstruction) can be particularly problematic in respiratory motion. Furthermore, stress FPP, typically performed through intravenous administration of a pharmacological agent such as adenosine, affects both cardiac [110] and respiratory motion [111]. Whilst motion-correction purely for the improvement of ROI drawing in quantitative perfusion analysis is beyond the scope of this review, issues of breath-hold versus non-breath-hold and cardiac motion directly affect parameters ranging from the required level of acceleration to the final image quality.

Cardiac motion

Whilst short acquisition windows per slice can be used in 2D FPP, potentially "freezing" motion for the duration of the acquisition, 3D acquisitions require extended acquisition windows within each cardiac cycle, making this assumption of minimal cardiac motion less valid. The largest impact is the introduction of cardiac blurring and DRA effects into the image [112].

Choosing a maximum appropriate acquisition window is difficult, despite its importance in trading off between potential cardiac blurring/reconstruction accuracy and required sequence acceleration. For example, the duration of the typical mid-diastolic quiescence is not only patient specific due to R-R interval, cardiac dysfunctions present, and many other factors, but has been shown to vary (even when normalised to the R-R interval) between cardiac cycles within the same person [113]. The introduction of a pharmacological stressor such as adenosine often increases the heart-rate, further reducing the durations of minimal cardiac movement, particularly in mid-diastole. This all potentially limits the duration of an acceptable typical acquisition window, although there is little literature on this topic in 3D FPP. The stated acquisition windows have varied in 3D FPP literature from 116 ms (with low spatial resolution) up to 380 ms (see Table 1), although some were only performed under resting conditions.

Arrhythmias and ECG triggering unreliability also present challenges, particularly in cases when multiple cardiac cycles are used in the reconstruction (k-t PI and some CS methods) as cardiac phase jitter reduces the temporal sparsity. This somewhat increases the difficulty of routine clinical application. Some transforms are less sensitive to irregular cardiac motion, such that 2D FPP ungated acquisitions have been reconstructed with high quality in patients with atrial fibrillation [114].

Respiratory motion

It is possible to instruct a patient to breath-hold just before the bolus arrival, and this will usually succeed in providing images of the same myocardial slices during peak enhancement. If an acceleration method depends on breath-hold, it may sometimes be unreliable in a routine clinical environment or where some patients under stress are unable to co-operate with breath-hold instructions. Free-breathing has the drawback for 2D FPP slices that different regions may be seen during the respiratory cycle, another motivation for 3D FPP imaging.

Breath-holding widens the range of sub-Nyquist reconstruction techniques that can be applied. Partial breath-holds, timed to coincide with the myocardial arrival of GBCA, or coached breath-holding may be used, with evident complications in clinical work. It is difficult to repeat FPP scans in the case of a failed breath-hold, and free-breathing robust FPP is therefore a topic of interest.

Motion correction and free-breathing 3D FPP

With the exceptions of Schmidt [58] and Akçakaya [105], there has been limited progress in making 3D FPP robust to free-breathing. This is owing to the fundamentally severe impact of respiratory motion when using reconstruction strategies that in any sense "share" information from multiple cardiac cycles. The ability to perform 3D FPP with free-breathing, given its dependence on some form of sub-Nyquist sampling, necessitates either mathematical modification to k-t PI/CS algorithms, correction to the data as it is collected or reconstruction strategies that make no use of temporal information.

Modifications to k-t PI methods for free-breathing or motion robustness correct the data or reconstruction into a state similar to some reference respiratory position. However, this involves a distinct step in complexity beyond the non-rigid image warping applied to conventional 2D FPP images [115, 116] or in correcting respiratory drift in a series of single-shot images (as in other applications such as T1-mapping [117]). Such non-rigid "rubber sheet" warping is performed on images that were already completed in separate cardiac cycles, where respiratory motion within the acquired raw data for each image is ignored. However, the modified advanced reconstruction methods must correct respiratory motion during the process of image reconstruction, a much more difficult challenge. This is the case in the "compartmental" and "motion-corrected" k-t PCA methods [58, 81] and adapted CS method [105] applied to 3D FPP discussed earlier, as well as others applied to 2D FPP, e.g. [41, 102, 108]. These

are currently popular as they enable the full power, and therefore acceleration, of k-t PI methods.

The challenge with the aforementioned approaches is that they attempt to compensate for raw data that is already 'corrupted' by motion; other potential methods may alternatively attempt to collect the data whilst prospectively compensating for the respiratory motion. This can give the additional benefit of correcting through-plane as well as in-plane motion. Diaphragm respiratory position "navigators" are used in CMR [118] for respiratory motion gating or adaptation while scanning. The traditional navigator accept/reject gating cannot be used with FPP because cardiac cycles cannot be omitted. However, the navigator has been used for 'slice tracking' the FPP slices to follow the respiratory motion of the heart. This was first demonstrated in FPP by Pedersen et al. [119] and improved with application of a 'navigator-restore' pulse to maintain sufficient navigator signal when combined with the FPP saturation recovery sequence [120]. However, as it has to prospectively shift the slice-excitation based on the navigator information, there will always be concerns over its reliability, and a motion-correction model between the typical right-hemidiaphragmatic navigator and the short-axis slices should be employed; this procedure cannot currently be regarded as clinically routine. A similar technique could in theory be used for 3D FPP where slab tracking might be less sensitive to tracking errors.

Finally, more basic undersampling and reconstruction techniques that do not directly utilise the dynamic nature of FPP series would eliminate inter-frame motion sensitivity. These have lower achievable acceleration factors and still require care to ensure that coil calibration methods, or similar, are not affected by respiratory motion. Without using temporal constraints, the challenge shifts for the most part from motion robustness to SNR considerations, due to the fundamental limitations of parallel imaging algorithms at such high accelerations. This could be, for example, the number of spatially significantly different receiver coils required to prevent an underdetermined PI solution. The high acceleration factors required and the prohibitive SNR losses to achieve successful reconstructions with non-k-t PI techniques make this approach less likely to succeed until new methods of accelerating the sequence or improving SNR are realised. Spatially constrained CS could potentially become more important in this way. Additionally, cardiac-specific coil arrays for optimal performance at high acceleration factors [121] would improve high-factor parallel imaging of the LV [122–124]; there are difficulties however in the transfer of these designs to a clinical setting, due to high production cost, variable body habitus, discomfort, or even simply fragility in routine use.

3D FPP literature overview

Much of the current 3D FPP literature was discussed above in the context of the advanced techniques used to realise whole-heart coverage. What follows is a more general overview of these evolving protocols, comparing and contrasting the results of these techniques and discussing novelties in their approaches, before taking a more detailed look at their clinical evaluations so far.

Developmental research review

Through examining Table 1 the development of 3D FPP results is clear, from early low-resolution images acquired at rest first demonstrating feasibility, up to the most recent higher resolution, shorter acquisition window protocols applied to populations with CAD.

The early work by Shin et al. focussed on demonstrating the feasibility and potential benefits of 3D FPP, first [70] comparing with 2D imaging inside an adjustable LV phantom, showing improved accuracy in estimation of defect size, as well as demonstrating in-vivo 3D use and examination of the time intensity curves. The in-vivo experiments included a slice by slice measurement of SNR and CNR in the 3D dataset, which exhibited the predicted losses in the edge slices due to imperfect slab excitation profile, a reason why many later works discard acquired edge slices. Also noticed was flickering in the time intensity curves, predicted to be an effect of the calibration method used in the simple temporal version of parallel imaging applied, as well as significant DRAs due to the low spatial resolution – both indicating need for new acceleration techniques in 3D FPP. The second paper by this group [19] used similar methods for early comparison between systolic and diastolic acquisitions, proposing end-systolic acquisition for 3D FPP in patients with severe arrhythmia. This was done through analysis of time intensity curves in healthy subjects and showed agreement, though increased DRAs were present at the reduced spatial resolution required to image in the shorter period of myocardial stasis in systole.

As previously discussed, the next body of work published made use of k-t PI methods, allowing improvements in many of the protocol parameters. Starting with the clinical application of the sequence [79] (Section Clinical research review) and compartment based improvement to the reconstruction [81], an isotropic in-plane spatial resolution of around 2.3 mm was first achieved and regularly applied thereafter. Alongside the implementation of the compartmental-based adaptation to k-t PCA (from Section Parallel imaging using joint spatiotemporal redundancy) and comparison with conventional k-t PCA using time intensity curves, this paper also examined performance due to number of k-t PCA training profiles and principal components, and various respiratory motion types. However, protocols during a series of clinical research papers [56, 125, 126] and recent examination with parallel transmit [21], continue to use standard k-t PCA without yet including the compartment-based extension. The more recent development of motion-corrected k-t PCA for 3D FPP [58], may possibly require further work before becoming clinically routine. Cartesian-based work from other groups have utilised CS algorithms to investigate motion-sensitivity of the technique [105] and partition ordering effects [45], as discussed in their respective sections.

Implementations of 3D FPP through non-Cartesian approaches began with the use of radial sequences, with the first focussing on application of an ungated sequence [25] and the latter testing the feasibility of radial in a more standard gated approach [44] (results in Fig. 9). Alongside numerical simulations to optimise parameters

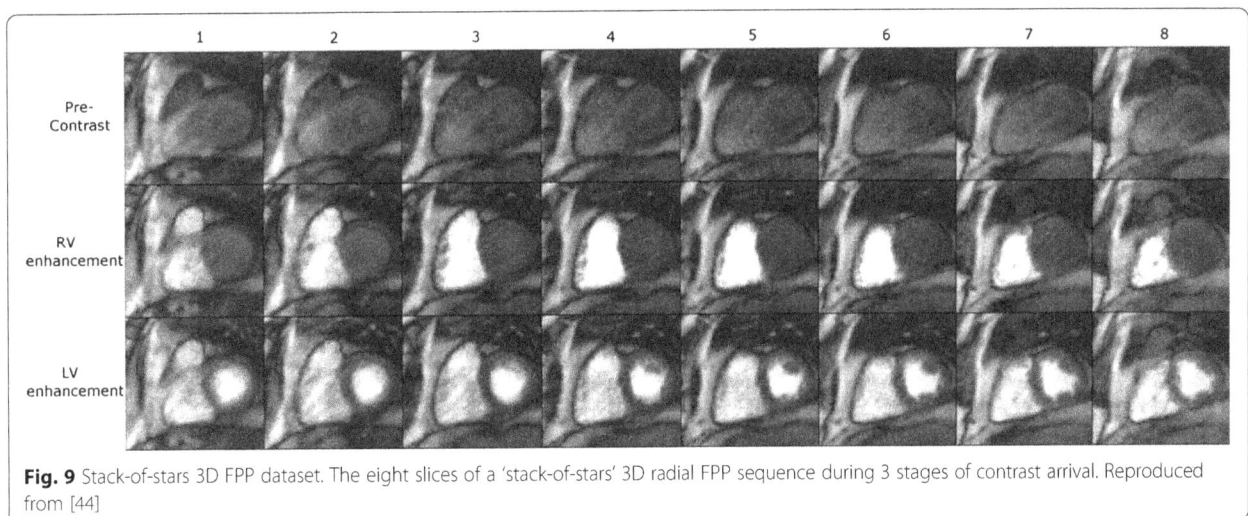

Fig. 9 Stack-of-stars 3D FPP dataset. The eight slices of a 'stack-of-stars' 3D radial FPP sequence during 3 stages of contrast arrival. Reproduced from [44]

of the sequence as mentioned in Section Alternative k-space coverage, this gated stack-of-stars approach varied the FOV as appropriate, therefore reporting a wider range of resolutions than in other 3D FPP work. With an altered sampling strategy combining higher acceleration and a slightly extended acquisition window, the ungated method gave one of the highest in-plane resolutions so far.

In work examining the optimisation of the first spiral 3D FPP sequence [39] (see Fig. 10), the higher efficiency of this k-space traversal permitted acquisition windows closer to those applied in the k-t clinical studies, at the smallest undersampling factor applied with a CS/k-t PI technique. With the stack-of-spiral acquisition placed during mid-diastole, a 2D single-slice Cartesian acquisition was also acquired each cardiac cycle allowing comparison of this 2D and 3D approach through analysis of the myocardial signal-time curves (Fig. 10). Finally, alongside the ungated radial approach just mentioned, one of the more novel attempts was continuous acquisition SSFPP [24]. With much of the paper focussing on the SFPP technique in 2D, the 3D initial experience only used a small amount of undersampling and other acceleration techniques, which explains the long acquisition window, nevertheless providing proof of concept.

Clinical research review

With the widening array of acceleration techniques increasing the feasibility of 3D FPP, a small amount of clinical research has begun. Papers that focus on investigating the clinical potential of 3D FPP rather than protocol design or other topics are examined here in more detail. Table 2 summarises the more clinically relevant aspects of studies containing a population of patients with known or suspected CAD that, among other investigations, compare 3D FPP against a reference standard. The more technical details of the protocols used in these studies can be viewed in their respective entries in Table 1.

In 2011, Manka et al. [79] first investigated the diagnostic ability of 3D FPP, comparing accuracy in identifying significant CAD against quantitative coronary angiography (QCA), as well as demonstrating the potential for volumetry of defect-induced hypointense regions. Compared against QCA, in 146 consecutively recruited patients, the sensitivity, specificity and accuracy were 92 %, 74 % and 83 % respectively, comparing favourably with CMR values in studies using 2D FPP [127, 128]. In a subgroup of 48 patients, who went on to have coronary stenting, repeat stress 3D FPP was performed within 24 h of the procedure. It was in these patients that volumetric analysis of the inducible perfusion defects was

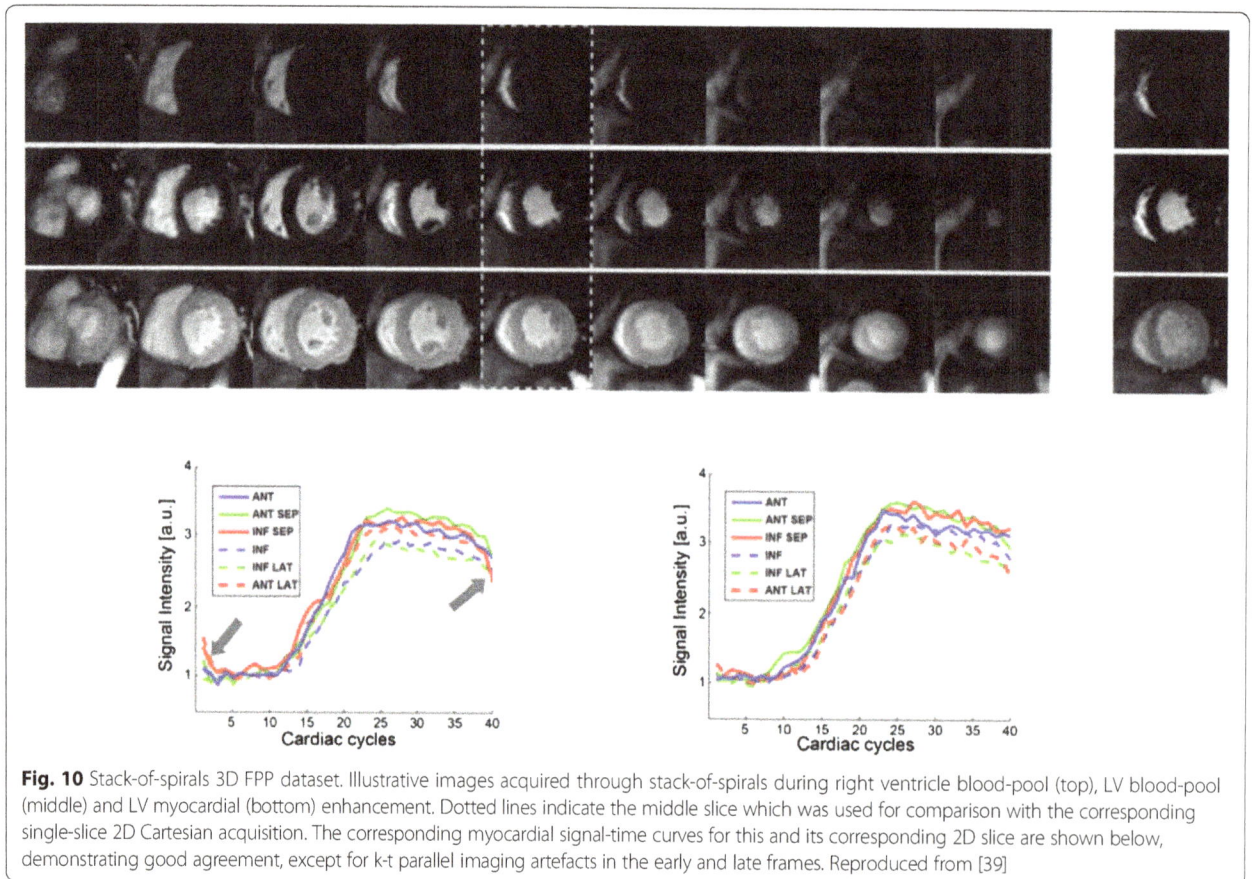

Fig. 10 Stack-of-spirals 3D FPP dataset. Illustrative images acquired through stack-of-spirals during right ventricle blood-pool (top), LV blood-pool (middle) and LV myocardial (bottom) enhancement. Dotted lines indicate the middle slice which was used for comparison with the corresponding single-slice 2D Cartesian acquisition. The corresponding myocardial signal-time curves for this and its corresponding 2D slice are shown below, demonstrating good agreement, except for k-t parallel imaging artefacts in the early and late frames. Reproduced from [39]

Table 2 Key parameters of clinical 3D whole-heart first-pass perfusion literature

Lead Author	Year	# of Patients	CMR Centres	CMR Observers	Reference Standards	QCA/%			FFR/%		
						Sensitivity	Specificity	Accuracy	Sensitivity	Specificity	Accuracy
Manka [79]	2011	146	Single	Single	QCA	92 CI[85 99]	74 CI[64 85]	83 CI[76 89]	N/A	N/A	N/A
Manka [125]	2012	120	Dual	Single	QCA & FFR	88 CI[77 95]	75 CI[61 83]	81 CI[73 88]	90 CI[82 98]	82 CI[71 94]	87 CI[80 93]
Jogiya [126]	2012	53	Single	Dual†	QCA & FFR	88 CI[71 96]	80 CI[56 93]	85	91 CI[75 98]	90 CI[66 98]	91 CI[83 95]
Jogiya [57]	2014	45	Single	Single	QCA & MPS‡	94 CI[71 100]	81 CI[54 95]	88	N/A	N/A	N/A
Manka [130]	2015	150	Five	Multiple	QCA & FFR	77 CI[67 85]	94 CI[84 99]	83 CI[76 88]	85 CI[75 92]	91 CI[81 97]	87 CI[81 92]

†3rd observer used when consensus could not be reached
‡For corresponding sensitivity, specificity and accuracy - see text
CI = 95 % confidence interval

performed, with comparison of pre and post procedure showing the predicted large effect of treatment. Further investigations of note, repeated in some of the more recent 3D FPP studies, were on image quality and whole-heart versus 3-slice CMR coverage. Artefacts were split into breathing related, k-t PI reconstruction related and DRA related, which were present in 12 %, 10 % and 8 % respectively. Whilst all images were deemed diagnostic in quality, this relatively high percentage of artefacts, along with their categorisation, highlights many of the problems already discussed in 3D FPP. Examination of 3 slices chosen from the 3D dataset produced a lower sensitivity than for the 3D dataset due to an increase in false-negatives. Whilst this agrees with a predicted advantage of 3D FPP over its 2D counterpart, this method of comparison is not a full test of the two as true 2D acquisitions have different properties, as noted in a later study [57]. That study [57] also included indication of the improved determination of ischaemic burden in 3D over 2D FPP via the same method of using a subset of the 3D dataset's slices.

With the limitation of poor correlation between the haemodynamic effect of a coronary stenosis and QCA [129], Manka et al. [125] further compared 3D FPP to fractional flow reserve (FFR). The study was also extended to two centres and included a subgroup undergoing repeat examination for inter-study reproducibility, which resulted in excellent correlation. Sensitivity, specificity and accuracy compared to QCA were similar to that in [79], whilst values were improved when using FFR as reference. This trend was also seen in [126], which provided some of the highest accuracy values, using two observers at a single centre and use of the Duke Jeopardy Score to complement FFR. Most recently [130] extension on the dual-centre investigation has been made with a multi-centre evaluation of a similar protocol across five (single vendor) European sites. With 155 patients recruited and 150 successfully examined, this is the largest 3D FPP study to date. With all CMR perfusion analysed in a central laboratory, measured image quality remained good and mean specificity compared against QCA and FFR were the highest of all studies in Table 2, although there was a decrease in sensitivity against the QCA reference.

Also recently [57], the measurement of ischaemic burden by 3D FPP was compared with that by myocardial perfusion scintigraphy (MPS), with sensitivities, specificities and accuracies of the two methods calculated for a subgroup undergoing coronary angiography. These values were 94 %, 81 % and 88 % respectively for CMR 3D FPP and 94 %, 63 % and 79 % for MPS. Comparison of ischaemic burden between the two showed no significant differences. Other clinically focussed work has investigated quantitative 3D FPP,

which is of increasing interest [104, 131], including a study of 35 patients that estimated myocardial blood flow and myocardial perfusion reserve in systole and diastole [56].

With all of the clinical studies thus far coming from related centres, parameters are understandably similar. In-plane spatial resolution is 2.3 × 2.3 mm in all cases with through plane resolution being changed from 10 mm to 5 mm after the first study. The first two studies in Table 2 were at 1.5 T, whilst the latest three were at 3 T and state that images were acquired during systole (cardiac phase not described in the first two). Unlike in [79], which used k-t SENSE as the k-t PI reconstruction technique, the latter studies employed k-t PCA. This goes some way to explaining a reduction in the number of k-t PI related artefacts in Jogiya '12 and Jogiya'14. Due to the limited variation in implementation, including protocols, reconstruction methods and breath-hold methods (not always stated), extrapolation of results to different CMR systems or non-specialist CMR sites is not yet possible, but these are positive early findings and validate many of the proposed benefits of 3D FPP.

Future considerations

Various combinations of acceleration methods, that allow total acceleration factors approaching those necessary for 3D FPP have been presented. Further acceleration would be desirable as the image acquisition time within each cardiac cycle remains too long, requiring some care in setup, and the current spatial resolution is also known to be vulnerable to imaging artefacts. Clear evidence for clinical advantages of 3D FPP over 2D would be required before proceeding to expensive large multi-centre, multi-vendor trials. Some of the reviewed 3D FPP methods require improved reliability and computational efficiency before they would be suitable for clinical trials.

Reliability and accuracy

The highly accelerated dynamic acquisition for 3D FPP is a particularly difficult problem. Some issues lowering the reliability were mentioned for techniques reviewed above, and are addressed further in this section.

Reliability can be an issue with Non-Cartesian trajectories. Such trajectories are a potential approach to 3D FPP sequences, but despite a long period of development there is a scarcity in their routine clinical usage. This can be largely attributed to their reliability depending on extra complications (e.g. requirement of field-map off-resonance corrections, scanner-specific adjustments of sequence timings, and more complex reconstructions) in comparison to what is realistic in a more routine clinical environment. Furthermore, where a long readout is used after each RF excitation, as in EPI and spiral methods, the nominal spatial resolution can be impacted by cumulative off-resonance phase errors during the readout.

Similarly, slice-tracking and other prospective motion-correction algorithms can be unreliable and damage irreparably an acquisition which might otherwise have been of clinically usable quality even if suboptimal. The majority of the presented techniques are in their early research stages and so the consistency of their performance is as yet uncertain. The non-Cartesian work so far has been developmental, applied at rest and requires some evaluation or improvement for stress before even approaching clinical utility. The use of dynamic information to support sub-Nyquist sampling reconstruction schemes has delivered clear improvement in performance. However, study is required over more subtle temporal effects that may arise with these techniques. Temporal smoothing is known in some PI methods that use temporal calibration of coil sensitivity data as well as k-t PI techniques, though methods to improve these issues have been proposed [132]. It is suggested more recent algorithms have shown less of this effect in FPP [80], but careful examination of the effect on dynamic regions of the image in particular may be important in techniques utilising temporal sparsity, even when all of the supporting conditions are perfectly satisfied.

The availability of 3 T, although sometimes of controversial benefit in clinical CMR compared to 1.5 T, is likely to be important for 3D FPP. As many of the acceleration methods sample fewer raw data points, which has a direct effect on SNR, the property of greater SNR at increased field strength becomes desirable. This SNR gain is not always straightforwardly delivered by 3 T for cardiac applications [10, 133]. However, if based on low flip-angles and short sampling trajectories after each RF pulse, especially at peak contrast-agent T1 reduction, as most GBCA relaxivities are not greatly reduced at 3 T vs 1.5 T [134] some SNR enhancement is predictable in 3D FPP. With traditional PI causing reduced SNR proportional to the square root of the acceleration, the increased SNR of higher field strengths can partially compensate. In addition, the coil sensitivity profiles at the higher frequencies of increased field strengths may improve parallel imaging performance (beyond a typical 'critical limit' of approximately 4) although this improvement only becomes significant at field strengths typically referred to as 'ultra-high field' [135]. Issues with higher field strengths are well known, with increased main field inhomogeneities of particular pertinence for longer raw data sampling after each RF pulse. These may increase some of the unreliability issues in non-Cartesian trajectories, therefore limiting achievable acceleration with these methods, and are responsible for increased

artefacts even in standard sequence designs [136]. A comparison of FPP in 2D between 1.5 T and 3 T, using k-t SENSE and other acceleration methods to achieve high spatial resolution acquisitions, showed similar artefacts and diagnostic quality between images acquired at the two field strengths [137].

As with all 3D CMR the slab profile must be optimised to minimise contamination of the edge partitions ("partition aliasing") while also exciting sufficient signal towards the edges of the slab (Fig. 11). As in 3D CE-MRA, this problem is exacerbated for FPP because of the fast repeat time of RF excitations, and is commonly concealed by clinical CMR protocols not displaying the edge slices. The 1D-selective slab-excitation RF pulse can potentially be 'truncated', enabling a shorter acquisition window within each cardiac cycle by the shorter TE and hence TR of the pulse sequence, as used in [105].

For assessing the clinical reliability of sequences utilising these techniques, large scale clinical trials have shown promise, with good results in large consecutive patient studies (Section Motion challenges). Further studies, including multi-vendor, multi-centre trials, are still required.

Computational efficiency

Virtually immediate reconstruction of images acquired with standard CMR protocols has become the expectation in the clinical environment. However, the acceleration methods required for 3D FPP demand greatly increased computation for reconstruction, and meeting this expectation of near-immediate results becomes a strong challenge.

Whilst the original version of many parallel imaging and k-t PI methods have an analytical solution, this does not apply to PI methods that involve non-linear components, CS, and some methods modified for motion correction or improved performance. Fundamentally, these methods require a computationally demanding iterative search for the optimised solution (i.e. the images). Further to the choices of search method, of what variables are searched over, and of exactly what types of "constraint" are applied, there are generally also weights controlling how strongly the constraints are enforced, and a stopping criterion for when the search is allowed to conclude (which may in some implementations simply be after a fixed number of iterations). These parameters are clearly crucial to the implementation and affect reconstruction times.

Using non-Cartesian trajectories, regardless of other applied acceleration techniques, also increases the complexity of the reconstruction and with it the computational workload. Gridding prior to fast Fourier transform (FFT), for which various techniques of differing accuracy and complexity exist (very popular is the so-called non-uniform FFT (NUFFT) [138]), is required due to non-uniform spacing of data points in k-space. Trade-offs must often be made between reconstruction accuracy and computational cost, but accurate reconstructions can typically be achieved in reasonable times. When combined with sub-Nyquist methods the reconstructions are further complicated and again require 'iterative solutions' as above. This computational strain of advanced reconstructions is especially pertinent for multi-frame 3D FPP sequences with numerous coil channels. For many methods, the reconstruction remains too slow for the images to be viewed while the patient stays in the scanner. Although there may sometimes be little prospect of re-acquiring for other reasons, such slow reconstructions are undesirable and potentially obstructive if a result is poor and an improved re-acquisition is feasible.

Many reconstruction algorithms used in 3D FPP are implemented only in prototype software that requires raw data to be exported from the scanner's standard clinical software reconstruction system. Such algorithms may be written in MATLAB (MathWorks, Natwick, MA) or similar and are far from optimised in terms of reconstruction time. Whilst this may be acceptable for initial "proof-of-concept" studies, improvements would be required for clinical application, and may be enabled by open-source reconstruction frameworks such as the Gadgetron [139], at least until manufacturers have implemented the more successful approaches.

Many attempts have been made to improve reconstruction times of advanced acceleration algorithms [140–142] and making more efficient use of available hardware such as graphical processing units (GPUs) can reduce reconstruction times [143]. This has been shown for non-Cartesian reconstructions [144] and PI/k-t PI techniques [145], but depends on specialised programming to optimise GPU performance.

Conclusions

While its clinical utility in comparison to multi-slice 2D remains hypothetical, advances in acceleration methods have opened up the feasibility of achieving 3D whole-heart coverage in FPP. The vast amount of data acquired and the short acquisition window within each cardiac cycle have required the application of multiple techniques simultaneously. Furthermore, the novelty of many of these methods requires further testing of their properties both individually and combined, and few of them are close to routine clinical application, unlike 2D FPP. Challenges with motion remain a real concern, as do reliability and reconstruction times. There is however promise in 3D FPP and with future improvements and careful evaluation of the effects of the applied acceleration

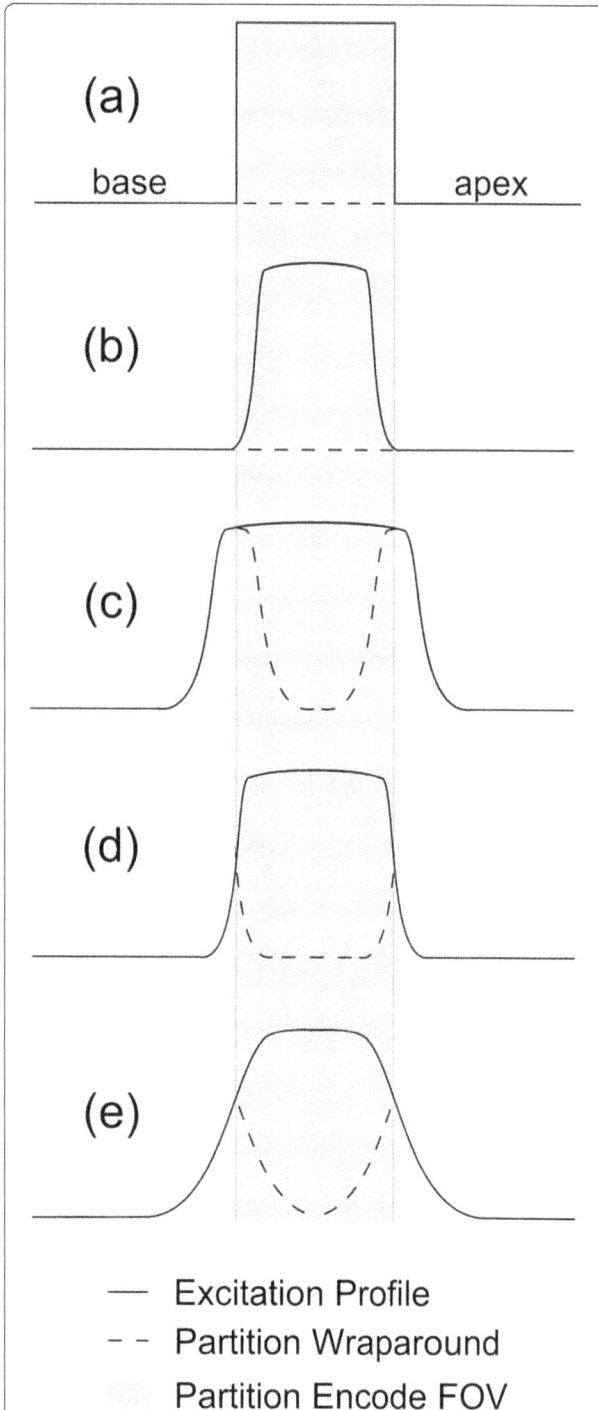

Fig. 11 'Partition-encoding aliasing' in 3D imaging. Demonstration of partition-encoding aliasing (or "wraparound") due to slab excitation profile imperfections. An ideal but impossible excitation profile would be as in (**a**), exactly matching the FOV in the slab direction. Using a narrower excitation pulse (**b**) loses SNR in the edge partitions, whilst in (**c**) exciting signal outside the FOV leads to wraparound contamination of many more partitions. A more realistic ideal scenario than (**a**) is shown in (**d**) whereby only the outermost partitions are affected by wraparound and these are usually not displayed. Due to timing constraints in 3D FPP, and therefore the short RF pulses used, avoiding results such as (**e**) is a distinct challenge

techniques, robust 3D FPP may soon be ready for multi-centre, multi-vendor trials to investigate its clinical utility of 3D FPP, both cross-modality and compared with 2D FPP.

Appendix

Timings of a 3D FPP sequences, given imaging parameters mentioned in Section Imaging parameters for FPP, estimated for typical FLASH, h-EPI and spiral sequences. With no other acceleration techniques applied to reduce these timings, and given the proposed allowed acquisition time, these should allow the reader an idea of approximate relative acceleration achievable through these sequence types and the level of acceleration still required through other methods. Care has been taken to choose values appropriate to the application, but with adjustment of these parameters a topic unto itself the examples provided are clearly only for illustrative purposes.

T_{RF} – duration of single RF excitation pulse.
T_{RO} – duration of single ADC readout.
T_{DEAD} – other time per TR, not due to T_{RF} or T_{RO}.

Desired Parameters

FOV/mm	(300×225)
Acquired in-plane resolution/mm	(2.3×2.3)
Acquired phase-encodes, N_Y	98
Acquired partition-encodes, N_Z	12 (to give 100 mm coverage at 10 mm resolution + 1 partition oversampling either side)
Allowed acquisition window in the cardiac cycle, T_A/ms	150

Calculations

	FLASH	h-EPI	Spiral
TR/ms	$T_{RF} + T_{DEAD} + T_{RO}$	$T_{RF} + T_{DEAD} + T_{RO}$	$T_{RF} + T_{DEAD} + T_{RO}$
Total Acquisition Time/ms	$TR*N_Y*N_Z$	$TR*N_Y*N_Z/N_E$	$TR*N_Z*N_{INT}$

Examples

T_{RF}/ms	0.6	0.6	0.6
T_{RO}/ms	0.6	Echo train length, N_E, dependent. E.g $N_E = 4$ giving 2.4	Number of interleaves, N_{INT}, dependent. E.g. $N_{INT} = 16$ giving 4.4
T_{DEAD}/ms	1.2	1.2	1.2
Total Acquisition Time/ms	2820	1230	1190
Required Acceleration = Total Acquisition Time/T_A	~19	~9	~8

Abbreviations
ADC: Analogue-to-digital converter; BLOSM: Block low-rank sparsity with motion-guidance; b-SSFP: Balanced steady state free precession; CAD: Coronary artery disease; CE-MRA: Contrast -enhanced magnetic resonance angiography; CMR: Cardiovascular magnetic resonance; CNR: Contrast to noise ratio; CS: Compressed sensing; DCE: Dynamic contrast enhanced; DRA: Dark-rim artefact; EPI: Echo planar imaging; ETL: Echo train length; FFT: Fast Fourier transform; FLASH: Fast low-angle shot; FOV: Field of view; FPP: First-pass perfusion; GBCA: Gadolinium based contrast agent; GPU: Graphical processing unit; GRAPPA: Generalized autocalibrating partially parallel acquisitions; h-EPI: Hybrid echo planar imaging; MPS: Myocardial perfusion scintigraphy; NLINV: Non-linear inversion; NUFFT: Non-uniform fast Fourier transform; PCA: Principal component analysis; PET: Positron emission tomography; PI: Parallel imaging; PROPELLER: Periodically rotated overlapping parallel lines with enhanced reconstruction; PSF: Point spread function; QCA: Quantitative coronary angiography; RF: Radiofrequency; SAR: specific absorption rate; SENSE: Sensitivity encoding; SGRE: Spoiled gradient echo; SNR: Signal to noise ratio; SPECT: Single photon emission computed tomography; SSFPP: Steady state free precession perfusion; T1: Longitudinal relaxation time; T2: Transverse relaxation time; TWIRL: Twisting radial lines; TWIST: Time-resolved angiography with interleaved stochastic trajectories; UNFOLD: Unaliasing by Fourier-encoding the overlaps using the temporal dimension; VIPR: Vastly undersampled isotropic projection reconstruction.

Competing interests
The authors have no competing interests to disclose.

Authors' contributions
All authors contributed in the design, intellectual conception, and revision. All authors read and approved the submitted manuscript.

Acknowledgements
This work was supported by the NIHR Cardiovascular Biomedical Research Unit of Royal Brompton and Harefield NHS Foundation Trust and Imperial College London, UK.
MF is funded by a British Heart Foundation (BHF) PhD Studentship Grant - FS/13/21/30143.

Author details
[1]National Heart & Lung Institute, Imperial College London, London, UK. [2]Cardiovascular Magnetic Resonance Unit, Royal Brompton Hospital, Sydney Street, London SW3 6NP, UK. [3]Utah Center for Advanced Imaging Research, University of Utah, Salt Lake City, UT, USA.

References
1. Schwitter J. Myocardial perfusion. J Magn Reson Imaging. 2006;24:953–63.
2. Skinner JS, Smeeth L, Kendall JM, Adams PC, Timmis A. NICE guidance. Chest pain of recent onset: assessment and diagnosis of recent onset chest pain or discomfort of suspected cardiac origin. Heart. 2010;96:974–8.
3. Atkinson DJ, Burstein D, Edelman RR. First-pass cardiac perfusion: evaluation with ultrafast MR imaging. Radiology. 1990;174(3 Pt 1):757–62.
4. Ebersberger U, Makowski MR, Schoepf UJ, Platz U, Schmidtler F, Rose J, et al. Magnetic resonance myocardial perfusion imaging at 3.0 Tesla for the identification of myocardial ischaemia: comparison with coronary catheter angiography and fractional flow reserve measurements. Eur Heart J Cardiovasc Imaging. 2013;14:1174–80.
5. Thom H, West NEJ, Hughes V, Dyer M, Buxton M, Sharples LD, et al. Cost-effectiveness of initial stress cardiovascular MR, stress SPECT or stress echocardiography as a gate-keeper test, compared with upfront invasive coronary angiography in the investigation and management of patients with stable chest pain: mid-term outcomes from the CECaT randomised controlled trial. BMJ Open. 2014;4, e003419.
6. Vogel-Claussen J. Will 3D at 3-T Make Myocardial Stress Perfusion Magnetic Resonance Imaging Even More Competitive? J Am Coll Cardiol. 2012;60:766–7.
7. Di Bella EV, Parker DL, Sinusas AJ. On the dark rim artifact in dynamic contrast-enhanced MRI myocardial perfusion studies. Magn Reson Med. 2005;54:1295–9.

8. Plein S, Ryf S, Schwitter J, Radjenovic A, Boesiger P, Kozerke S. Dynamic contrast-enhanced myocardial perfusion MRI accelerated with k-t sense. Magn Reson Med. 2007;58:777–85.

9. Fair M, Gatehouse P, Firmin D. Through-plane dark-rim artefacts in 3D first-pass myocardial perfusion. J Cardiovasc Magn Reson. 2015;17(Suppl 1):P100.

10. Gerber B, Raman S, Nayak K, Epstein F, Ferreira P, Axel L, et al. Myocardial first-pass perfusion cardiovascular magnetic resonance: history, theory, and current state of the art. J Cardiovasc Magn Reson. 2008;10:18.

11. Schwitter J, Nanz D, Kneifel S, Bertschinger K, Büchi M, Knüsel PR, et al. Assessment of myocardial perfusion in coronary artery disease by magnetic resonance a comparison with positron emission tomography and coronary angiography. Circulation. 2001;103:2230–5.

12. Biglands JD. Quanitifying myocardial blood flow using dynamic contrast enhanced cardiac magnetic resonance imaging. PhD Thesis. UK: University of Leeds; 2012.

13. Motwani M, Jogiya R, Kozerke S, Greenwood JP, Plein S. Advanced cardiovascular magnetic resonance myocardial perfusion imaging high-spatial resolution versus 3-dimensional whole-heart coverage. Circ Cardiovasc Imaging. 2013;6:339–48.

14. Shaw LJ, Berman DS, Maron DJ, Mancini GBJ, Hayes SW, Hartigan PM, et al. Optimal medical therapy with or without percutaneous coronary intervention to reduce ischemic burden results from the Clinical Outcomes Utilizing Revascularization and Aggressive Drug Evaluation (COURAGE) Trial Nuclear Substudy. Circulation. 2008;117:1283–91.

15. Cerqueira MD, Weissman NJ, Dilsizian V, Jacobs AK, Kaul S, Laskey WK, et al. Standardized myocardial segmentation and nomenclature for tomographic imaging of the heart a statement for healthcare professionals from the Cardiac Imaging Committee of the Council on Clinical Cardiology of the American Heart Association. Circulation. 2002;105:539–42.

16. Edelstein WA, Glover GH, Hardy CJ, Redington RW. The intrinsic signal-to-noise ratio in NMR imaging. Magn Reson Med. 1986;3:604–18.

17. Huang T-Y, Tseng Y-S, Chuang T-C. Automatic calibration of trigger delay time for cardiac MRI. NMR Biomed. 2014;27:417–24.

18. Motwani M, Fairbairn TA, Larghat A, Mather AN, Biglands JD, Radjenovic A, et al. Systolic versus diastolic acquisition in myocardial perfusion MR imaging. Radiology. 2012;262:816–23.

19. Shin T, Pohost GM, Nayak KS. Systolic 3D first-pass myocardial perfusion MRI: comparison with diastolic imaging in healthy subjects. Magn Reson Med. 2010;63:858–64.

20. Chung CS, Karamanoglu M, Kovács SJ. Duration of diastole and its phases as a function of heart rate during supine bicycle exercise. Am J Physiol - Heart Circ Physiol. 2004;287:H2003–8.

21. Jogiya R, Schuster A, Zaman A, Motwani M, Kouwenhoven M, Nagel E, et al. Three-dimensional balanced steady state free precession myocardial perfusion cardiovascular magnetic resonance at 3T using dual-source parallel RF transmission: initial experience. J Cardiovasc Magn Reson. 2014;16:90.

22. Kellman P, Arai AE. Imaging sequences for first pass perfusion –a review. J Cardiovasc Magn Reson Off J Soc Cardiovasc Magn Reson. 2007;9:525–37.

23. Mansfield P. Multi-planar image formation using NMR spin echoes. J Phys C Solid State Phys. 1977;10:L55–8.

24. Giri S, Xue H, Maiseyeu A, Kroeker R, Rajagopalan S, White RD, et al. Steady-state first-pass perfusion (SSFPP): A new approach to 3D first-pass myocardial perfusion imaging. Magn Reson Med. 2014;71:133–44.

25. DiBella EVR, Chen L, Schabel MC, Adluru G, McGann CJ. Myocardial perfusion acquisition without magnetization preparation or gating. Magn Reson Med. 2012;67:609–13.

26. Ding S, Wolff SD, Epstein FH. Improved coverage in dynamic contrast-enhanced cardiac MRI using interleaved gradient-echo EPI. Magn Reson Med. 1998;39:514–9.

27. Edelman RR, Li W. Contrast-enhanced echo-planar MR imaging of myocardial perfusion: preliminary study in humans. Radiology. 1994;190:771–7.

28. Panting JR, Gatehouse PD, Yang GZ, Jerosch-Herold M, Wilke N, Firmin DN, et al. Echo-planar magnetic resonance myocardial perfusion imaging: Parametric map analysis and comparison with thallium SPECT. J Magn Reson Imaging. 2001;13:192–200.

29. Ferreira P, Gatehouse P, Firmin D. Myocardial first-pass perfusion imaging with hybrid-EPI: frequency-offsets and potential artefacts. J Cardiovasc Magn Reson. 2012;14:44.

30. Takase B, Nagata M, Kihara T, Kameyawa A, Noya K, Matsui T, et al. Whole-Heart Dipyridamole Stress First-Pass Myocardial Perfusion MRI for the Detection of Coronary Artery Disease. Jpn Heart J. 2004;45:475–86.

31. Kellman P, Derbyshire JA, Agyeman KO, McVeigh ER, Arai AE. Extended coverage first-pass perfusion imaging using slice-interleaved TSENSE. Magn Reson Med. 2004;51:200–4.

32. Likes RS. Moving gradient zeugmatography. In: US Patent, #4307343. 1981.

33. Ljunggren S. A simple graphical representation of fourier-based imaging methods. J Magn Reson. 1983;54:338–43.

34. Yudilevich E, Stark H. Spiral sampling in magnetic resonance imaging-the effect of inhomogeneities. IEEE Trans Med Imaging. 1987;6:337–45.

35. Salerno M, Sica CT, Kramer CM, Meyer CH. Optimization of spiral-based pulse sequences for first-pass myocardial perfusion imaging. Magn Reson Med. 2011;65:1602–10.

36. Wong STS, Roos MS. A strategy for sampling on a sphere applied to 3D selective RF pulse design. Magn Reson Med. 1994;32:778–84.

37. Salerno M, Sica C, Kramer CM, Meyer CH. Improved first-pass spiral myocardial perfusion imaging with variable density trajectories. Magn Reson Med. 2013;70:1369–79.

38. Tsai C-M, Nishimura DG. Reduced aliasing artifacts using variable-density k-space sampling trajectories. Magn Reson Med. 2000;43:452–8.

39. Shin T, Nayak KS, Santos JM, Nishimura DG, Hu BS, McConnell MV. Three-dimensional first-pass myocardial perfusion MRI using a stack-of-spirals acquisition. Magn Reson Med. 2013;69:839–44.

40. Kholmovski EG, DiBella EVR. Perfusion MRI with radial acquisition for arterial input function assessment. Magn Reson Med. 2007;57:821–7.

41. Ge L, Kino A, Griswold M, Carr JC, Li D. Free-breathing myocardial perfusion MRI using SW-CG-HYPR and motion correction. Magn Reson Med. 2010;64:1148–54.

42. Lustig M, Donoho D, Pauly JM. Sparse MRI: The application of compressed sensing for rapid MR imaging. Magn Reson Med. 2007;58:1182–95.

43. Adluru G, McGann C, Speier P, Kholmovski EG, Shaaban A, DiBella EVR. Acquisition and reconstruction of undersampled radial data for myocardial perfusion magnetic resonance imaging. J Magn Reson Imaging. 2009;29:466–73.

44. Chen L, Adluru G, Schabel MC, McGann CJ, DiBella EVR. Myocardial perfusion MRI with an undersampled 3D stack-of-stars sequence. Med Phys. 2012;39:5204–11.

45. Wang H, Bangerter NK, Park DJ, Adluru G, Kholmovski EG, Xu J, et al. Comparison of centric and reverse-centric trajectories for highly accelerated three-dimensional saturation recovery cardiac perfusion imaging. Magn Reson Med 2014: doi: 10.1002/mrm.25478.

46. Glover GH, Pauly JM, Bradshaw KM. Boron-11 imaging with a three-dimensional reconstruction method. J Magn Reson Imaging. 1992;2:47–52.

47. Barger AV, Block WF, Toropov Y, Grist TM, Mistretta CA. Time-resolved contrast-enhanced imaging with isotropic resolution and broad coverage using an undersampled 3D projection trajectory. Magn Reson Med. 2002;48:297–305.

48. Mistretta CA. Undersampled radial MR acquisition and highly constrained back projection (HYPR) reconstruction: Potential medical imaging applications in the post-Nyquist era. J Magn Reson Imaging. 2009;29:501–16.

49. Jackson JI, Nishimura DG, Macovski A. Twisting radial lines with application to robust magnetic resonance imaging of irregular flow. Magn Reson Med. 1992;25:128–39.

50. Pipe JG. Motion correction with PROPELLER MRI: Application to head motion and free-breathing cardiac imaging. Magn Reson Med. 1999;42:963–9.

51. Bernstein MA, King KF, Zhou XJ. Handbook of MRI Pulse Sequences. Burlington, MA, USA: Elsevier Academic Press; 2004.

52. Haacke E, Brown R, Thompson M, Venkatesan R. Magnetic Resonance Imaging: Physical Principles and Dequence Design. Hoboken, NJ, USA: Wiley-Liss; 1999

53. Feinberg DA, Hale JD, Watts JC, Kaufman L, Mark A. Halving MR imaging time by conjugation: demonstration at 3.5 kG. Radiology. 1986;161:527–31.

54. Cuppen J, van Est A. Reducing MR imaging time by one-sided reconstruction. Magn Reson Imaging. 1987;5:526–7.
55. Haacke EM, Lindskogj ED, Lin W. A fast, iterative, partial-fourier technique capable of local phase recovery. J Magn Reson 1969. 1991;92:126–45.
56. Motwani M, Kidambi A, Sourbron S, Fairbairn TA, Uddin A, Kozerke S, et al. Quantitative three-dimensional cardiovascular magnetic resonance myocardial perfusion imaging in systole and diastole. J Cardiovasc Magn Reson. 2014;16:19.
57. Jogiya R, Morton G, Silva KD, Reyes E, Hachamovitch R, Kozerke S, et al. Ischemic Burden by Three-dimensional Myocardial Perfusion Cardiovascular Magnetic Resonance: Comparison with Myocardial Perfusion Scintigraphy. Circ Cardiovasc Imaging 2014: doi: 10.1161/CIRCIMAGING.113.001620.
58. Schmidt JFM, Wissmann L, Manka R, Kozerke S. Iterative k-t principal component analysis with nonrigid motion correction for dynamic three-dimensional cardiac perfusion imaging. Magn Reson Med. 2014;72:68–79.
59. Ferreira P, Gatehouse P, Kellman P, Bucciarelli-Ducci C, Firmin D. Variability of myocardial perfusion dark rim Gibbs artifacts due to sub-pixel shifts. J Cardiovasc Magn Reson. 2009;11:17.
60. Bernstein MA, Fain SB, Riederer SJ. Effect of windowing and zero-filled reconstruction of MRI data on spatial resolution and acquisition strategy. J Magn Reson Imaging. 2001;14:270–80.
61. Feinberg DA, Hoenninger JC, Crooks LE, Kaufman L, Watts JC, Arakawa M. Inner volume MR imaging: technical concepts and their application. Radiology. 1985;156:743–7.
62. Gatehouse PD, Panting JR, Grothues F, Firmin DN. Multislice Zonal EPI Myocardial Perfusion Imaging. In 8th Scientific Meeting of ISMRM. Colorado, USA; 2000.
63. Pauly J, Nishimura D, Macovski A. A k-space analysis of small-tip-angle excitation. J Magn Reson 1969. 1989;81:43–56.
64. Deshmane A, Gulani V, Griswold MA, Seiberlich N. Parallel MR imaging. J Magn Reson Imaging. 2012;36:55–72.
65. Larkman DJ, Nunes RG. Parallel magnetic resonance imaging. Phys Med Biol. 2007;52:R15–55.
66. Köstler H, Sandstede JJW, Lipke C, Landschütz W, Beer M, Hahn D. Auto-SENSE perfusion imaging of the whole human heart. J Magn Reson Imaging. 2003;18:702–8.
67. Kellman P, Epstein FH, McVeigh ER. Adaptive sensitivity encoding incorporating temporal filtering (TSENSE). Magn Reson Med. 2001;45:846–52.
68. Weiger M, Pruessmann KP, Boesiger P. 2D sense for faster 3D MRI. Magn Reson Mater Phys Biol Med. 2002;14:10–9.
69. Kellman P, Zhang Q, Larson AC, Simonetti OP, Mcveigh ER, Arai AE. Cardiac First-pass Perfusion MRI using 3d trueFISP Parallel Imaging using TSENSE. In Proceedings of the 12th Annual Meeting of ISMRM. Kyoto, Japan; 2004.
70. Shin T, Hu HH, Pohost GM, Nayak KS. Three dimensional first-pass myocardial perfusion imaging at 3T: feasibility study. J Cardiovasc Magn Reson. 2008;10:57.
71. Tsao J, Kozerke S. MRI temporal acceleration techniques. J Magn Reson Imaging. 2012;36:543–60.
72. Madore B, Glover GH, Pelc NJ. Unaliasing by Fourier-encoding the overlaps using the temporal dimension (UNFOLD), applied to cardiac imaging and fMRI. Magn Reson Med. 1999;42:813–28.
73. Chao T-C, Chung H-W, Hoge WS, Madore B. A 2D MTF approach to evaluate and guide dynamic imaging developments. Magn Reson Med. 2010;63:407–18.
74. Tsao J. On the UNFOLD method. Magn Reson Med. 2002;47:202–7.
75. Ablitt NA, Gatehouse PD, Firmin DN, Yang G-Z. Respiratory reordered UNFOLD perfusion imaging. J Magn Reson Imaging. 2004;20:817–25.
76. Tsao J, Boesiger P, Pruessmann KP. k-t BLAST and k-t SENSE: Dynamic MRI with high frame rate exploiting spatiotemporal correlations. Magn Reson Med. 2003;50:1031–42.
77. Vitanis V, Manka R, Boesiger P, Kozerke S. Accelerated cardiac perfusion imaging using k-t SENSE with SENSE training. Magn Reson Med. 2009;62:955–65.
78. Ponce IP, Blaimer M, Breuer FA, Griswold MA, Jakob PM, Kellman P. Auto-calibration approach for k–t SENSE. Magn Reson Med. 2014;71:1123–9.
79. Manka R, Jahnke C, Kozerke S, Vitanis V, Crelier G, Gebker R, et al. Dynamic 3-dimensional stress cardiac magnetic resonance perfusion imaging. J Am Coll Cardiol. 2011;57:437–44.
80. Pedersen H, Kozerke S, Ringgaard S, Nehrke K, Kim WY. k-t PCA: Temporally constrained k-t BLAST reconstruction using principal component analysis. Magn Reson Med. 2009;62:706–16.
81. Vitanis V, Manka R, Giese D, Pedersen H, Plein S, Boesiger P, et al. High resolution three-dimensional cardiac perfusion imaging using compartment-based k-t principal component analysis. Magn Reson Med. 2011;65:575–87.
82. Lustig M, Pauly JM. SPIRiT: Iterative self-consistent parallel imaging reconstruction from arbitrary k-space. Magn Reson Med. 2010;64:457–71.
83. Uecker M, Hohage T, Block KT, Frahm J. Image reconstruction by regularized nonlinear inversion—Joint estimation of coil sensitivities and image content. Magn Reson Med. 2008;60:674–82.
84. Knoll F, Clason C, Bredies K, Uecker M, Stollberger R. Parallel imaging with nonlinear reconstruction using variational penalties. Magn Reson Med. 2012;67:34–41.
85. Pruessmann KP, Weiger M, Börnert P, Boesiger P. Advances in sensitivity encoding with arbitrary k-space trajectories. Magn Reson Med. 2001;46:638–51.
86. Arunachalam A, Samsonov A, Block WF. Self-calibrated GRAPPA method for 2D and 3D radial data. Magn Reson Med. 2007;57:931–8.
87. Seiberlich N, Breuer F, Heidemann R, Blaimer M, Griswold M, Jakob P. Reconstruction of undersampled non-Cartesian data sets using pseudo-Cartesian GRAPPA in conjunction with GROG. Magn Reson Med. 2008;59:1127–37.
88. Codella NCF, Spincemaille P, Prince M, Wang Y. A Radial Self-Calibrated (RASCAL) GRAPPA method using Weight Interpolation. NMR Biomed. 2011;24:844–54.
89. Seiberlich N, Ehses P, Duerk J, Gilkeson R, Griswold M. Improved radial GRAPPA calibration for real-time free-breathing cardiac imaging. Magn Reson Med. 2011;65:492–505.
90. Seiberlich N, Lee G, Ehses P, Duerk JL, Gilkeson R, Griswold M. Improved temporal resolution in cardiac imaging using through-time spiral GRAPPA. Magn Reson Med. 2011;66:1682–8.
91. Hamilton JI, Barkauskas K, Seiberlich N. Accelerated 2D multi-slice first-pass contrast-enhanced myocardial perfusion using through-time radial GRAPPA. J Cardiovasc Magn Reson. 2014;16 (Suppl 1):P378.
92. Wright KL, Lee GR, Ehses P, Griswold MA, Gulani V, Seiberlich N. Three-dimensional through-time radial GRAPPA for renal MR angiography. J Magn Reson Imaging. 2014;40:864–74.
93. Donoho DL. Compressed sensing. IEEE Trans Inf Theory. 2006;52:1289–306.
94. Lustig M, Donoho DL, Santos JM, Pauly JM. Compressed Sensing MRI. IEEE Signal Process Mag. 2008;25:72–82.
95. Taubman D, Marcellin M. JPEG2000 Image Compression Fundamentals, Standards and Practice - Image Compression Fundamentals. 2002 [Kluwer International Series in Engineering and Computer Science].
96. Otazo R, Kim D, Axel L, Sodickson DK. Combination of compressed sensing and parallel imaging for highly accelerated first-pass cardiac perfusion MRI. Magn Reson Med. 2010;64:767–76.
97. Vitanis V, Gamper U, Boesiger P, Kozerke S. Compressed sensing cardiac perfusion imaging: feasibility and comparison to k-t BLAST. J Cardiovasc Magn Reson 2008, 10(Suppl 1):A268.
98. Lustig M, Santas JM, Donoho DL, Pauly JM. k-t SPARSE: High frame rate dynamic MRI exploiting spatio-temporal sparsity. In Proceedings of the 14th Annual Meeting of ISMRM. Seattle, Washington, USA; 2006.
99. Jung H, Sung K, Nayak KS, Kim EY, Ye JC. k-t FOCUSS: A general compressed sensing framework for high resolution dynamic MRI. Magn Reson Med. 2009;61:103–16.
100. Lingala SG, Hu Y, DiBella E, Jacob M. Accelerated dynamic MRI exploiting sparsity and low-rank structure: k-t SLR. IEEE Trans Med Imaging. 2011;30:1042–54.
101. Lingala SG, DiBella E, Adluru G, McGann C, Jacob M. Accelerating free breathing myocardial perfusion MRI using multi coil radial k-t SLR. Phys Med Biol. 2013;58:7309–27.
102. Usman M, Atkinson D, Odille F, Kolbitsch C, Vaillant G, Schaeffter T, et al. Motion corrected compressed sensing for free-breathing dynamic cardiac MRI. Magn Reson Med. 2013;70:504–16.
103. Chen X, Salerno M, Yang Y, Epstein FH. Motion-compensated compressed sensing for dynamic contrast-enhanced MRI using regional spatiotemporal sparsity and region tracking: Block low-rank sparsity with motion-guidance (BLOSM). Magn Reson Med. 2014;72:1028–38.

104. Yang Y, Chen X, Epstein FH, Meyer CH, Kramer CM, Salerno M. 3D whole-heart quantitative first-pass perfusion imaging with a stack-of-spirals trajectory. In Joint Annual Meeting ISMRM-ESMRMB 2014. Milan, Italy; 2014.

105. Akçakaya M, Basha TA, Pflugi S, Foppa M, Kissinger KV, Hauser TH, et al. Localized spatio-temporal constraints for accelerated CMR perfusion. Magn Reson Med. 2014;72:629–39.

106. Block KT, Uecker M, Frahm J. Undersampled radial MRI with multiple coils. Iterative image reconstruction using a total variation constraint. Magn Reson Med. 2007;57:1086–98.

107. Liang D, Liu B, Wang J, Ying L. Accelerating SENSE using compressed sensing. Magn Reson Med. 2009;62:1574–84.

108. Otazo R, Kim D, Axel L, Sodickson DK. Combination of compressed sensing and parallel imaging with respiratory motion correction for highly-accelerated cardiac perfusion MRI. J Cardiovasc Magn Reson. 2011;13 Suppl 1:O98.

109. Van Heeswijk RB, Bonanno G, Coppo S, Coristine A, Kober T, Stuber M. Motion compensation strategies in magnetic resonance imaging. Crit Rev Biomed Eng. 2012;40:99–119.

110. Ogilby JD, Iskandrian AS, Untereker WJ, Heo J, Nguyen TN, Mercuro J. Effect of intravenous adenosine infusion on myocardial perfusion and function. Hemodynamic/angiographic and scintigraphic study. Circulation. 1992;86:887–95.

111. Watt A, Routledge P. Adenosine stimulates respiration in man. Br J Clin Pharmacol. 1985;20:503–6.

112. Wang H, Bangerter NK, Kholmovski E, Taylor MI, DiBella EVR. Dark rim artifacts from motion in highly accelerated 3D cardiac perfusion imaging. In Joint Annual Meeting ISMRM-ESMRMB 2014. Milan, Italy; 2014.

113. Ravichandran L, Wick CA, Tridandapani S. Detection of quiescent phases in echocardiography data using non-linear filtering and boundary detection. Conf Proc Annu Int Conf IEEE Eng Med Biol Soc IEEE Eng Med Biol Soc Conf. 2012;2012:1562–5.

114. Harrison A, Adluru G, Damal K, Shaaban AM, Wilson B, Kim D, et al. Rapid ungated myocardial perfusion cardiovascular magnetic resonance: preliminary diagnostic accuracy. J Cardiovasc Magn Reson. 2013;15:26.

115. Li C, Sun Y. Nonrigid registration of myocardial perfusion MRI using pseudo ground truth. Med Image Comput Comput-Assist Interv MICCAI Int Conf Med Image Comput Comput-Assist Interv. 2009;12(Pt 1):165–72.

116. Xue H, Zuehlsdorff S, Kellman P, Arai A, Nielles-Vallespin S, Chefdhotel C, et al. Unsupervised inline analysis of cardiac perfusion MRI. Med Image Comput Comput-Assist Interv MICCAI Int Conf Med Image Comput Comput-Assist Interv. 2009;12(Pt 2):741–9.

117. Xue H, Shah S, Greiser A, Guetter C, Littmann A, Jolly M-P, et al. Motion correction for myocardial T1 mapping using image registration with synthetic image estimation. Magn Reson Med. 2012;67:1644–55.

118. Scott AD, Keegan J, Firmin DN. Motion in Cardiovascular MR Imaging. Radiology. 2009;250:331–51.

119. Pedersen H, Kelle S, Ringgaard S, Schnackenburg B, Nagel E, Nehrke K, et al. Quantification of myocardial perfusion using free-breathing MRI and prospective slice tracking. Magn Reson Med. 2009;61:734–8.

120. Basha TA, Roujol S, Kissinger KV, Goddu B, Berg S, Manning WJ, et al. Free-breathing cardiac MR stress perfusion with real-time slice tracking. Magn Reson Med. 2014;72:689–98.

121. Ohliger MA, Sodickson DK. An introduction to coil array design for parallel MRI. NMR Biomed. 2006;19:300–15.

122. Weiger M, Pruessmann KP, Leussler C, Röschmann P, Boesiger P. Specific coil design for SENSE: A six-element cardiac array. Magn Reson Med. 2001;45:495–504.

123. Schmitt M, Potthast A, Sosnovik DE, Polimeni JR, Wiggins GC, Triantafyllou C, et al. A 128-channel receive-only cardiac coil for highly accelerated cardiac MRI at 3 Tesla. Magn Reson Med. 2008;59:1431–9.

124. Schuppert M, Keil B, Guerin B, Fischer S, Rehner R, Wald LL, et al. A 64-channel cardiac receive-only phased array coil for cardiac imaging at 3T. In Joint Annual Meeting ISMRM-ESMRMB 2014. Milan, Italy; 2014.

125. Manka R, Paetsch I, Kozerke S, Moccetti M, Hoffmann R, Schroeder J, et al. Whole-heart dynamic three-dimensional magnetic resonance perfusion imaging for the detection of coronary artery disease defined by fractional flow reserve: determination of volumetric myocardial ischaemic burden and coronary lesion location. Eur Heart J. 2012;33:2016–24.

126. Jogiya R, Kozerke S, Morton G, De Silva K, Redwood S, Perera D, et al. Validation of dynamic 3-dimensional whole heart magnetic resonance myocardial perfusion imaging against fractional flow reserve for the detection of significant coronary artery disease. J Am Coll Cardiol. 2012;60:756–65.

127. Schwitter J, Wacker CM, van Rossum AC, Lombardi M, Al-Saadi N, Ahlstrom H, et al. MR-IMPACT: comparison of perfusion-cardiac magnetic resonance with single-photon emission computed tomography for the detection of coronary artery disease in a multicentre, multivendor, randomized trial. Eur Heart J. 2008;29:480–9.

128. Greenwood JP, Maredia N, Younger JF, Brown JM, Nixon J, Everett CC, et al. Cardiovascular magnetic resonance and single-photon emission computed tomography for diagnosis of coronary heart disease (CE-MARC): a prospective trial. Lancet. 2012;379:453–60.

129. White CW, Wright CB, Doty DB, Hiratza LF, Eastham CL, Harrison DG, et al. Does visual interpretation of the coronary arteriogram predict the physiologic importance of a coronary stenosis? N Engl J Med. 1984;310:819–24.

130. Manka R, Wissmann L, Gebker R, Jogiya R, Motwani M, Frick M, et al. Multicenter evaluation of dynamic three-dimensional magnetic resonance myocardial perfusion imaging for the detection of coronary artery disease defined by fractional flow reserve. Circ Cardiovasc Imaging 2015;8:10.1161/CIRCIMAGING.114.003061.

131. Wissmann L, Niemann M, Manka R, Kozerke S. Quantitative 3D myocardial perfusion imaging at high does with accurate arterial input function assessment. In Joint Annual Meeting ISMRM-ESMRMB 2014. Milan, Italy; 2014.

132. Blaimer M, Ponce IP, Breuer FA, Jakob PM, Griswold MA, Kellman P. Temporal filtering effects in dynamic parallel MRI. Magn Reson Med. 2011;66:192–8.

133. Hinton DP, Wald LL, Pitts J, Schmitt F. Comparison of cardiac MRI on 1.5 and 3.0 Tesla clinical whole body systems. Invest Radiol. 2003;38:436–42.

134. Sharma P, Socolow J, Patel S, Pettigrew RI, Oshinski JN. Effect of Gd-DTPA-BMA on blood and myocardial T1 at 1.5T and 3T in humans. J Magn Reson Imaging. 2006;23:323–30.

135. Wiesinger F, Van de Moortele P-F, Adriany G, De Zanche N, Ugurbil K, Pruessmann KP. Potential and feasibility of parallel MRI at high field. NMR Biomed. 2006;19:368–78.

136. Bernstein MA, Huston J, Ward HA. Imaging artifacts at 3.0T. J Magn Reson Imaging. 2006;24:735–46.

137. Plein S, Schwitter J, Suerder D, Greenwood JP, Boesiger P, Kozerke S. k-Space and Time Sensitivity Encoding–accelerated Myocardial Perfusion MR Imaging at 3.0 T: Comparison with 1.5 T1. Radiology. 2008;249:493–500.

138. Fessler JA, Sutton BP. Nonuniform fast Fourier transforms using min-max interpolation. IEEE Trans Signal Process. 2003;51:560–74.

139. Hansen MS, Sørensen TS. Gadgetron: an open source framework for medical image reconstruction. Magn Reson Med. 2013;69:1768–76.

140. Murphy M, Alley M, Demmel J, Keutzer K, Vasanawala S, Lustig M. Fast-SPIRiT Compressed Sensing Parallel Imaging MRI: scalable parallel implementation and clinically feasible runtime. IEEE Trans Med Imaging. 2012;31:1250–62.

141. Smith DS, Gore JC, Yankeelov TE, Welch EB. Real-Time Compressive Sensing MRI Reconstruction Using GPU Computing and Split Bregman Methods. Int J Biomed Imaging. 2012;2012:e864827.

142. Cauley SF, Xi Y, Bilgic B, Xia J, Adalsteinsson E, Balakrishnan V, et al. Fast reconstruction for multichannel compressed sensing using a hierarchically semiseparable solver. Magn Reson Med. 2015;73:1034–40.

143. Stone SS, Haldar JP, Tsao SC, Hwu W-MW, Sutton BP, Liang Z-P. Accelerating advanced MRI reconstructions on GPUs. J Parallel Distrib Comput. 2008;68:1307–18 [General-Purpose Processing Using Graphics Processing Units].

144. Sorensen TS, Schaeffter T, Noe KO, Hansen MS. Accelerating the Nonequispaced fast Fourier transform on commodity graphics hardware. IEEE Trans Med Imaging. 2008;27:538–47.

145. Hansen MS, Atkinson D, Sorensen TS. Cartesian SENSE and k-t SENSE reconstruction using commodity graphics hardware. Magn Reson Med. 2008;59:463–8.

5

Impact of arrhythmia on diagnostic performance of adenosine stress CMR in patients with suspected or known coronary artery disease

Simon Greulich, Hannah Steubing, Stefan Birkmeier, Stefan Grün, Kerstin Bentz, Udo Sechtem and Heiko Mahrholdt[*]

Abstract

Background: The diagnostic performance of adenosine stress cardiovascular magnetic resonance (CMR) in patients with arrhythmias presenting for work-up of suspected or known CAD is largely unknown, since most CMR studies currently available exclude arrhythmic patients from analysis fearing gating problems, or other artifacts will impair image quality. The primary aim of our study was to evaluate the diagnostic performance of adenosine stress CMR for detection of significant coronary stenosis in patients with arrhythmia presenting for 1) work-up of suspected coronary artery disease (CAD), or 2) work-up of ischemia in known CAD.

Methods: Patients with arrhythmia referred for work-up of suspected CAD or work-up of ischemia in known CAD undergoing adenosine stress CMR were included if they had coronary angiography within four weeks of CMR.

Results: One hundred fifty-nine patients were included ($n = 64$ atrial fibrillation, $n = 87$ frequent ventricular extrasystoles, $n = 8$ frequent supraventricular extrasystoles). Of these, $n = 72$ had suspected CAD, and $n = 87$ had known CAD. Diagnostic accuracy of the adenosine stress CMR for detection of significant CAD was 73 % for the entire population (sensitivity 72 %, specificity 76 %). Diagnostic accuracy was 75 % (sensitivity 80 %, specificity 74 %) in patients with suspected CAD, and 74 % (sensitivity 71 %, specificity 79 %) in the group with known CAD. For different types of arrhythmia, diagnostic accuracy of CMR was 70 % in the atrial fibrillation group, and 79 % in patients with ventricular extrasystoles. On a per coronary territory analysis, diagnostic accuracy of CMR was 77 % for stenosis of the left and 82 % for stenosis of the right coronary artery.

Conclusion: The present data demonstrates good diagnostic performance of adenosine stress CMR for detection of significant coronary stenosis in patients with arrhythmia presenting for work-up of suspected CAD, or work-up of ischemia in known CAD. This holds true for a per patient, as well as for a per coronary territory analysis.

Keywords: CMR, Adenosine stress, Arrhythmia, Coronary artery disease, Risk stratification

* Correspondence: Heiko.Mahrholdt@rbk.de
Department of Cardiology, Robert Bosch Medical Center, Auerbachstrasse 110, 70376 Stuttgart, Germany

Background

Coronary artery disease (CAD) is the leading cause of death in the western world [1]. Current clinical practice guidelines recommend noninvasive stress testing for 1) work-up of suspected CAD [2], and 2) work-up of ischemia in known CAD [3].

Adenosine stress cardiovascular magnetic resonance (CMR) is a noninvasive stress-testing modality offering high diagnostic accuracy without need for radiation or acoustic window [4–7]. However, up to 90 % of patients with CAD suffer from frequent ventricular ectopic beats [8], and/or other arrhythmias [9, 10]. Unfortunately, the diagnostic performance of adenosine stress CMR in this important subgroup is widely unknown, since most CMR studies currently available exclude arrhythmic patients from analysis [6, 11–13] fearing gating problems, or other artifacts will impair image quality [14].

Thus, our primary aim was to evaluate the diagnostic performance of adenosine stress CMR for detection of significant coronary stenosis in patients with arrhythmia presenting for 1) work-up of suspected CAD, or 2) work-up of ischemia in known CAD. In addition, we aimed to assess the diagnostic performance of adenosine stress CMR for different types of arrhythmia and for different coronary territories.

Methods

Patient population

All patients referred for 1) work-up of suspected CAD, and 2) work-up of ischemia in known CAD undergoing adenosine stress CMR at our institution between January 2011 and June 2014 were prospectively screened for study enrolment on a consecutive basis. We included all patients with arrhythmia during the stress CMR procedure (see definition of arrhythmia below), who underwent invasive coronary angiography within 4 weeks before or after the stress CMR, and who gave written informed consent to the protocol, which was approved by the local institutional review board (University of Tübingen, Germany). Exclusion criteria for the analysis were collateralized total occlusions revealed by coronary angiography, since in those cases no ischemia may be present despite occlusion, nondiagnostic images due to breathing artifacts, withdrawal of consent before completion of procedure, or other technical problems (Fig. 1). Baseline characteristics of the patient population can be viewed in Table 1.

Definitions

Relevant coronary stenosis/CAD was defined as ≥70 % narrowing of the luminal diameter in at least one projection of at least one major epicardial artery, or ≥50 % narrowing of the left main [2].

Suspected CAD: Patients without prior history of CAD.

Known CAD: Patients with prior myocardial infarction and/or revascularization procedure(s) such as percutaneous coronary intervention (PCI) or coronary artery bypass graft (CABG).

CAD-type late gadolinium enhancement (LGE): Subendocardial or transmural LGE consistent with prior myocardial infarction [15].

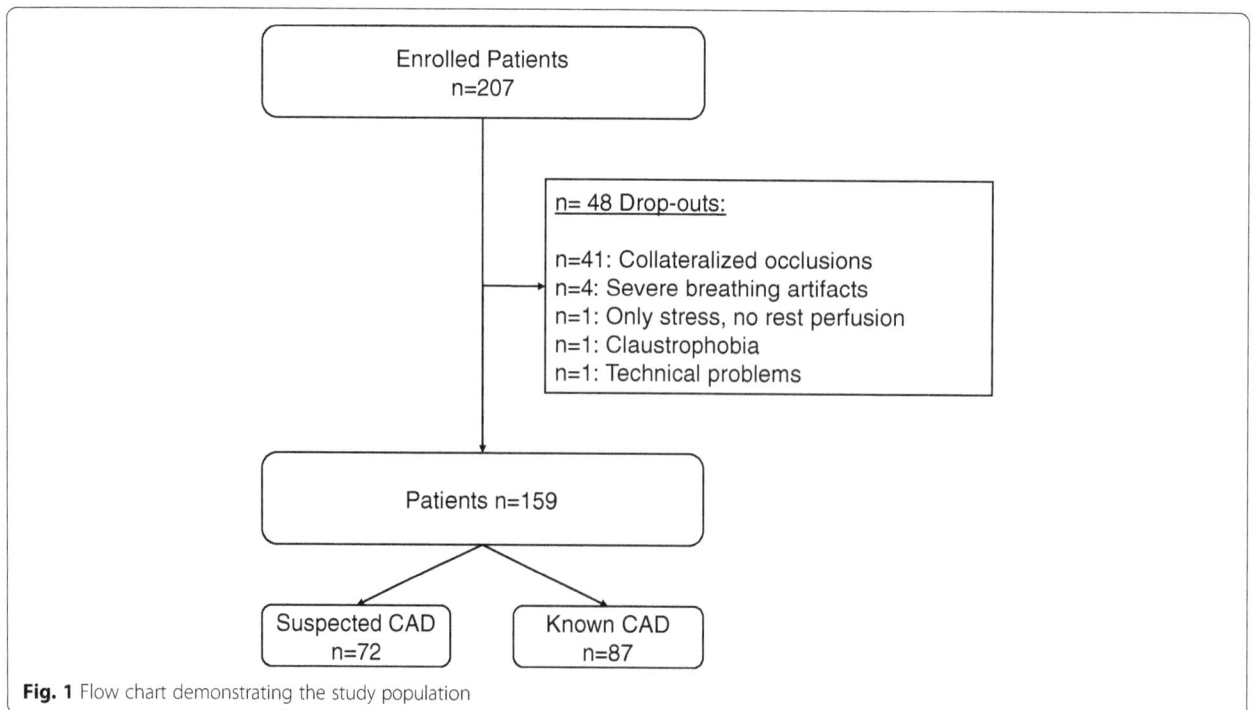

Fig. 1 Flow chart demonstrating the study population

Table 1 Baseline characteristics

	Entire group (n = 159)	Suspected CAD (n = 72)	Known CAD (n = 87)	p
Age (yrs)	71.1 ± 10	69.9 ± 10.4	72.2 ± 9.6	0.17
Gender (female)	55 (35 %)	39 (54 %)	16 (18 %)	<0.05
CAD Risk Factors				
Diabetes	51 (32 %)	20 (28 %)	31 (36 %)	0.31
Hypertension	127 (80 %)	58 (81 %)	69 (79 %)	1
Smoking[a]	49 (31 %)	18 (25 %)	31 (36 %)	0.17
Hyperlipidemia	105 (66 %)	39 (54 %)	66 (76 %)	0.004
Family history of CVD	55 (35 %)	24 (33 %)	31 (36 %)	0.74
Menopause[b]	52 (95 %)[b]	37 (95 %)[b]	15 (94 %)[b]	1
Obesity (BMI ≥ 30 kg/m^2)	30 (19 %)	17 (24 %)	13 (15 %)	0.15
Number of risk factors	2.9 ± 1.2	2.9 ± 1.3	3.0 ± 1.2	0.53
Cardiac Arrhythmia				
Heart rate at rest (beats/min.)	67 [60–78]	68 [60–80]	66 [59–78]	0.71
Heart rate at stress (beats/min.)	85 [77–99]	85 [78–101]	85 [77–98]	0.89
Atrial fibrillation	64 (40 %)	32 (44 %)	32 (37 %)	0.34
VES	87 (55 %)	35 (49 %)	52 (60 %)	0.20
Couplets	15 (9 %)	4 (6 %)	11 (13 %)	0.18
Triplets	6 (4 %)	2 (3 %)	4 (5 %)	0.69
Bigeminus	32 (20 %)	12 (17 %)	20 (23 %)	0.43
Trigeminus	6 (4 %)	3 (4 %)	3 (3 %)	1
SVES	8 (5 %)	5 (7 %)	3 (3 %)	0.47
Medication				
Statins	92 (58 %)	34 (47 %)	58 (67 %)	0.03
Beta-blockers	100 (63 %)	38 (53 %)	62 (71 %)	0.03
Aspirin	93 (59 %)	34 (47 %)	59 (68 %)	0.02
ARB	105 (66 %)	41 (57 %)	64 (74 %)	0.06
Nitrates	37 (23 %)	12 (17 %)	25 (29 %)	0.13
Diuretics	77 (48 %)	31 (43 %)	46 (53 %)	0.33
Symptoms (multiple possible)				
Chest pain	107 (67 %)	43 (60 %)	64 (74 %)	0.43
Dyspnea	87 (55 %)	46 (64 %)	41 (47 %)	0.04
Palpitations	16 (10 %)	9 (13 %)	7 (8 %)	0.09
Syncope	10 (6 %)	5 (7 %)	5 (6 %)	0.75
Reduced LV-EF	56 (35 %)	23 (32 %)	33 (38 %)	0.61
ECG abnormality	105 (66 %)	37 (51 %)	68 (78 %)	<0.001
Wall motion abnormality	46 (29 %)	12 (17 %)	34 (39 %)	0.02

Values are n (%), mean ± SD or median [IQR]

suspected CAD CMR work-up of suspected CAD in patients without history of CAD, *known CAD* CMR work-up of ischemia in patients with prior myocardial infarction and/or revascularization procedure (PCI or CABG), *CAD* coronary artery disease, *PCI* percutaneous coronary intervention, *CABG* coronary artery bypass graft, *CVD* cardiovascular disease, *BMI* body mass index, *VES* ventricular extrasystoles, *SVES* supraventricular extrasystoles, *ARB* angiotensin receptor blocker, *CMR* cardiac magnetic resonance, *LV-EF* left ventricular ejection fraction, *ECG* electrocardiography

[a]Current or ever-smokers

[b]Calculated for females

Arrhythmia was defined as atrial fibrillation, and/or frequent ectopic beats >20/min (of ventricular or supra-ventricular origin) [13]. All arrhythmias were detected by ECG and/or Holter ECG, and had to be present during both adenosine stress and rest perfusion.

Analysis per coronary territory was made on a 17 segment model basis according to AHA guidelines as previously described [16]. Left coronary artery (LCA) included the following coronary arteries: left main (LM), left anterior descending (LAD) and left circumflex artery (LCX).

CMR protocol

Electrocardiogram (ECG) gated CMR imaging was performed in breath-hold using a 1.5 T Magnetom Aera (Siemens-Healthcare, Germany) in line with recommendations of the Society of Cardiac Magnetic Resonance, and the European Society of Cardiology Working Group EuroCMR, respectively [17].

Details of the CMR protocol have been reported previously [18]. In brief, steady-state free-precession cine images for assessment of LV function were acquired in multiple short-axis (every 10 mm throughout the LV) and three long-axis views. Adenosine (140 $\mu g \cdot kg^{-1} \cdot min^{-1}$) was infused under continuous electrocardiography and blood pressure monitoring for approximately 3 min. At 2.5 min into the infusion, gadolinium (0.07 mmol/kg Gadodiamide or Gadopentetate-Dimeglumine) first-pass imaging for assessment of stress perfusion was performed in three short axis views (basal, mid, apical, matched to cine locations excluding most basal and apical slices) using a saturation-recovery, single-shot, gradient-echo sequence (90° pre-pulse before each slice; echo time, 1.1 ms; delay time, 85–100 ms; temporal resolution, 110–125 ms; voxel size, $3.0 \times 1.8 \times 8.0$ mm). In order to speed up imaging parallel imaging with 2-fold acceleration was employed. Repeat first-pass images without adenosine 15 min later were performed for assessment of rest perfusion. Five minutes after rest perfusion (additional 0.07 mmol/kg Gadodiamide or Gadopentetate-Dimeglumine), late gadolinium enhancement was performed using a segmented inversion-recovery technique in the identical views as cine-CMR. The image acquisition protocol was completed in about 45 min.

CMR analysis

Scans were analyzed by consensus of two experienced observers (S.G., H.M.), who were blinded to patient identity, clinical information, and the angiography results. A perfusion defect was defined as a regional dark area, that 1) persisted for >2 beats while other regions enhanced during the first-pass of contrast through the myocardium, and 2) involved the subendocardium [19, 20]. Dark rim artifact was not regarded as perfusion deficit using previously described criteria [21].

Cine and contrast images were evaluated as described elsewhere [22]. In brief, endocardial and epicardial borders were outlined on the short axis cine images. Volumes and ejection fraction were derived by summation of epicardial and endocardial contours.

In patients referred for work-up of suspected CAD the Duke algorithm was used for diagnosis of CAD [18]: Patients were diagnosed having relevant stenosis/CAD if they had 1) evidence of LGE consistent with a prior myocardial infarction, or 2) no evidence of prior myocardial infarction, but perfusion defects present with adenosine that were absent or reduced at rest (reversible perfusion defect). If patients showed a matched perfusion defect under stress and rest perfusion, patients were considered having no relevant stenosis/CAD [18].

In patients referred for work-up of ischemia in known CAD two different algorithms were used depending on the presence of ischemic scar: 1) In the absence of ischemic scar on LGE images relevant stenosis/ischemia was defined as the presence of a reversible perfusion defect as described above [18]. 2) In the presence of ischemic scar on LGE images ischemia was defined as a mismatch between the first-pass stress perfusion defect and enhancement seen on LGE sequences, whereas a match between the first-pass stress perfusion defect and LGE was considered as chronic myocardial infarction with no additional reversible ischemia [23].

Coronary angiography and analysis by coronary artery territory

Coronary angiography was performed by standard techniques [24] and analyzed masked to identity, clinical information, and CMR results. Significant CAD was defined as ≥70 % narrowing of the luminal diameter in at least one projection of at least one major epicardial artery, or ≥50 % narrowing of the left main [2]. Native vessels with a diameter smaller than 2 mm were excluded from the analysis. Two experienced interventional cardiologists (S.G, H.M.) blinded to the results of the CMR imaging visually evaluated the coronary angiograms by consensus.

Statistical analysis

Absolute numbers and percentages were computed to describe the patient population. All continuous variables were tested for normality. Normally distributed continuous variables were expressed as means (with standard deviation) and skewed variables were presented as medians (with quartiles). Comparisons between groups were made using the Mann-Whitney U test or the Fisher's exact test, as appropriate. Statistical tests were two-tailed; p-value < 0.05 was considered significant. Positive and negative likelihood ratios (LR) were calculated. All statistical analyses were performed using SPSS, version 22.0 (IBM Corp., Armonk, NY, USA).

Results
Patient characteristics
In total 159 patients were included in the final analysis (Fig. 1). Table 1 summarizes the patient characteristics. At inclusion, patients were 71 ± 10 years of age and predominantly male (65 %). Atrial fibrillation was present in 64 patients (40 %), 87 patients (55 %) suffered from frequent ventricular extrasystoles (VES), and 8 patients (5 %) showed frequent supraventricular extrasystoles (SVES). The majority (67 %) had chest pain as primary reason to suspect significant CAD, followed by dyspnea (55 %), and palpitations (10 %).

Seventy-two patients were referred for work-up of suspected CAD, and 87 patients were referred for work-up of ischemia in known CAD. The group with known CAD was older (72.2 ± 9.6) with fewer females (18 %) than the group with suspected CAD (age 69.9 ± 10.4, $p = 0.17$; 54 % females, $p < 0.05$). Patients presenting with known CAD had a higher prevalence of hyperlipidemia ($p = 0.004$), and wall motion abnormalities ($p = 0.02$) than patients with suspected CAD. Of note, the prevalence of the different types of arrhythmia was similar between the two groups.

General CMR findings
General CMR results are displayed in Table 2. Left ventricular ejection fraction (LV-EF) in the study population was mildly impaired (median 54 %) with normal mean cardiac volumes. Overall, CMR perfusion revealed LCA ischemia in 31 %, and RCA ischemia in 23 % of patients. CAD-type LGE was present in 47 % of patients.

Among patients with known CAD, LV-EF was significantly lower compared to the suspected CAD group, $p = 0.04$. Conversely, left ventricular end-diastolic volumes (LV-EDV) and left ventricular end-systolic volumes (LV-ESV) were significantly larger in the known CAD group (LV-EDV $p = 0.01$, LV-ESV $p = 0.007$ respectively). In addition, patients with known CAD were diagnosed with relevant stenosis/ischemia more frequently than patients with suspected CAD ($p = 0.001$, $p < 0.001$, respectively). CAD-type LGE was also more common in the known CAD group (68 vs. 21 %, $p < 0.001$).

Diagnostic performance of CMR
Entire population
Overall diagnostic accuracy of adenosine stress CMR for the detection of ≥ 70 % stenosis on coronary angiography was 73 % (sensitivity 72 %, specificity 76 %) for patients with suspected or known CAD (Table 3). On a per coronary territory basis the diagnostic accuracy of CMR was 77 % for LCA stenosis (sensitivity 78 %, specificity 77 %) and 82 % for detection of RCA stenosis (sensitivity 63 %, specificity 88 %).

Table 2 CMR results

Parameter	Entire group (n = 159)	Suspected CAD (n = 72)	Known CAD (n = 87)	p
LV-EF (%)	54 [39–66]	61 [45–67]	50 [34–64]	0.04
LV-EDV (ml)	124 [101–168]	116 [91–145]	133 [106–181]	0.01
LV-ESV (ml)	54 [32–98]	49 [28–69]	68 [40–109]	0.007
LA (cm^2)	26 [21–35]	27 [22–38]	26 [21–34]	0.43
IVS (mm)	12 [10–13]	11 [10–13]	12 [10–14]	0.58
Ischemia LCA	49 (31 %)	13 (18 %)	36 (41 %)	0.001
Ischemia RCA	36 (23 %)	7 (10 %)	29 (33 %)	<0.001
CAD-type LGE	74 (47 %)	15 (21 %)	59 (68 %)	<0.001

Values are median [IQR], or n (%)

CAD coronary artery disease, *suspected CAD* CMR work-up of suspected CAD in patients without history of CAD, *known CAD* CMR work-up of ischemia in patients with prior myocardial infarction and/or revascularization procedure (PCI or CABG), *LV* left ventricular, *EF* ejection fraction, *EDV* end-diastolic volume, *ESV* end-systolic volume, *LA* left atrium, *IVS* interventricular septum, *LCA* LM + LAD + LCX, *LCA* left coronary artery, *LM* left main, *LAD* left anterior descending, *LCX* left circumflex artery, *LGE* late gadolinium enhancement

Table 3 Diagnostic performance of CMR stress testing for the detection of ≥ 70 % stenosis on coronary angiography in all patients ($n = 159$)

	Per patient	LCA[a]	RCA
All Types of Arrhythmia[b]			
Sensitivity	72 % (49/68)	78 % (53/68)	63 % (24/38)
Specificity	76 % (69/91)	77 % (70/91)	88 % (107/121)
Diagnostic Accuracy	73 % (118/159)	77 % (123/159)	82 % (131/159)
LR+	3.00	3.39	5.25
LR-	0.37	0.29	0.42
AFib Only			
Sensitivity	71 % (25/35)	81 % (22/27)	63 % (10/16)
Specificity	69 % (20/29)	76 % (28/37)	88 % (42/48)
Diagnostic Accuracy	70 % (45/64)	78 % (50/64)	81 % (52/64)
LR+	2.29	3.38	5.25
LR-	0.42	0.25	0.42
VES Only			
Sensitivity	74 % (23/31)	75 % (30/40)	65 % (13/20)
Specificity	82 % (46/56)	81 % (38/47)	90 % (61/67)
Diagnostic Accuracy	79 % (69/87)	78 % (68/87)	85 % (74/87)
LR+	4.11	3.95	6.05
LR-	0.32	0.31	0.39

Values are % (n)

AFib atrial fibrillation, *VES* ventricular extrasystoles, *SVES* supraventricular extrasystoles, *LR+* positive likelihood ratio, *LR-* negative likelihood ratio

[a]LCA = LM + LAD + LCX, abbreviations see Table 2

[b]All types of arrhythmia: $n = 64$ AFib + $n = 87$ VES + $n = 8$ SVES

Looking at patients presenting with atrial fibrillation ($n = 64$) revealed a diagnostic accuracy of 70 % for CMR (sensitivity 71 %, specificity 69 %), which is lower than in the 87 patients presenting with VES (diagnostic accuracy 79 %, sensitivity 74 %, specificity 82 %). On a per coronary territory basis, the diagnostic accuracy for detection of LCA and RCA stenosis was good in patients with atrial fibrillation (78 %, 81 % respectively), and in patients with VES (78 %, 85 % respectively).

Considering the low number of patients with SVES ($n = 8$), these patients were included in the entire population analysis. Five of those patients were in the suspected CAD group, and three out of five were classified correctly as negative by CMR. The other three patients had known CAD, two of them had coronary stenosis on coronary angiography, one of them was correctly identified by CMR.

Patients with suspected CAD

Diagnostic accuracy of CMR stress testing for the detection of ≥70 % stenosis in patients with suspected CAD was 75 % (sensitivity 80 %, specificity 74 %), positive likelihood ratio (LR) 3.08, negative LR 0.27 (Table 4). The prevalence of significant coronary stenosis on coronary angiography was 14 % (10 out of 72 patients with suspected CAD).

CMR identified 80 % of the patients with suspected CAD and stenosis of the LCA correctly, yielding to a diagnostic accuracy of 76 % (specificity 76 %), positive LR 3.33 and negative LR 0.26. For the RCA, CMR revealed a diagnostic accuracy of 89 %, with a sensitivity of 100 %, and a specificity of 89 %, positive LR 8.33, negative LR 0. Figure 2 demonstrates two typical patients with suspected CAD and different types of arrhythmia.

Patients with known CAD

The diagnostic accuracy of CMR stress for detection of ≥70 % stenosis in patients with known CAD was 74 % (sensitivity 71 %, specificity 79 %), positive LR 3.38,

negative LR 0.37, see Table 5. The prevalence of significant coronary stenosis on coronary angiography was 67 % (58 out of 87 patients with known CAD).

CMR identified 78 % of patients with known CAD and stenosis ≥70 % in the LCA correctly, yielding a diagnostic accuracy of 78 % and a specificity of 79 %, positive LR 3.71, and negative LR 0.28. For the RCA, CMR revealed a diagnostic accuracy of 77 %, with a sensitivity of 62 %, and a specificity of 88 %, positive LR 5.17, negative LR 0.43. Typical CMR results are displayed in Fig. 3

Discussion

To the best of our knowledge, this is the first study evaluating the diagnostic performance of adenosine stress CMR for detection of significant coronary stenosis in patients with different types of arrhythmia. Our data indicate that adenosine stress CMR performs well for detection of relevant coronary stenosis in patients with suspected CAD (diagnostic accuracy 75 %), and also in patients with known CAD (diagnostic accuracy 74 %), despite the presence of various arrhythmias during the CMR procedure. These results underscore the increasing value of adenosine stress CMR in the real world clinical routine.

Patient characteristics

The average patient age and gender distribution are similar to previous stress CMR studies in which patients with arrhythmia where usually excluded from analysis [5]. This also holds true for the clinical symptoms leading to CMR referral in the present population [25]. Types of arrhythmia found in our patients include atrial fibrillation, frequent VES and frequent SVES, which are known to be associated with CAD [8–10]. As to expect, the subgroup with known CAD was older (72.2 ± 9.6 years), with fewer females (18 %) and higher prevalence of hyperlipidemia than the group with suspected CAD (69.9 ± 10.4 years, $p = 0.17$; 54 % females, $p < 0.05$).

General CMR findings

Median LV-EF of all patients was 54 %, which is comparable to other studies evaluating the diagnostic performance of adenosine stress CMR in a mixed patient population comprising patients with suspected and known CAD [23]. Patients with known CAD had a lower LV-EF and larger end-diastolic and end-systolic volumes, most likely explained by the higher prevalence of ischemic scar represented by CAD-type LGE (68 vs. 21 % in the suspected CAD group), resulting in reduced LV-EF and ventricular remodeling. Ischemia was also more common in patients with known CAD than in the group with suspected CAD, respectively.

Table 4 Diagnostic performance of CMR stress testing for the detection of ≥70 % stenosis on coronary angiography in patients with suspected CAD by use of the Duke algorithm[a]

	Per patient	LCA[b]	RCA
Sensitivity	80 % (8/10)	80 % (8/10)	100 % (1/1)
Specificity	74 % (46/62)	76 % (47/62)	89 % (63/71)
Diagnostic Accuracy	75 % (54/72)	76 % (55/72)	89 % (64/72)
LR+	3.08	3.33	8.33
LR-	0.27	0.26	0

Values are % (n)

suspected CAD CMR work-up of suspected CAD in patients without history of CAD

[a]Presence of CAD-type LGE or stress induced perfusion defect

[b]LCA = LM + LAD + LCX; $n = 32$ AFib + $n = 35$ VES + $n = 5$ SVES; other abbreviations see Table 3

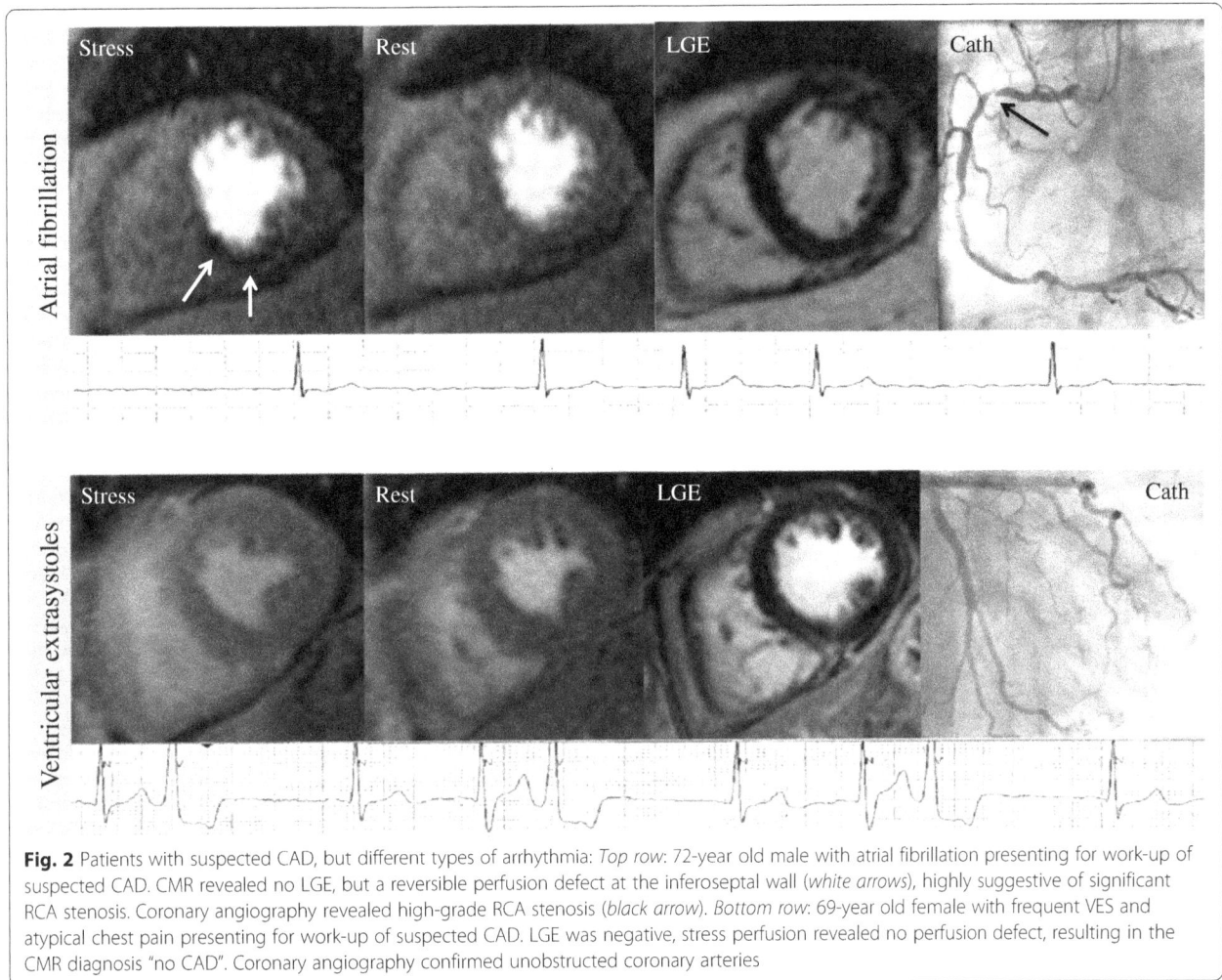

Fig. 2 Patients with suspected CAD, but different types of arrhythmia: *Top row*: 72-year old male with atrial fibrillation presenting for work-up of suspected CAD. CMR revealed no LGE, but a reversible perfusion defect at the inferoseptal wall (*white arrows*), highly suggestive of significant RCA stenosis. Coronary angiography revealed high-grade RCA stenosis (*black arrow*). *Bottom row*: 69-year old female with frequent VES and atypical chest pain presenting for work-up of suspected CAD. LGE was negative, stress perfusion revealed no perfusion defect, resulting in the CMR diagnosis "no CAD". Coronary angiography confirmed unobstructed coronary arteries

Diagnostic performance of CMR

Entire population

Looking at the entire population, the diagnostic accuracy of stress CMR for the detection of ≥70 % stenosis on coronary angiography was 73 % (sensitivity 72 %, specificity 76 %) for all 159 patients with suspected or known CAD, and different types of arrhythmia. This is lower than reported in a large meta-analysis [5] calculating a sensitivity of 90 % and a specificity of 81 %. However, many studies of this meta-analysis excluded patients with arrhythmia to improve image quality, which most likely explains the difference to our data based on patients presenting with arrhythmia only.

Analyzing our entire population data per coronary territory demonstrate CMR to yield a diagnostic accuracy of 77 % for the LCA (sensitivity 78 %, specificity 77 %), and of 82 % for the RCA (sensitivity 63 %, specificity 88 %). This is also lower than in the meta-analysis mentioned above, demonstrating sensitivities of 83, 76 and 78 % and specificities of 83, 87, and 87 % for LAD, LCX and RCA, respectively. However, patients with arrhythmias were excluded in most studies of this meta-analysis [5].

Comparing patients with atrial fibrillation to patients with VES (Table 3) reveals a good diagnostic accuracy for LCA and RCA (78 and 81 %) in the atrial fibrillation group, and in patients with VES (78 and 85 %). However, the sensitivities for detecting relevant RCA stenosis were

Table 5 Diagnostic performance of CMR stress testing for the detection of ≥70 % stenosis on coronary angiography in patients with known CAD

	Per patient	LCA[a]	RCA
Sensitivity	71 % (41/58)	78 % (45/58)	62 % (23/37)
Specificity	79 % (23/29)	79 % (23/29)	88 % (44/50)
Diagnostic Accuracy	74 % (64/87)	78 % (68/87)	77 % (67/87)
LR+	3.38	3.71	5.17
LR-	0.37	0.28	0.43

Values are % (n)

known CAD CMR work-up of ischemia in patients with prior myocardial infarction and/or revascularization procedure (PCI or CABG)

[a]LCA = LM + LAD + LCX, $n = 32$ AFib + $n = 52$ VES + $n = 3$ SVES, abbreviations see Table 3

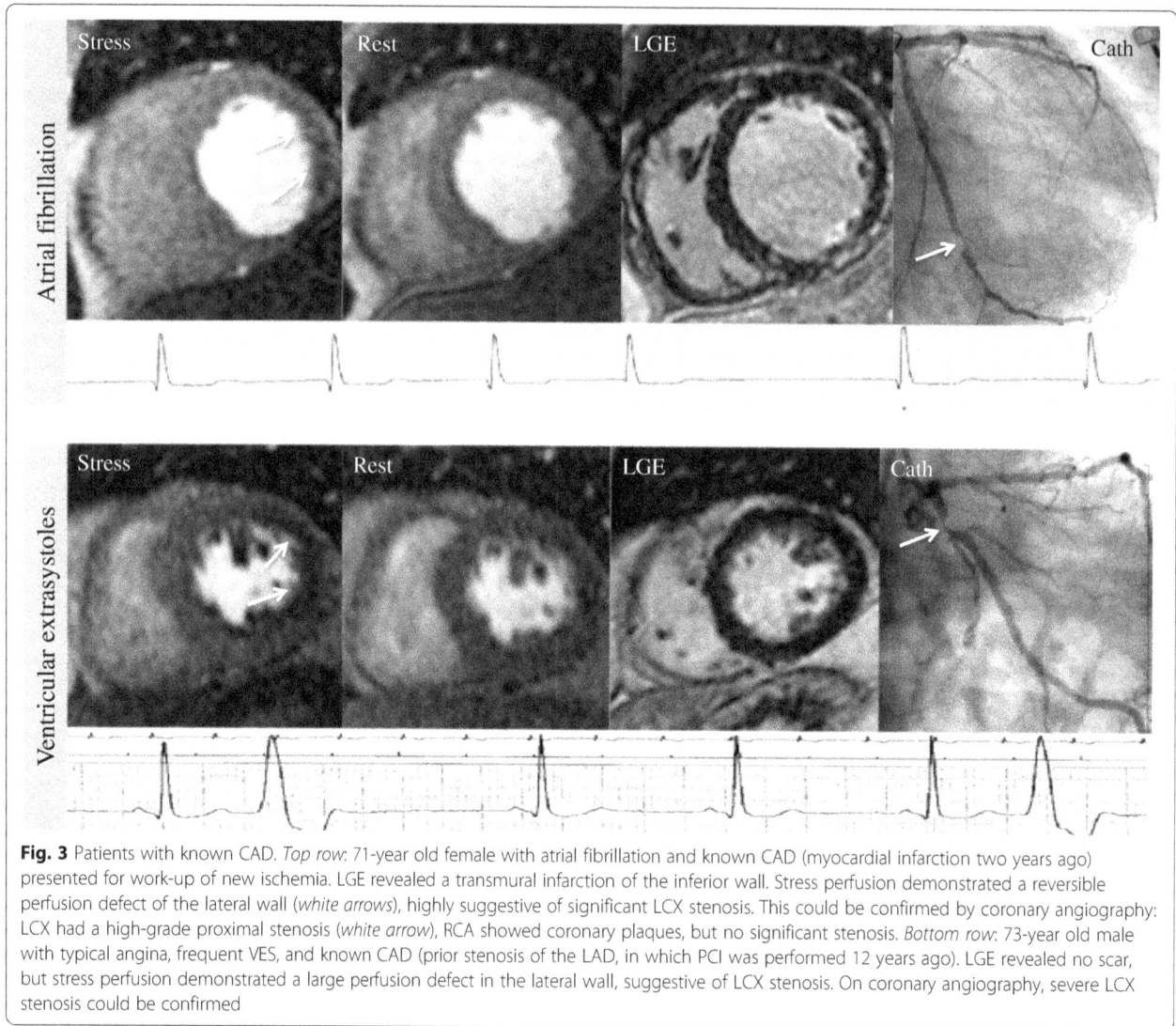

Fig. 3 Patients with known CAD. *Top row*: 71-year old female with atrial fibrillation and known CAD (myocardial infarction two years ago) presented for work-up of new ischemia. LGE revealed a transmural infarction of the inferior wall. Stress perfusion demonstrated a reversible perfusion defect of the lateral wall (*white arrows*), highly suggestive of significant LCX stenosis. This could be confirmed by coronary angiography: LCX had a high-grade proximal stenosis (*white arrow*), RCA showed coronary plaques, but no significant stenosis. *Bottom row*: 73-year old male with typical angina, frequent VES, and known CAD (prior stenosis of the LAD, in which PCI was performed 12 years ago). LGE revealed no scar, but stress perfusion demonstrated a large perfusion defect in the lateral wall, suggestive of LCX stenosis. On coronary angiography, severe LCX stenosis could be confirmed

lower in both groups when compared to the LCA (atrial fibrillation 63 vs. 81 %, VES 65 vs. 75 %). This is in accordance with other studies [5], reporting a higher sensitivity for detection of stenosis in the LAD when compared to LCX and RCA, most likely due to the surface radiofrequency coil receiving lower signal intensities from the inferior and lateral segments [5].

Patients with suspected CAD

Evaluating the subgroup presenting for work-up of suspected CAD the diagnostic accuracy was 75 % (sensitivity 80 %, specificity 74 %). This is less than reported by Klem et al. [18], who first described the Duke algorithm for work-up of suspected CAD by combining LGE and perfusion sequences in 92 patients. However, in contrast to the present data, the Klem population only included one patient with atrial fibrillation and two patients with VES.

Among our 72 patients with suspected CAD the prevalence of significant coronary stenosis was low (14 %), underscoring the need of noninvasive imaging in patients with arrhythmia before undergoing coronary angiography. One reason for the low prevalence of CAD might be that patients with arrhythmia are at an "increased risk" to be referred to coronary angiography due to previous inconclusive exercise tests, or the presence of arrhythmia itself in combination with risk factors and complaints. Interestingly, this finding nicely matches the results of Smit et al. who performed a myocardial perfusion single photon emission computed tomography (SPECT) analysis in patients with atrial fibrillation and suspected CAD. The prevalence of CAD ($\geq$70 % stenosis) in this group was 13 % [26].

In a per coronary territory analysis, the diagnostic accuracy for the LCA was 76 % (sensitivity 80 %, specificity

76 %). For the RCA our data revealed a diagnostic accuracy of 89 % (sensitivity 100 %, specificity 89 %), completely in line with the results of Klem et al. [18]. However, it must be noted that only one patient with suspected CAD had ≥70 % RCA stenosis.

Patients with known CAD

Focusing on the subgroup with known CAD the diagnostic accuracy of CMR stress testing for the detection of ≥70 % stenosis was 74 % (sensitivity 71 %, specificity 79 %). A study by Klein et al. investigated the diagnostic performance of adenosine perfusion CMR in 78 patients [27] reporting a diagnostic accuracy of 82 % for detection of ≥50 % stenosis (sensitivity 77 %, specificity 90 %), excluding patients with atrial fibrillation.

Per coronary territory the diagnostic accuracy for the LCA was 78 and 77 % for the RCA, which is also quite in line with other reports [23, 27]. Figure 4 demonstrates the feasibility of adenosine stress CMR in a patient presenting with frequent VES (bigeminus).

Limitations

Limitations of the present study are, that adenosine stress CMR was compared with invasive coronary angiography, which is not the perfect gold standard for comparison as functional significance of coronary obstruction and luminal diameter stenosis are known to show only moderate correlation. Furthermore, it is important to keep in mind that the algorithm used for CMR analysis of patients with suspected CAD is intended to detect significant obstruction of the epicardial coronaries compared to invasive coronary angiography (>70 % stenosis). Thus, perfusion defects that were considered as artifacts according to the algorithm used in this analysis may be a surrogate parameter for microvascular dysfunction. Hence, it might be possible that these patients who suffer partly from distinct anginal symptoms were classified as healthy by CMR, which could be confirmed by coronary angiography. Another limitation is the selection bias introduced by excluding patients with collateralized occlusions and CMR studies with severe breathing artifacts. Despite introducing a bias, we believe that the exclusion of collateralized occlusions is favorable in order to keep the data consistent, since in those cases no ischemia may be present despite occlusion of the vessel. Furthermore, removal of CMR data sets due to severe breathing artifacts seems reasonable since aim of our study was to evaluate the impact of arrhythmia (and not of severe breathing artifacts) on the diagnostic accuracy of an adenosine stress CMR test. Moreover, it should be stated that only a few patients (4 out of 163 patients, =0.02 %) were excluded due to severe breathing artifacts.

Clinical implications

On the basis of the data presented it may be safe to assume that the diagnostic performance of adenosine stress CMR for detection of significant coronary stenosis is somewhat impaired in patients presenting with

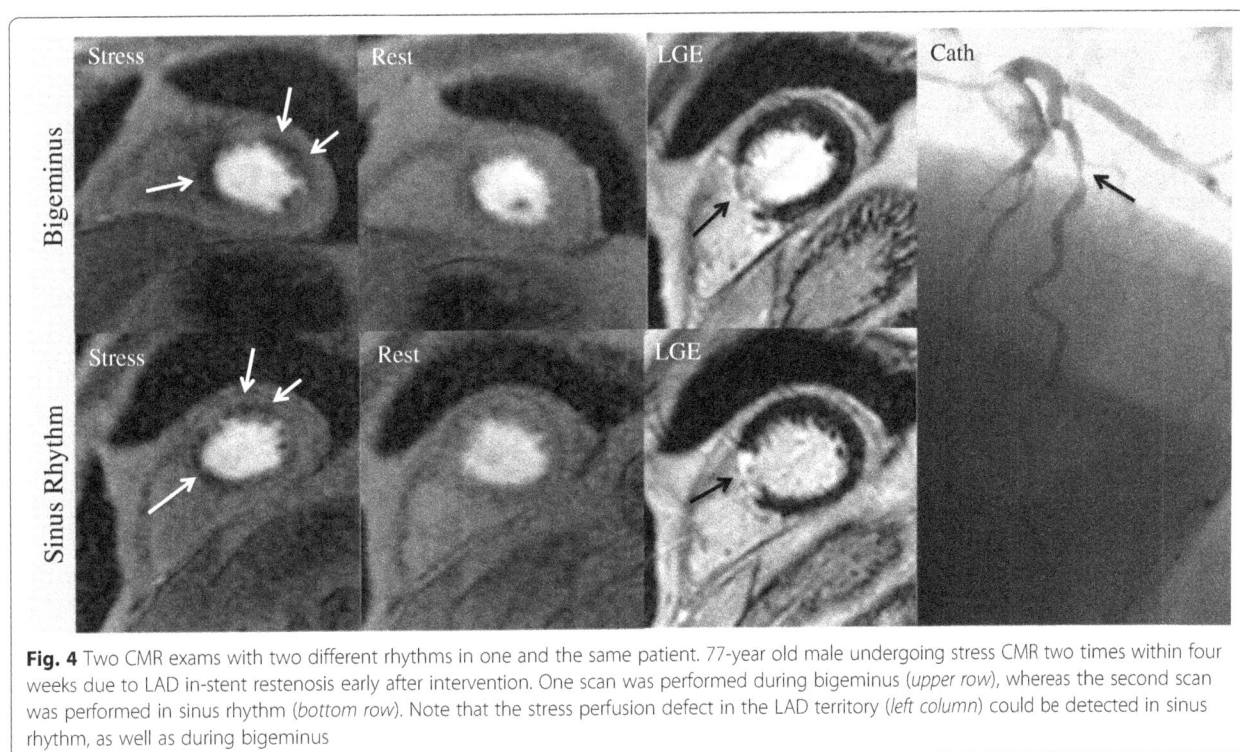

Fig. 4 Two CMR exams with two different rhythms in one and the same patient. 77-year old male undergoing stress CMR two times within four weeks due to LAD in-stent restenosis early after intervention. One scan was performed during bigeminus (*upper row*), whereas the second scan was performed in sinus rhythm (*bottom row*). Note that the stress perfusion defect in the LAD territory (*left column*) could be detected in sinus rhythm, as well as during bigeminus

arrhythmias compared to patients without arrhythmias (75 vs. 88 % for suspected CAD [18] and 74 vs. 82 % in known CAD [27]), but still sufficient for clinical routine use. In fact, with a sensitivity of 72 %, and specificity of 76 % (overall diagnostic accuracy of 73 %) adenosine stress CMR in patients with arrhythmias performs well in comparison to other stress testing modalities (SPECT: sensitivity 73–92 %, specificity 63–87; stress echocardiography: sensitivity 80–85 %, specificity 80–88 %; exercise ECG: sensitivity 45–50 %, specificity 85–90 %) [2], underscoring the value of adenosine stress CMR in a real world clinical setting.

Unfortunately, the current study was not designed to evaluate the prognostic value of stress CMR in patients with arrhythmias. However, given the encouraging results with regard to the diagnostic performance in those patients, and the results of the EuroCMR Registry demonstrating a good prognostic value of adenosine stress CMR in patients presenting for work-up of suspected CAD [28], including those with arrhythmias, it is likely that adenosine stress CMR also has a good prognostic value in arrhythmic patients. Nevertheless, additional data is needed to underscore this important point.

Conclusions

The present data demonstrates a good diagnostic performance of adenosine stress CMR for detection of significant coronary stenosis in patients with arrhythmia presenting for 1) work-up of suspected CAD, or 2) work-up of ischemia in known CAD. This holds true in the entire population for a per patient, as well as a per coronary territory analysis.

Abbreviations

AFib: Atrial fibrillation; CABG: Coronary artery bypass graft; CAD: Coronary artery disease; CMR: Cardiovascular magnetic resonance; ECG: Electrocardiogram; IQR: Interquartile range; LA: Left atrial; LCA: Left coronary artery; LCX: Left circumflex artery; LGE: Late gadolinium enhancement; LR: Likelihood ratio; LV: Left ventricle; LV-EDV: Left ventricular end-diastolic volume; LV-ESV: Left ventricular end-systolic volume; LV-EF: Left ventricular ejection fraction; PCI: Percutaneous coronary intervention; RCA: Right coronary artery; SPECT: Single photon emission computed tomography; SVES: Supraventricular extrasystoles; VES: Ventricular extrasystoles.

Competing interests

The authors declare that they have no competing interests.

Authors' contributions

SG and HS contributed to the idea and design of the study, acquired and analyzed the data, and wrote the report. SB, SG, KB, US contributed to the idea and design of the study, analysis of the data, and revision of the report. HM designed the study, contributed to the acquisition and analysis of the data, and wrote the report. All authors read and approved the final manuscript.

Funding sources

This work was funded in part by the Robert Bosch Foundation 1) clinical research grant for CMR risk stratification in HCM and 2) clinical research grant for inflammatory heart disease KKF-11-18, KKF-13-2.

References

1. Lloyd-Jones D, Adams RJ, Brown TM, Carnethon M, Dai S, De Simone G, et al. Heart disease and stroke statistics–2010 update: a report from the American Heart Association. Circulation. 2010;121:e46–e215.
2. Montalescot G, Sechtem U, Achenbach S, Andreotti F, Arden C, Budaj A, et al. 2013 ESC guidelines on the management of stable coronary artery disease: the Task Force on the management of stable coronary artery disease of the European Society of Cardiology. Eur Heart J. 2013;34:2949–3003.
3. Windecker S, Kolh P, Alfonso F, Collet JP, Cremer J, Falk V, et al. 2014 ESC/EACTS Guidelines on myocardial revascularization: The Task Force on Myocardial Revascularization of the European Society of Cardiology (ESC) and the European Association for Cardio-Thoracic Surgery (EACTS)Developed with the special contribution of the European Association of Percutaneous Cardiovascular Interventions (EAPCI). Eur Heart J. 2014;35:2541–619.
4. Nandalur KR, Dwamena BA, Choudhri AF, Nandalur MR, Carlos RC. Diagnostic performance of stress cardiac magnetic resonance imaging in the detection of coronary artery disease: a meta-analysis. J Am Coll Cardiol. 2007;50:1343–53.
5. Hamon M, Fau G, Nee G, Ehtisham J, Morello R, Hamon M. Meta-analysis of the diagnostic performance of stress perfusion cardiovascular magnetic resonance for detection of coronary artery disease. J Cardiovasc Magn Reson : Off J Soc Cardiovascular Magnetic Resonance. 2010;12:29.
6. Schwitter J, Wacker CM, Wilke N, Al-Saadi N, Sauer E, Huettle K, et al. MR-IMPACT II: Magnetic Resonance Imaging for Myocardial Perfusion Assessment in Coronary artery disease Trial: perfusion-cardiac magnetic resonance vs. single-photon emission computed tomography for the detection of coronary artery disease: a comparative multicentre, multivendor trial. Eur Heart J. 2013;34:775–81.
7. Greenwood JP, Maredia N, Younger JF, Brown JM, Nixon J, Everett CC, et al. Cardiovascular magnetic resonance and single-photon emission computed tomography for diagnosis of coronary heart disease (CE-MARC): a prospective trial. Lancet. 2012;379:453–60.
8. Bigger Jr JT, Dresdale FJ, Heissenbuttel RH, Weld FM, Wit AL. Ventricular arrhythmias in ischemic heart disease: mechanism, prevalence, significance, and management. Prog Cardiovasc Dis. 1977;19:255–300.
9. AFFIRM Investigator, Atrial Fibrillation Follow-up Investigation of Rhythm Management. Baseline characteristics of patients with atrial fibrillation: the AFFIRM Study. Am Heart J. 2002;143:991_1001.
10. Hohnloser SH, Crijns HJ, van Eickels M, Gaudin C, Page RL, Torp-Pedersen C, et al. Effect of dronedarone on cardiovascular events in atrial fibrillation. N Engl J Med. 2009;360:668–78.
11. Giang TH, Nanz D, Coulden R, Friedrich M, Graves M, Al-Saadi N, et al. Detection of coronary artery disease by magnetic resonance myocardial perfusion imaging with various contrast medium doses: first European multi-centre experience. Eur Heart J. 2004;25:1657–65.
12. Merkle N, Wohrle J, Grebe O, Nusser T, Kunze M, Kestler HA, et al. Assessment of myocardial perfusion for detection of coronary artery stenoses by steady-state, free-precession magnetic resonance first-pass imaging. Heart. 2007;93:1381–5.
13. Schwitter J, Wacker CM, van Rossum AC, Lombardi M, Al-Saadi N, Ahlstrom H, et al. MR-IMPACT: comparison of perfusion-cardiac magnetic resonance with single-photon emission computed tomography for the detection of coronary artery disease in a multicentre, multivendor, randomized trial. Eur Heart J. 2008;29:480–9.
14. Kohli P, Waters DD. Looking for coronary disease in patients with atrial fibrillation. Can J Cardiol. 2014;30:861–3.
15. Mahrholdt H, Wagner A, Judd RM, Sechtem U, Kim RJ. Delayed enhancement cardiovascular magnetic resonance assessment of non-ischaemic cardiomyopathies. Eur Heart J. 2005;26:1461–74.
16. Cerqueira MD, Weissman NJ, Dilsizian V, Jacobs AK, Kaul S, American Heart Association Writing Group on Myocardial Segmentation and Registration for Cardiac Imaging, et al. Standardized myocardial segmentation and nomenclature for tomographic imaging of the heart. A statement for healthcare professionals from the cardiac imaging committee of the council on clinical cardiology of the american heart association. Circulation. 2002;105(4):539–42.
17. Kramer CM, Barkhausen J, Flamm SD, Kim RJ, Nagel E. Standardized cardiovascular magnetic resonance imaging (CMR) protocols, society for cardiovascular magnetic resonance: board of trustees task force on standardized protocols. J Cardiovasc Magn Reson: Off J Soc Cardiovascular Magnetic Resonance. 2008;10:35.

18. Klem I, Heitner JF, Shah DJ, Cawley P, Behar V, Weinsaft J, et al. Improved detection of coronary artery disease by stress perfusion cardiovascular magnetic resonance with the use of delayed enhancement infarction imaging. J Am Coll Cardiol. 2006;47:1630–8.

19. Greulich S, Bruder O, Parker M, Schumm J, Grün S, Schneider S, et al. Comparison of exercise electrocardiography and stress perfusion CMR for the detection of coronary artery disease in women. J Cardiovasc Magn Reson : Off J Soc Cardiovascular Magnetic Resonance. 2012;14:36.

20. Klem I, Greulich S, Heitner JF, Kim H, Vogelsberg H, Kispert EM, et al. Value of cardiovascular magnetic resonance stress perfusion testing for the detection of coronary artery disease in women. JACC Cardiovasc Imaging. 2008;1:436–45.

21. Di Bella EV, Parker DL, Sinusas AJ. On the dark rim artifact in dynamic contrast-enhanced MRI myocardial perfusion studies. Magn Reson Med: Off J Soc Magnetic Resonance Med Soc Magnetic Resonance Med. 2005;54:1295–9.

22. Mahrholdt H, Goedecke C, Wagner A, Meinhardt G, Athanasiadis A, Vogelsberg H, et al. Cardiovascular magnetic resonance assessment of human myocarditis: a comparison to histology and molecular pathology. Circulation. 2004;109:1250–8.

23. Bernhardt P, Spiess J, Levenson B, Pilz G, Höfling B, Hombach V, et al. Combined assessment of myocardial perfusion and late gadolinium enhancement in patients after percutaneous coronary intervention or bypass grafts: a multicenter study of an integrated cardiovascular magnetic resonance protocol. JACC Cardiovasc Imaging. 2009;2:1292–300.

24. Scanlon PJ, Faxon DP, Audet AM, Carabello B, Dehmer GJ, Eagle KA, et al. ACC/AHA guidelines for coronary angiography: executive summary and recommendations. A report of the american college of cardiology/american heart association task force on practice guidelines (committee on coronary angiography) developed in collaboration with the society for cardiac angiography and interventions. Circulation. 1999;99:2345–57.

25. Bingham SE, Hachamovitch R. Incremental prognostic significance of combined cardiac magnetic resonance imaging, adenosine stress perfusion, delayed enhancement, and left ventricular function over preimaging information for the prediction of adverse events. Circulation. 2011;123:1509–18.

26. Smit MD, Tio RA, Slart RH, Zijlstra F, Van Gelder IC. Myocardial perfusion imaging does not adequately assess the risk of coronary artery disease in patients with atrial fibrillation. Europace. 2010;12:643–8.

27. Klein C, Nagel E, Gebker R, Kelle S, Schnackenburg B, Graf K, et al. Magnetic resonance adenosine perfusion imaging in patients after coronary artery bypass graft surgery. JACC Cardiovasc Imaging. 2009;2:437–45.

28. Bruder O, Wagner A, Lombardi M, Schwitter J, Pilz G, Nothnagel D, et al. European Cardiovascular Magnetic Resonance (EuroCMR) registry–multi national results from 57 centers in 15 countries. J Cardiovasc Magn Reson. 2013;15:9.

6

Positive contrast high-resolution 3D-cine imaging of the cardiovascular system in small animals using a UTE sequence and iron nanoparticles at 4.7, 7 and 9.4 T

Aurélien J. Trotier, William Lefrançois, Kris Van Renterghem, Jean-michel Franconi, Eric Thiaudière and Sylvain Miraux[*]

Abstract

Background: To show that 3D sequences with ultra-short echo times (UTEs) can generate a positive contrast whatever the magnetic field (4.7, 7 or 9.4 T) and whatever Ultra Small Particles of Iron Oxide (USPIO) concentration injected and to use it for 3D time-resolved imaging of the murine cardiovascular system with high spatial and temporal resolutions.

Methods: Three different concentrations (50, 200 and 500 μmol Fe/kg) of USPIO were injected in mice and static images of the middle part of the animals were acquired at 4.7, 7 and 9.4 T pre and post-contrast with UTE (TE/TR = 0.05/4.5 ms) sequences. Signal-to-Noise Ratio (SNR) and Contrast-to-Noise Ratio (CNR) of blood and static tissus were evaluated before and after contrast agent injection. 3D-cine images (TE/TR = 0.05/3.5 ms, scan time < 12 min) at 156 μm isotropic resolution of the mouse cardiopulmonary system were acquired prospectively with the UTE sequence for the three magnetic fields and with an USPIO dose of 200 μmol Fe/kg. SNR, CNR and signal homogeneity of blood were measured. High spatial (104 μm) or temporal (3.5 ms) resolution 3D-cine imaging (scan time < 35 min) isotropic resolution were also performed at 7 T with a new sequence encoding scheme.

Results: UTE imaging generated positive contrast and higher SNR and CNR whatever the magnetic field and the USPIO concentration used compared to pre-contrast images. Time-resolved 3D acquisition enables high blood SNR (66.6 ± 4.5 at 7 T) and CNR (33.2 ± 4.2 at 7 T) without flow or motion artefact. Coronary arteries and aortic valve were visible on images acquired at 104 μm resolution.

Conclusions: We have demonstrated that by combining the injection of iron nanoparticles with 3D-cine UTE sequences, it was possible to generate a strong positive contrast between blood and surrounding tissues. These properties were exploited to produce images of the cardiovascular system in small animals at high magnetic fields with a high spatial and temporal resolution. This approach might be useful to measure the functional cardiac parameters or to assess anatomical modifications to the blood vessels in cardio-vascular disease models.

Keywords: UTE (Ultra-short Echo Time), Iron based nanoparticles, Positive contrast, Cine 3D, Mouse models, Cardio-vascular

* Correspondence: miraux@rmsb.u-bordeaux2.fr
Centre de Résonance Magnétique des Systèmes Biologiques, UMR 5536
CNRS/Université de Bordeaux, 146 rue Léo Saignat, Cedex 33076 Bordeaux,
France

Background

In clinical practice, magnetic resonance angiography (MRA) enhanced by a gadolinium-based contrast agent is the gold standard for many applications [1–3] (MRA of the lower limbs, supra-aortic MRA, dynamic MRA, etc.).

However, the use of this type of contrast agent has two major disadvantages: 1) intra-venous injection entails a risk for the patient to develop nephrogenic systemic fibrosis [4]; 2) first pass extraction and rapid redistribution into the extracellular space limits the time-window of imaging enhanced vasculature [5]. One way to overcome this limitation is to use contrast agents with higher blood half-life. Some gadolinium-based contrast agents have been developed and validated in preclinical models [6].

The use of ultrasmall superparamagnetic iron oxides (USPIOs) can also appear as a good alternative [7, 8]. In patients, numerous studies at 1.5 T described the use of USPIO-based contrast agents for contrast-enhanced angiography [5, 9] and coronary MR angiography [10]. Similar positive contrast was also obtained at low field strength (0.5 T) [11]. Recently, ferumoxytol was used at 3 T for contrast-enhanced high resolution imaging of the cardio-vascular system [12, 13].

In small animals, the use of USPIO-type contrast agents is even more common, but is rarely applied to vascular imaging. In fact, they are mostly used for cell tracking [14, 15] or molecular imaging [16–19]. In these domains, and for reasons of sensitivity, they are rather used as T_2^* negative contrast agents and at high field strength. Nevertheless, several methods, like off-resonance saturation (ORS) techniques [20–22], have been developed to provide a positive contrast with USPIO-type agents.

These methods use the disturbances of the magnetic field induced by USPIOs. Their limitation, however, is that such disturbances can arise from other sources (air/tissue interface, imperfections in B0 field homogeneity, etc.). Furthermore, these effects are even more prevalent at high magnetic fields. They may prevent the use of these methods for highly resolved angiography at high magnetic fields commonly used in preclinical studies.

Iron-based contrast agents can produce a positive effect at high fields for angiography if the T2 and T_2^* effects are limited, and their slight T1 effect availed of. To do this, it is necessary to limit the signal decay caused by the phase-shifts of the spins surrounding the USPIOs. This phenomenon is enhanced by significant and turbulent blood flows in some blood vessels. The best way to limit this signal decay is to drastically reduce the echo times (TEs) of the MRI sequences.

Ultrashort TE (UTE) pulse sequences allow for signal acquisition with little T2 influence [23] and have been used to probe the T1 effect generated by USPIO. This approach has shown great promise for in vivo applications particularly in the field of quantitative imaging [24, 25].

The aim of this study was to show that 3D imaging with ultra-short echo times (TE < 0.050 ms) can generate a positive contrast for blood other a wide range of magnetic fields (4.7, 7 or 9.4 T) and USPIO concentrations injected. This method was combined to a new 3D cine UTE encoding scheme, to provide 3D time-resolved images of the murine cardiovascular system with either very high spatial or very high temporal resolutions.

Methods

Magnets and gradient systems

Experiments were performed on 4.7, 7 and 9.4-Tesla Bruker Biospec Systems (Ettlingen, Germany) equipped with gradient systems capable of 660 mT/m maximum strength and 110-µs rise time. Two different coil systems were used, depending on experiments: (a) a mouse-dedicated probe (birdcage resonator, 35 mm in diameter and 60 mm long at 4.7 T (static images), 7 T (static images) and 9.4 T (static and cine images); (b) a volume resonator (75.4 mm inner diameter, active length 70 mm) operating in quadrature mode was used for transmission, and a four-element (2 × 2) phased array surface coil (outer dimensions of one coil element: $12 × 16$ mm^2; total outer dimensions: $26 × 21$ mm^2) was used for signal reception at 4.7 and 7 T for cine imaging.

In-vivo MR experiments

Contrast agents

Three concentrations of Sinerem contrast agent (Guerbet, Aulnay-sous-bois, France) were used: 50 µmol Fe/kg - 2.8 mg Fe/kg, 200 µmol Fe/kg - 11.2 mg Fe/kg, and 500 µmol Fe/kg - 28 mg Fe/kg. The r1 and r2 for Sinerem measured in saline were $1.14 ± 0.06$ mM^{-1}.sec^{-1} and $36.46 ± 3.03$ mM^{-1}.sec^{-1} at 4.7 T, $1.13 ± 0.09$ mM^{-1}.sec^{-1} and $65.21 ± 4.23$ mM^{-1}.sec^{-1} at 7 T and $1.14 ± 0.1$ mM^{-1}.sec^{-1} and $86.23 ± 3.81$ mM^{-1}.sec^{-1} at 9.4 T, respectively.

Animal preparation

All experimental procedures were approved by the Institutional Ethics committee for Animal Care and Use at Bordeaux university, France (Approval No. 5012032-A).

Static imaging

Mice (C57BL/6, $n = 3$ for each condition, body weights: 21-25 g) were anesthetized with isoflurane (1.0 % in air) and 100 µL of contrast agent was injected through the tail vein. Imaging was performed before and after injection of the contrast agent; total imaging duration was 1 h.

Cine imaging

Mice (C57BL/ 6, $n = 12$, body weights: 21–25 g) were anesthetized with isoflurane (1.0 % in air). The ECG signal was picked up using electrodes wrapped around the forelimbs. This signal was converted into a square trigger pulse by a specific monitoring and gating system (SA Instruments, Inc., NY, USA) connected to the spectrometer. A respiratory sensor was placed under the animal's thorax. ECG and respiratory signals were visualized on a user-interface; cardiac rhythm was stabilized (380–420 beats/min) and anesthesia was regulated by modifying the proportion of isoflurane inhaled. A 100-μL volume of 200 μmol Fe/kg was injected through the tail vein. Images were acquired pre and post injection of the contrast agents.

MRI parameters
Static imaging

To determine the signal-to-noise ratio and contrast-to-noise ratio obtained before and after injection of the three USPIO concentrations at 4.7, 7 and 9.4 T, non-synchronized images were acquired with 3D UTE sequences on a large field-of-view (FOV) (extending from liver to neck). Imaging parameters are indicated in Table 1.

Cine imaging

3D cine UTE images were acquired at 4.7, 7 and 9.4 T with an isotropic resolution of 156 μm, hereafter called "mid-resolution UTE" and at 7 T with an isotropic resolution of 104 μm, hereafter called "high-resolution UTE".

The acquisition scheme of the triggered prospective sequence is shown on Fig. 1. The proposed encoding scheme allows to reconstruct with the same acquisition datas, either Ncine = R-Rinterval/(4 x TR) High Spatial Resolution images (HSR), or Ncine = R-Rinterval/TR High Temporal Resolution (HTR) images.

Half-projections were sampled in a distribution previously described [26–28], with sampling starting at a pole of the sphere and spiraling down to the other pole as the scan progressed.

To reconstruct HSR images, block of 4 consecutive k-spaces trajectories (named « 1-2-3-4 » for the first R-R interval, « 5-6-7-8 » for the second R-R interval, …) were combined to describe a sphere with the maximum numbers of projections (52540 per cine). The same encoding was used for each cine HSR images (HSR1, HSR2, …, HSR10).

By using each projections per RR-interval individually, four-times more cine HTR images could be reconstructed with 4 times-less projections (13135). It corresponds to the sampling trajectory with the same color code described in Fig. 1c (blue). HTR1, HTR5, … HTR37 have the same sampling trajectory which slightly differs from the HTR2, HTR6, … HTR38 red trajectories, HTR3 to HTR 39 green trajectories and HTR4 to HTR40 magenta trajectories.

This method allows to homogeneously distribute projections on the surface of the sphere, both in HSR and HTR images.

Imaging parameters are indicated in Table 1.

Reconstruction procedure

All the UTE data where reconstructed using the following procedure: k-space data were regridded with an oversampling ratio of 2 using a Kaiser-Bessel kernel [29]. Data were transformed by applying a conventional fast Fourier transform (FFT). Each phased array receiver magnitude image was reconstructed using the

Table 1 Imaging parameters used for static and cine images

Imaging parameters	Static imaging UTE	Cine-imaging Mid resolution UTE	High resolution UTE
Coil/Magnetic Field	Volumetric/ 4.7, 7, 9.4 T	Volumetric/9.4 T phased array/ 4.7, 7 T	phased array/7 T
TR/TE (ms)	4.5/0.031	3.5/0.031	3.5/0.031
Excitation Pulse/ duration (ms) / FA°	square / 0.05 / 15°	square / 0.05 / 15°	square / 0.05 / 15°
Field of view (mm)	$30 \times 30 \times 30$	$20 \times 20 \times 20$	$20 \times 20 \times 20$
Matrix	$128 \times 128 \times 128$	$128 \times 128 \times 128$	$192 \times 192 \times 192$
Number of projections	51360	18144/cine	52540/cine
Resolution (μm)	$234 \times 234 \times 234$	$156 \times 156 \times 156$	$104 \times 104 \times 104$
Bandwith (Hz/Pixel)	781	781	520
Triggering	No	ECG	ECG
Cine images (N)	-	10	10
Excitations (N)	1	1	1
Total acquisition time	3 min 51 s	11 min 20 s	32 min 50 s

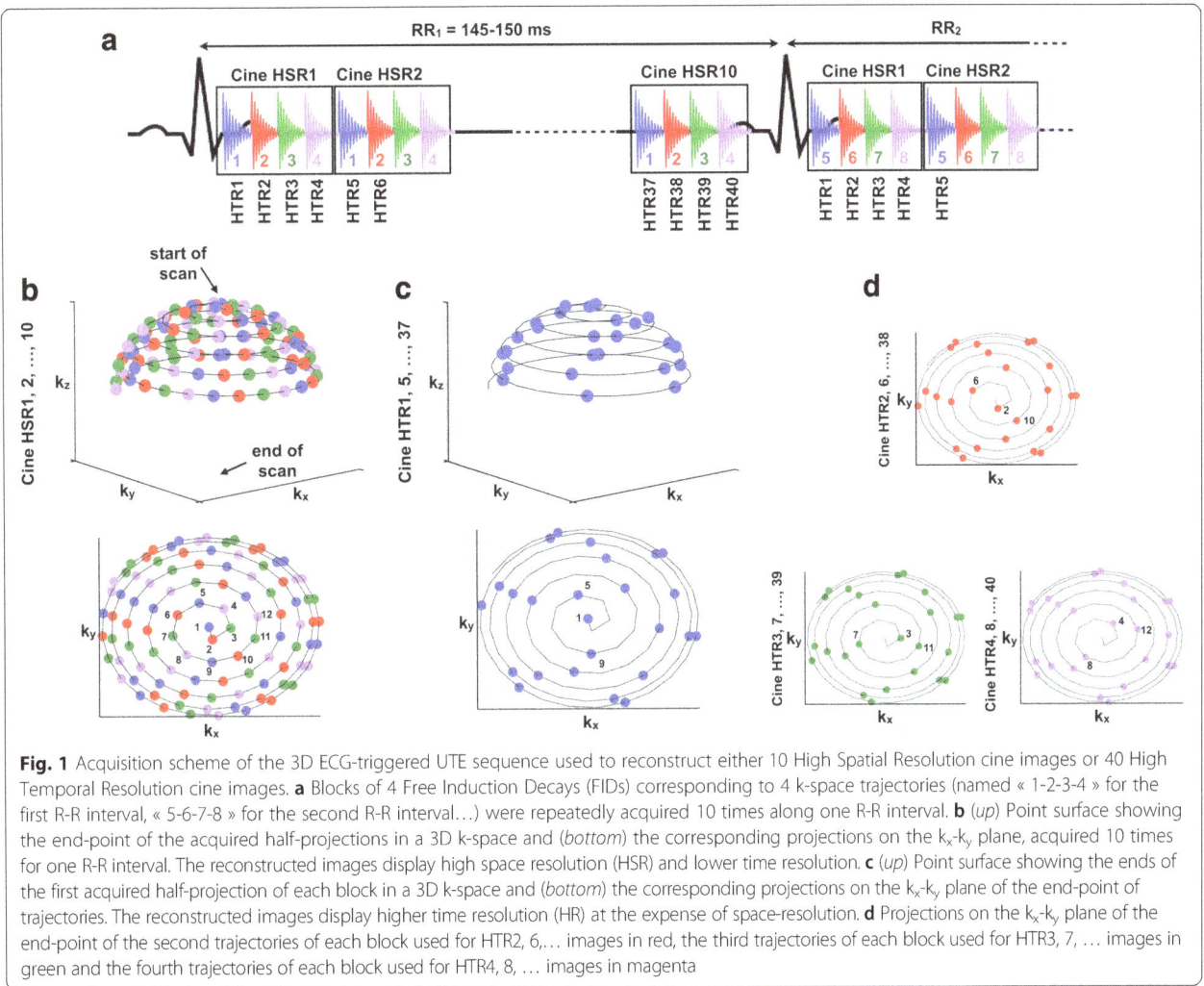

Fig. 1 Acquisition scheme of the 3D ECG-triggered UTE sequence used to reconstruct either 10 High Spatial Resolution cine images or 40 High Temporal Resolution cine images. **a** Blocks of 4 Free Induction Decays (FIDs) corresponding to 4 k-space trajectories (named « 1-2-3-4 » for the first R-R interval, « 5-6-7-8 » for the second R-R interval...) were repeatedly acquired 10 times along one R-R interval. **b** (*up*) Point surface showing the end-point of the acquired half-projections in a 3D k-space and (*bottom*) the corresponding projections on the k_x-k_y plane, acquired 10 times for one R-R interval. The reconstructed images display high space resolution (HSR) and lower time resolution. **c** (*up*) Point surface showing the ends of the first acquired half-projection of each block in a 3D k-space and (*bottom*) the corresponding projections on the k_x-k_y plane of the end-point of trajectories. The reconstructed images display higher time resolution (HR) at the expense of space-resolution. **d** Projections on the k_x-k_y plane of the end-point of the second trajectories of each block used for HTR2, 6,... images in red, the third trajectories of each block used for HTR3, 7, ... images in green and the fourth trajectories of each block used for HTR4, 8, ... images in magenta

method described above, and then combined by a sum of squares reconstruction.

Image analysis
Signal-to-noise ratio, contrast-to-noise ratio and signal homogeneity measurements
Igor Pro (Wavemetrics, Lake Oswego, OR) data processing software was used to calculate the apparent signal-to-noise ratio (SNR) for blood, myocardium and muscle. Apparent SNR was defined as the signal intensity for the Region Of Interest (ROI) divided by the standard deviation of the noise (measured for an ROI positioned outside the mouse body).

The contrast-to-noise ratio (CNR) for blood compared to stationary tissue was defined as CNR = SNR (blood) – SNR (myocardium or muscle). CNR was measured at the level of the aortic arch and jugular veins for static imaging, and in the ventricles for cine imaging.

Signal homogeneity of blood throughout the cycle was assessed using the measurements of the standard deviation for the blood signal in the left and right ventricles and in the aortic arch.

Statistical analysis
Results were compared using an Anova-test. $P < 0.05$ was considered for a significant difference.

Volume analysis
Volume analysis was performed on 6 mice with a semi-automated segmentation procedure on Amira (Visage Imaging GmbH, Germany) to calculate left ventricular end-diastolic volume, left ventricular end-systolic volume, left ventricular stroke volume (LVSV), left ventricular ejection fraction (LVEF), right ventricular end-diastolic volume, right ventricular end-systolic volume, right ventricular stroke volume (RVSV), and right ventricular ejection fraction (RVEF).

Results

Static imaging – pre and post contrast with UTE sequences

Images were acquired in a zone extending from the liver to the neck. Three different concentrations of contrast agents were used, and the images acquired at 9.4 T pre- and post contrast agent injection with UTE sequences are shown in Fig. 2. Before injecting the contrast agent, the blood vessels and the blood inside the ventricles were not readily visible. After injection of the contrast agent, whatever the concentration injected, the blood in the various blood vessels was visible with the UTE sequence with an intense signal. This signal was highly homogeneous, whether in zones with high turbulence, such as the aortic arch (Fig. 2, small arrow), or in blood vessels with slow-flow, such as the jugular veins. No artefact related to blood flow or movement was visible on the images.

It should also be noted that the liver (Fig. 2, dashed arrow) always appears with a positive contrast and that its signal increases with USPIO concentration.

The same experiments were performed at 4.7 T, 7.0 T and 9.4 T, and the signal-to-noise ratio was measured for blood (aortic arch, jugular vein) and for the muscles. The blood-to-muscle contrast-to-noise ratios under the different conditions are indicated in Fig. 3.

Before contrast agent injection, contrast-to-noise ratio was very low (in the range of -2). After injection, whatever the magnetic field and the concentration of nanoparticles used, the contrast-to-noise ratio was always positive, and greater than or equal to 18. Increasing the concentration raised the contrast-to-noise ratio, at all magnetic fields ($p < 0.05$ for 200 µmol Fe/kg vs. 500 µmol Fe/kg). The highest concentration gave a better contrast-to-noise ratio, always greater than 40, whatever the magnetic field. Increasing the magnetic field slightly decreased the contrast-to-noise ratio, but this change was not significant.

It must be noted that for the lowest Sinerem concentration (50 µmol Fe/kg), the contrast varied slightly during the experiment (data not shown). This tended to decrease about 30 % over one hour with the UTE sequence. In contrast, the CNR measurements remained stable for at least one hour after injection for the two highest concentrations of contrast agent.

Cine imaging
Mid-resolution UTE

3D-cine images at 156 µm isotropic resolution were acquired prospectively with the UTE sequence for the three magnetic fields tested before and after contrast agent injection. The intermediate concentration of contrast agent (200 µmol Fe/kg) was used for the images shown in Fig. 4, but similar results were obtained with the highest concentration. Slices were extracted during systole and diastole in two orientations (short axis and long axis) and are shown for the three magnetic fields. The acquisition times for these images were around 12 min.

Before injection, a contrast to noise ratio around -3 was obtained. After injection, and whatever the magnetic field, a positive contrast between myocardial blood and the myocardial wall was obtained at all times throughout the cardiac cycle (Table 2). The signal was also highly homogeneous, in both the blood vessels and in the heart cavities. For example, during a given experiment at 7 T, the standard deviation of the signal measured in the ventricles and the aortic arch during

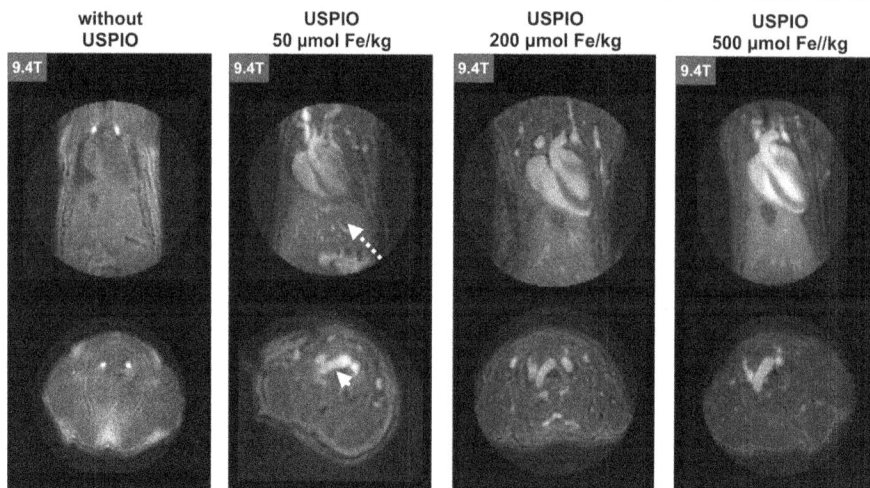

Fig. 2 3D UTE images at 9.4 T showing the heart and the liver of a mouse. Images were acquired before and after injection of USPIO at 50, 200 and 500 µmol Fe/kg, without cardiac or respiratory synchronization. The small arrow indicates the aortic arch and the dashed arrow indicates the liver

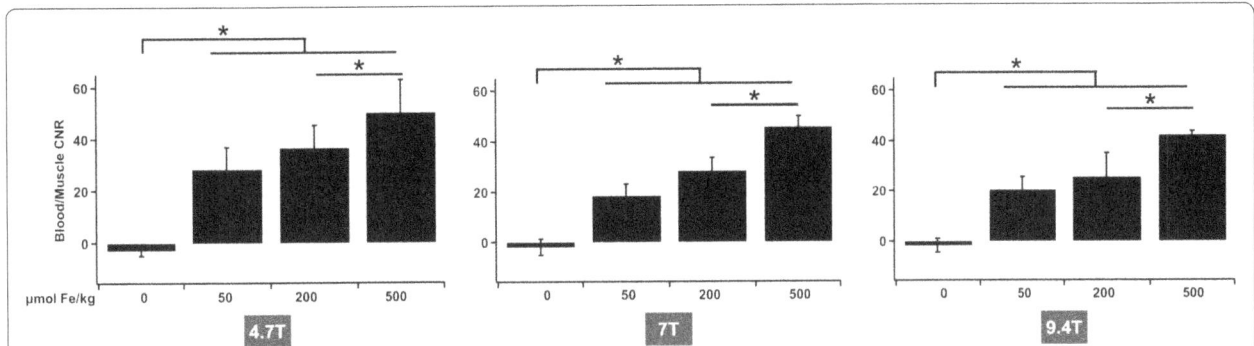

Fig. 3 Contrast-to-noise ratio between blood in the aortic arch and muscle, obtained with UTE sequences before and after injection of USPIO at 4.7, 7 and 9.4 T and for different injection doses (200 and 500 µmol Fe/kg). p values lower than 0.05 are indicated by an asterisk

the cardiac cycle gave a value between 1.43 and 2.2 with an apparent SNR of 70.

The images at 4.7 T and 7 T were of comparable quality, while at 9.4 T the signal-to-noise ratio and the contrast-to-noise ratio were lower. This discrepancy can be explained by the use of dedicated 4-channel receiver coils at 4.7 and 7 T only.

High-resolution UTE

Images at 104-µm isotropic resolution were acquired at 7 T (Fig. 5). Such a resolution necessitated 35 min acquisition. As expected, the concentration of contrast agent was sufficient during the experiment to enable a very good apparent signal-to-noise ratio for the blood (40.2 ± 2.3) and a good contrast-to-noise ratio between the blood and the myocardium (15.8 ± 2.0).

The spatial resolution appears to be effectively improved compared to images acquired at a resolution of 156 µm. This improvement in resolution can be used to perform precise volumetry (LVSV (µL) = 27.1 ± 3.2; LVEF (%) = 64.1 ± 4.2; RVSV (µL) = 27.4 ± 3.6; RVEF (%) = 61.8 ± 5.2).

It can also be used to better appreciate the deformations of the aortic arch during the cardiac cycle and to distinguish aortic valve (arrowheads, Fig. 5a N°6) and to track the left and right coronary arteries (arrows, Fig. 5b).

Movies showing the 4D-cine images are available as Additional file 1, Additional file 2, Additional file 3 and Additional file 4.

Finally, with the acquisition method used, although it decreases the spatial resolution and the signal-to-noise ratio due to 4 times less number of projections per cine, it is also possible to reconstruct a greater number of images per cardiac cycle. In the videos shown in Additional file 3 and Additional file 4, forty images were reconstructed per R-R interval.

Discussion

This article demonstrates that by combining the use of a UTE 3D imaging sequence with USPIO-based contrast agents it is possible to achieve a strong Signal-to-Noise Ratio and a strong positive contrast at high magnetic fields (4.7 and 9.4 T), and thus to generate highly temporally

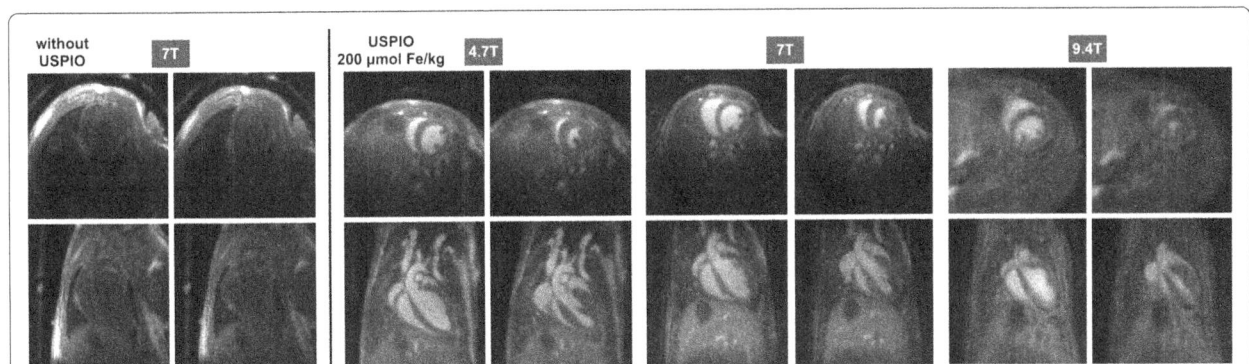

Fig. 4 3D ECG-gated cine image of a mouse heart at 156 µm isotropic resolution obtained before (at 7 T) and after injection of USPIO at 200 µmol Fe/kg (at 4.7, 7 and 9.4 T). Ten images per cardiac cycle were generated, the images at the end of diastole (*left*) and systole (*right*) are shown in two orientations (*short axis: upper panels; long axis: lower panels*). No respiratory gating was used

Table 2 CNR values between the blood in the ventricles and the myocardial wall obtained with the UTE sequence at 156 μm isotropic resolution without USPIO and after injection of USPIO at 200 μmol Fe/kg

CNR (left ventricule - left myocardium)		End-diastole	End-systole
UTE 4.7 T	without USPIO	−2.6 ± 0.6	−4.0 ± 0.9
	USPIO 200 μmol Fe/kg	31.4 ± 3.8	30.2 ± 2.2
UTE 7 T	without USPIO	−2.5 ± 0.7	−3.9 ± 0.6
	USPIO 200 μmol Fe/kg	33.2 ± 4.2	29.2 ± 2.5
UTE 9.4 T	without USPIO	−2.1 ± 0.5	−3.9 ± 0.9
	USPIO 200 μmol Fe/kg	16.3 ± 5.8	15.2 ± 3.2

and spatially resolved images of the cardiovascular system in small animals.

The term "apparent SNR" instead of SNR was used in this article because the method of SNR calculation did not take into account the spatial variance of noise of phased-array coils. However, as mentioned by Kellman et al. [30], this spatial variation is important only when parallel reconstruction is used which was not the case in our experiments.

We believe that the contrast obtained here is greater than those described to date in the literature on mouse cardiac MRI [31–34].

Up to now, iron nanoparticles have mainly been used through their T2* effect, which allows their presence to be detected at high magnetic fields (≥4.7 T), in particular in the field of cellular imaging. Recently, Strobel et al. [35] exploited the T1 effect of iron oxide particles to detect pulmonary inflammation. However, in these experiments, the increase in signal for the lung appears weak, probably due to a low concentration of contrast agent in the observed zone.

At 3 T, Girard et al. [24] showed that, with a subUTE sequence, it is possible to have a positive T1 effect and to exploit it to demonstrate tumor targeting *in vivo*. At lower magnetic fields (< 3 T) [6, 36, 37], and recently at 3 T [12, 13], iron nanoparticles have been shown to be good contrast agents for angiography with classical gradient echo sequences.

In these studies, to limit the susceptibility effect, contrast agent was injected at doses between 50 and 100 μmol Fe/kg. At high magnetic fields, as used here, a dose of 50 μmol Fe/kg gives a positive contrast with a UTE sequence. However, this contrast is lower than with other concentrations and decreases over time. It can therefore limit the acquisition of high-resolution images because a high contrast is necessary during more than 30 min.

With higher doses of injections, the contrast-to-noise ratio was significantly increased for all magnetic fields,

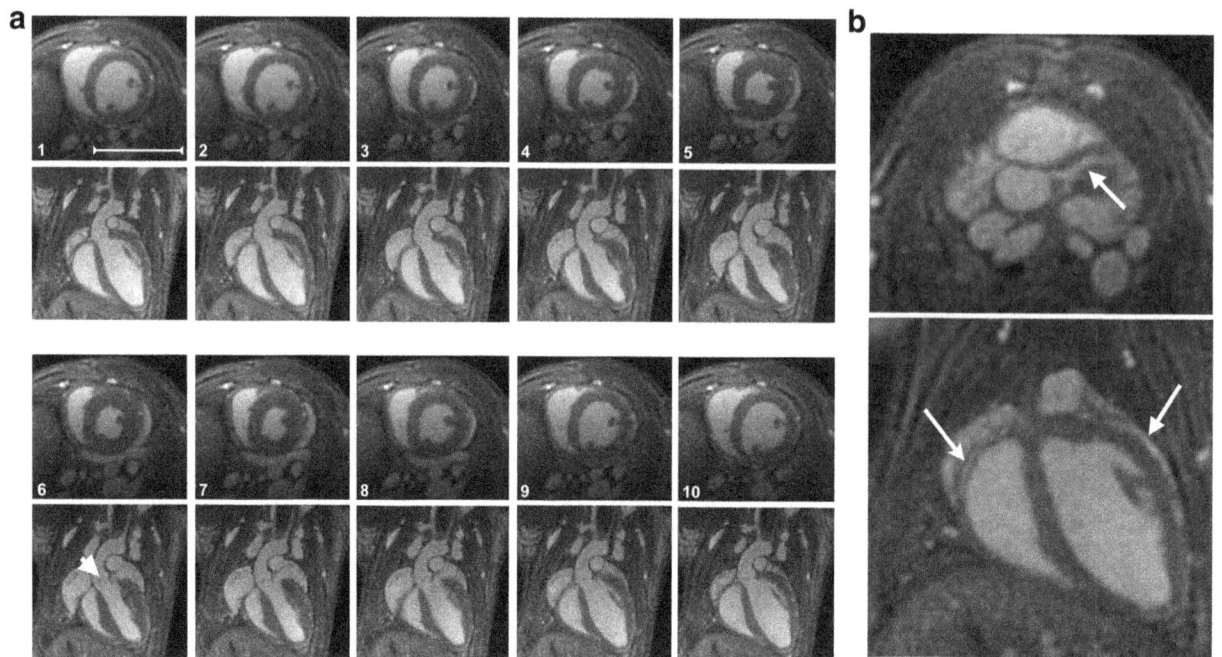

Fig. 5 a 3D ECG-gated cine image as a function of cardiac cycle, obtained at 7 T at 104 μm isotropic resolution after injection of USPIO at 200 μmol Fe/kg. Short axis: upper panel; long axis: lower panel. No respiratory gating was used. The arrow (*image 6*) indicates the aortic valve. **b** Slices extracted from a 3D volume showing the coronary arteries (*right coronary arteries: arrow in upper image; right coronary arteries and left coronary arteries: arrows lower image*). The scale-bar represents 1 cm

Positive contrast high-resolution 3D-cine imaging of the cardiovascular system in small animals using...

75

and it remained constant for a duration compatible with high-resolution cardiac cine image acquisition (> 40 min). Although the doses injected in this study were higher than the doses used for clinical angiography, they remained significantly lower than the doses used for *in-vivo* targeting imaging (1000 µmol Fe/kg) [37].

Compared to gadolinium chelate-type contrast agents, the major advantage of iron nanoparticles is their much longer half-life in the blood, which permits 3D-cine acquisition in small animal. Other gadolinium-based contrast agents have been developed which have a longer half-life. For example, reports are given for p846 [6], a blood pool contrast agent consisting of a single gadolinium ion in a macrocyclic 3-armed chelate, developed by Guerbet (Aulnay-sous-bois, France), or gadolinium-loaded liposomes [31, 32]. However, none of these agents has been approved for clinical use, and their long-term innocuousness has yet to be confirmed. In contrast, a large variety of iron-based nanoparticles has been developed with various sizes, coating compounds and surface charges (Sinerem °, Endorem °, P904 ° from Guerbet, Resovist ° and Supravist ° from Bayer Schering, Clariscan ° from Amersham Health and Ferumoxytol ° from AMAG Pharmaceuticals, ...) [38] and tested on small animals or humans. Among them, P904 is still available for preclinical imaging (Chematech, Dijon, France). Ferumoxitol has recently gained in interest in clinical MRI [39] due to its U.S. FDA approval as an iron supplement for patients with chronic kidney disease. Moreover, its higher relaxivity compared to Sinerem ($r1 = 2$ mM^{-1} s^{-1} at 7 T [25]) combined with a prolonged circulating half-life (14–15 h), should make it an excellent contrast agent for high field MRI.

Since such contrast agents are strongly paramagnetic, ultra-short echo times are needed to achieve significant positive contrast. The UTE sequence used in this study has several advantages. The use of radial encoding with sampling from the center of the k-space, combined with 3D imaging without slice selection and the use of a short excitation pulse (50 µs) makes it possible to generate extremely short TEs, less than 0.05 ms in this study. In small animals, this type of sequence has already been used for 2D-cine cardiac imaging and makes it possible to observe a time-of-flight effect. However, resolution of 2D MRI is often limited in the third dimension of space, and the TE is increased (> 0.3 ms), which can limit its usefulness when a contrast agent with a strong susceptibility effect is injected.

The other advantage of UTE sequences is their low sensitivity to several artefacts due to motion or blood flow. Thus, the signal from blood in areas particularly prone to turbulent flow appears quite homogeneous. This makes it possible to unambiguously measure the volume of the ventricles, whereas in conventional bright-blood images measurements can be affected by errors due to signal loss caused by significant phase-shifts of the spins in blood. The method presented here (UTE + USPIO) could thus be used for phase imaging in regions of extremely turbulent blood flow. Kadbi et al. [40] have already demonstrated the efficacy of UTE sequences to measure blood flow. However, to obtain a significant time-of-flight effect, they had to introduce a slice selection into the UTE sequence, thus increasing the value of TE. The method used here, using both non-selective volume excitation and USPIO injection, allows shorter TE and would be also useful for blood flow quantification.

Finally, we have shown that the combination of the 3D UTE sequence with the injection of an USPIO-type contrast agent makes it possible to generate very high spatial resolution, even though iron-based nanoparticles are known to diminish this resolution, particularly at high magnetic fields. Thus, by using significantly lower voxel sizes than those used to date in the literature [34, 41], a particularly precise ventricular volume can be determined (with semi-automated segmentation) in a relatively short acquisition time (around 12 min for a resolution of 156 µm, and around 35 min for a resolution of 104 µm). This should make it possible to study numerous models of heart diseases. In addition, the coronary arteries (right and left) are clearly visible at high resolution (Fig. 5b) as a function of the heart rate, whereas previous coronary images in small animals were acquired only during diastole [42, 43].

Among the limitations of the method proposed, the acquisition time for radial UTE images appears long compared to classical Cartesian methods, particularly when high spatial resolutions are necessary. However, as previously shown [44], radial methods are favorable to the use of compressed sensing reconstruction algorithms which can be used to limit the acquisition time.

One caveat of this study is that the doses of contrast agent used are higher than those commonly used for USPIO-based angiography in humans. However, they remain lower than those used in targeting imaging. In the absence of additional data, it is not possible today to use these doses as a first-pass agent for angiography in humans. However, doses between 50 and 100 µmol Fe/kg combined with 3D UTE imaging sequences, particularly at magnetic fields of 3 T or higher, should make it possible to image human vascular systems with temporal and spatial resolution which could be higher than those currently used in the clinical practice.

Conclusion

In conclusion, we have demonstrated that by combining the injection of iron nanoparticles with 3D-cine UTE sequences, it was possible to generate a strong positive contrast between the blood and surrounding tissues. These signals and their high contrast were exploited to produce images of the cardiovascular system in small animals at high magnetic fields with a high spatial and temporal resolution. It can be useful for measuring the functional cardiac parameters or for assessing anatomical modifications to the blood vessels in disease models.

Additional files

Additional file 1: Movie generated from the ten 3D cine images at 104 μm isotropic resolution. Transverse orientation. The slices go from the aortic arch to the apex of the heart.

Additional file 2: Movie generated from the ten 3D cine images at 104 μm isotropic resolution. The slices go in the direction of the coronal plane.

Additional file 3: Movie of the heart in the direction of the short axis. The same data are used for the images at 104 μm isotropic resolution, but here, forty images per cycle were reconstructed with high temporal resolution encoding scheme.

Additional file 4: Movie of the heart in the direction of the long axis. The same data are used for the images at 104 μm isotropic resolution, but here, forty images per cycle were reconstructed with high temporal resolution encoding scheme.

Abbreviations

UTE: Ultra-short echo time; FID: Free induction decay; ROI: Region-of-interest; TE: Echo time; TR: Repetition time.

Competing interests

The authors declare that they have no competing interests.

Authors' contributions

AJT and SM designed 3D UTE sequence, acquired and reconstructed in vivo data. WL, KVR and SM have participated to the design of experiments and collection of data. SM and AJT have analyzed and interpreted data and performed statistical analysis. SM, ET and JMF have helped to draw the manuscript. All authors read and approved the final manuscript.

Acknowledgements

This work was supported by a public grant, Translational Research and Advanced Imaging Laboratory, which is part of the French National Research Agency's Investments for the Future Program ("NewFISP"; ANR- 10-LABX-57). The authors thank Dr Julie Magat for technical assistance at 9.4 T.

References

1. Nielsen YW, Thomsen HS. Contrast-enhanced peripheral MRA: technique and contrast agents. Acta Radiol. 2012;53:769–77.
2. Kramer JH, Arnoldi E, François CJ, Wentland AL, Nikolaou K, Wintersperger BJ, et al. Dynamic and static magnetic resonance angiography of the supra-aortic vessels at 3.0 T: intraindividual comparison of gadobutrol, gadobenate dimeglumine, and gadoterate meglumine at equimolar dose. Invest Radiol. 2013;48:121–8.
3. Gaens ME, Backes WH, Rozel S, Lipperts M, Sanders SN, Jaspers K, et al. Dynamic contrast-enhanced MR imaging of carotid atherosclerotic plaque: model selection, reproducibility, and validation. Radiology. 2013;266:271–9.
4. Kaewlai R, Abujudeh H. Nephrogenic systemic fibrosis. AJR Am J Roentgenol. 2012;199:W17–23.
5. Prince MR, Zhang HL, Chabra SG, Jacobs P, Wang Y. A pilot investigation of new superparamagnetic iron oxide (ferumoxytol) as a contrast agent for cardiovascular MRI. J Xray Sci Technol. 2003;11:231–40.
6. Kinner S, Maderwald S, Parohl N, Albert J, Corot C, Robert P, et al. Contrast-enhanced magnetic resonance angiography in rabbits:

evaluation of the gadolinium-based agent p846 and the iron-based blood pool agent p904 in comparison with gadoterate meglumine. Invest Radiol. 2011;46:524–9.
7. Neuwelt EA, Hamilton BE, Varallyay CG, Rooney WR, Edelman RD, Jacobs PM, et al. Ultrasmall superparamagnetic iron oxides (USPIOs): a future alternative magnetic resonance (MR) contrast agent for patients at risk for nephrogenic systemic fibrosis (NSF)? Kidney Int. 2009;75:465–74.
8. Corot C, Robert P, Idée J, Port M. Recent advances in iron oxide nanocrystal technology for medical imaging. Adv Drug Deliv Rev. 2006;58:1471–504.
9. Bremerich J, Bilecen D, Reimer P. MR angiography with blood pool contrast agents. Eur Radiol. 2007;17:3017–24.
10. Wagner M, Wagner S, Schnorr J, Schellenberger E, Kivelitz D, Krug L, et al. Coronary MR angiography using citrate-coated very small superparamagnetic iron oxide particles as blood-pool contrast agent: initial experience in humans. J Magn Reson Imaging. 2011;34:816–23.
11. Clarke SE, Weinmann HJ, Dai E, Lucas AR, Rutt BK. Comparison of two blood pool contrast agents for 0.5-T MR angiography: experimental study in rabbits. Radiology. 2000;214:787–94.
12. Han F, Rapacchi S, Khan S, Ayad I, Salusky I, Gabriel S, et al. Four-dimensional, multiphase, steady-state imaging with contrast enhancement (MUSIC) in the heart: A feasibility study in children. Magn Reson Med. 2014, doi: 10.1002/mrm.25491.
13. Ruangwattanapaisarn N, Hsiao A, Vasanawala SS. Ferumoxytol as an off-label contrast agent in body 3T MR angiography: a pilot study in children. Pediatr Radiol. 2015;45(6):831–9. doi:10.1007/s00247-014-3226-3.
14. Josephson L, Tung CH, Moore A, Weissleder R. High-efficiency intracellular magnetic labeling with novel superparamagnetic-Tat peptide conjugates. Bioconjug Chem. 1999;10:186–91.
15. Lewin M, Carlesso N, Tung CH, Tang XW, Cory D, Scadden DT, et al. Tat peptide-derivatized magnetic nanoparticles allow in vivo tracking and recovery of progenitor cells. Nat Biotechnol. 2000;18:410–4.
16. Peng XH, Qian X, Mao H, Wang AY. Targeted magnetic iron oxide nanoparticles for tumor imaging and therapy. Int J Nanomedicine. 2008;3:311–21.
17. Weinstein JS, Varallyay CG, Dosa E, Gahramanov S, Hamilton B, Rooney WD, et al. Superparamagnetic iron oxide nanoparticles: diagnostic magnetic resonance imaging and potential therapeutic applications in neurooncology and central nervous system inflammatory pathologies, a review. J Cereb Blood Flow Metab. 2010;30:15–35.
18. Qiao J, Li S, Wei L, Jiang J, Long R, Mao H, et al. HER2 targeted molecular MR imaging using a de novo designed protein contrast agent. PLoS One. 2011;6:e18103.
19. Sun C, Lee JS, Zhang M. Magnetic nanoparticles in MR imaging and drug delivery. Adv Drug Deliv Rev. 2008;60:1252–65.
20. Farrar CT, Dai GP, Novikov M, Rosenzweig A, Weissleder R, Rosen BR, et al. Impact of field strength and iron oxide nanoparticle concentration on the linearity and diagnostic accuracy of off-resonance imaging. NMR Biomed. 2008;21:453–63.
21. Stuber M, Gilson WD, Schar M, Kedziorek DA, Hofmann LV, Shah S, et al. Positive contrast visualization of iron oxide-labeled stem cells using inversion-recovery with ON-resonant water suppression (IRON). Magn Reson Med. 2007;58:1072–7.
22. Zurkiya O, Hu XP. Off-resonance saturation as a means of generating contrast with superparamagnetic nanoparticles. Magn Reson Med. 2006;56:726–32.
23. Tyler DJ, Robson MD, Henkelman RM, Young IR, Bydder GM. Magnetic resonance imaging with ultrashort TE (UTE) PULSE sequences: technical considerations. J Magn Reson Imaging. 2007;25:279–89. Review.
24. Girard OM, Du J, Agemy L, Sugahara KN, Kotamraju VR, Ruoslahti E, et al. Optimization of iron oxide nanoparticle detection using ultrashort echo time pulse sequences: comparison of T1, T2*, and synergistic T1-T2* contrast mechanisms. Magn Reson Med. 2011;65:1649–60.
25. Gharagouzloo CA, McMahon PN, Sridhar S. Quantitative contrast-enhanced MRI with superparamagnetic nanoparticles using ultrashort time-to-echo pulse sequences. Magn Reson Med. 2014, doi: 10.1002/mrm.25426.
26. Saff EB, Kuijlaars ABJ. Distributing many points on a sphere. Math Intell. 1997;19:5–11.
27. Nielles-Vallespin S, Weber MA, Bock M, Bongers A, Speier P, Combs SE, et al. 3D radial projection technique with ultrashort echo times for sodium MRI: clinical applications in human brain and skeletal muscle. Magn Reson Med. 2007;57:74–81.

28. Koktzoglou I. 4D Dark blood arterial wall magnetic resonance imaging: methodology and demonstration in the carotid arteries. Magn Reson Med. 2013;69:956–65.
29. Beatty PJ, Nishimura DG, Pauly JM. Rapid gridding reconstruction with a minimal oversampling ratio. IEEE Trans Med Imaging. 2005;24:799–808.
30. Kellman P, McVeigh ER. Image reconstruction in SNR units: a general method for SNR measurement. Magn Reson Med. 2005;54:1439–47.
31. Bucholz E, Ghaghada K, Qi Y, Mukundan S, Johnson GA. Four-dimensional MR microscopy of the mouse heart using radial acquisition and liposomal gadolinium contrast agent. Magn Reson Med. 2008;60:111–8.
32. Bucholz E, Ghaghada K, Qi Y, Mukundan S, Rockman HA, Johnson GA. Cardiovascular phenotyping of the mouse heart using a 4D radial acquisition and liposomal Gd-DTPA-BMA. Magn Reson Med. 2010;63:979–87.
33. Hoerr V, Nagelmann N, Nauerth A, Kuhlmann MT, Stypmann J, Faber C. Cardiac-respiratory self-gated cine ultra-short echo time (UTE) cardiovascular magnetic resonance for assessment of functional cardiac parameters at high magnetic fields. J Cardiovasc Magn Reson. 2013;15:59.
34. Feintuch A, Zhu Y, Bishop J, Davidson L, Dazai J, Bruneau BG, et al. 4D cardiac MRI in the mouse. NMR Biomed. 2007;20:360–5.
35. Strobel K, Hoerr V, Schmid F, Wachsmuth L, Löffler B, Faber C. Early detection of lung inflammation: exploiting T1-effects of iron oxide particles using UTE MRI. Magn Reson Med. 2012;68:1924–31.
36. Ersoy H, Jacobs P, Kent CK, Prince MR. Blood pool MR angiography of aortic stent-graft endoleak. AJR Am J Roentgenol. 2004;182:1181–6.
37. Sigovan M, Boussel L, Sulaiman A, Sappey-Marinier D, Alsaid H, Desbleds-Mansard C, et al. Rapid-clearance iron nanoparticles for inflammation imaging of atherosclerotic plaque: initial experience in animal model. Radiology. 2009;252:401–9.
38. Neuwelt EA, Hamilton BE, Varallyay CG, Rooney WR, Edelman RD, Jacobs PM, et al. Ultrasmall superparamagnetic iron oxides (USPIOs): a future alternative magnetic resonance (MR) contrast agent for patients at risk for nephrogenic systemic fibrosis (NSF)? Kidney Int. 2009;75:465–74. Review.
39. Bashir MR, Bhatti L, Marin D, Nelson RC. Emerging applications for ferumoxytol as a contrast agent in MRI. J Magn Reson Imaging. 2015;41:884–98.
40. Kadbi M, Wang H, Negahdar M, Warner L, Traughber M, Martin P, et al. A novel phase-corrected 3D cine ultra-short te (UTE) phase-contrast MRI technique. In: Proceeding of the Engineering in Medicine and Biology Society (EMBC). San Diego, USA: 2012 Annual International Conference of the IEEE; 2012. p. 77–81.
41. Miraux S, Calmettes G, Massot P, Lefrançois W, Parzy E, Muller B, et al. 4D retrospective black blood trueFISP imaging of mouse heart. Magn Reson Med. 2009;62:1099–105.
42. Ruff J, Wiesmann F, Lanz T, Haase A. Magnetic resonance imaging of coronary arteries and heart valves in a living mouse: techniques and preliminary results. J Magn Reson. 2000;146:290–6.
43. Cochet H, Montaudon M, Laurent F, Calmettes G, Franconi JM, Miraux S, et al. In vivo MR angiography and velocity measurement in mice coronary arteries at 9.4 T: assessment of coronary flow velocity reserve. Radiology. 2010;254:441–8.
44. Nam S, Akçakaya M, Basha T, Stehning C, Manning WJ, Tarokh V, et al. Compressed sensing reconstruction for whole-heart imaging with 3D radial trajectories: a graphics processing unit implementation. Magn Reson Med. 2013;69:91–102.

7

Value of additional strain analysis with feature tracking in dobutamine stress cardiovascular magnetic resonance for detecting coronary artery disease

Christopher Schneeweis[1*], Jianxing Qiu[2], Bernhard Schnackenburg[3], Alexander Berger[1], Sebastian Kelle[1], Eckart Fleck[1] and Rolf Gebker[1]

Abstract

Background: Dobutamine stress cardiovascular magnetic resonance (DS-CMR) has been established for the detection of coronary artery disease (CAD). The novel technique feature tracking (FT) analyses left ventricular circumferential strain (Ecc) thus offering detailed information about myocardial deformation. The purpose of this study was to evaluate FT based Ecc for the detection of myocardial ischemia during DS-CMR.

Methods: A total of 25 patients (18 males; mean age 64 ± 10 years) with suspected or known CAD underwent a standardized high-dose DS-CMR protocol at 1.5 T. For FT analysis cine short axis (SAX) views (apical, medial, basal) at rest and during maximum dobutamine stress were used. None of the patients had wall motion abnormalities (WMAs) or impaired left ventricular function at rest or scar tissue. For analysis of Ecc the three SAX planes were divided into 16 segments (n = 400 segments). During stress 15 patients (34 segments) developed WMAs as assessed by visual analysis. All patients underwent x-ray coronary angiography for clinical reasons which served as the reference standard. Patients without WMAs during DS-CMR and exclusion of stenotic CAD were defined as normal (10 patients, 160 segments). In patients with significant CAD segments that were supplied by a vessel of >70% narrowing were defined as stenotic (n = 64). The remaining segments in patients with significant CAD were considered as remote (n = 176).

Results: At rest no differences in Ecc were observed between normal, stenotic and remote segments. High-dose dobutamine stress revealed highly significant differences between Ecc of normal and stenotic segments ($p < 0.001$), as well as between remote and stenotic segments ($p < 0.001$). The same observation took place for the absolute change of Ecc ($p < 0.001$ and $p = 0.01$). ROC analysis of Ecc during maximum DS-CMR differentiated normal from stenotic segments with a sensitivity of 75% and specificity of 67% using a cutoff -33.2% with an area under the curve of 0.78. Additional analysis of intermediate-dose dobutamine also showed a significant difference between normal and stenotic segments ($p = 0.001$).

Conclusion: FT based analysis of Ecc during intermediate- and high-dose DS-CMR was feasible and differentiated between stenotic, remote and normal segments. Quantitative assessment of Ecc with FT may improve the diagnostic accuracy of DS-CMR for detection of ischemia.

Keywords: Dobutamine stress cardiovascular magnetic resonance, Coronary artery disease, Feature tracking, Circumferential strain, Wall motion abnormality

* Correspondence: christopher.schneeweis@googlemail.com
[1]Department of Internal Medicine/Cardiology, German Heart Institute Berlin, Augustenburger Platz 1, 13353 Berlin, Germany
Full list of author information is available at the end of the article

Background

High-dose dobutamine stress cardiovascular magnetic resonance (DS-CMR) has been established as a method with high diagnostic accuracy for the evaluation of patients with suspected myocardial ischemia [1,2]. Steady state free precession (SSFP) cine imaging during DS-CMR provides a high contrast between intracavitary blood and the endocardium, resulting in a consistently high capability to evaluate myocardial thickening and detection of wall motion abnormalities (WMAs). The assessment of WMAs tends to be subjective as it is based on visual analysis and the clinical experience of the observer. Futhermore, WMAs appear relatively late during the ischemic cascade. Therefore, newer techniques which provide quantitative information about myocardial deformation may be helpful to detect deteriorating myocardial motion at an earlier point in time. Myocardial tagging has shown promising results to improve the detection of ischemia [3], but has been limited by acquiring additional sequences and time consuming post processing. The novel technique feature tracking (FT) analyses left ventricular myocardial strain [4] on the basis of conventional cine images. It was shown that FT is able to detect quantitative changes of wall motion at rest and during low dose dobutamine in healthy volunteers [5] as well as in patients with ischemic cardiomyopathy [6]. However, data on the utility of myocardial strain during high-dose DS-CMR are limited to a few tagging studies [7] and most of them are based on visual or semi-quantitative assessment only [8]. Currently no information exists about the capability of FT for the detection of ischemia during high-dose DS-CMR. Hence, the purpose of this study was to assess FT based left ventricular circumferential strain (Ecc) during DS-CMR and to test its ability to differentiate between stenotic, remote and normal segments.

Methods

Patient population

In this retrospective study we included DS-CMR examinations of 25 patients (18 males; mean age 64 ± 10 years) examined for suspicion or progression of known CAD (1 patient). The study was conducted in accordance with the ethical standards defined by local law. In general, written informed consent from patients was obtained before their inclusion in the study. In addition, all participants gave a signature, that their data could be used in anonymized form for scientific work. Further information on patients is given in Table 1. Patients with impaired left ventricular ejection fraction (LVEF), a history of heart surgery, WMA at rest, atrial fibrillation, premature beats, glomerular filtration rate <30 ml/min and/or myocardial scar on Late Gadolinium Enhancement (LGE) were excluded, as well as patients who met contraindications for cardiovascular magnetic resonance (CMR) (e.g. pacemaker, ICD,

Table 1 Shows demographic details of patients, hemodynamic data and main CMR measurements

	Positive DSMR (n = 15)	Negative DSMR (n = 10)
Age (years)	66 ± 8	59 ± 12
Female	3	4
Hypertension	15	7
Diabetes mellitus	3	5
Hyperlipedemia	12	4
Known CAD	1	0
Time between DSMR and coronary angiogramm (weeks)	4 ± 12	8 ± 20
Hemodynamic data		
Peak heart rate (bpm)	136 ± 12	143 ± 9
Heart rate at rest (bpm)	66 ± 9	70 ± 9
Peak BP (mmHg)	146/73 ± 28/13	131/68 ± 17/9
BP at rest (mmHg)	141/76 ± 22/14	129/71 ± 15/13
Maximum dobutamine dose (µg/kg/min)	36 ± 7	37 ± 5
Atropin dose (ml)	0.6 ± 0.3	0.25 ± 0.04
MRI parameter		
LVEF (%)	61 + 4	62 ± 4
LVEDV (ml)	154 ± 31	143 ± 32
LVESV (ml)	60 ± 14	54 ± 14

claustrophobia). Examinations with severe artefacts and low image quality were not considered for this study.

Coronary angiography

Coronary angiography served as reference standard to define stenotic CAD. All patients underwent coronary angiography within 8 ± 20 weeks (no WMA during DS-CMR) and 4 ± 12 weeks (WMA during DS-CMR) after DS-CMR. Patients without WMAs underwent coronary angiography due to clinical indications. Angiograms were evaluated visually for stenosis of all major epicardial coronary arteries and their branches by a highly experienced interventional cardiologist. The severity of coronary stenosis was derived from one single view showing the maximal reduction in absolute luminal diameter. A significant coronary stenosis was defined as $\geq 70\%$ luminal diameter reduction in vessels with ≥ 2 mm diameter. In addition, myocardial segments were assigned to the supplying coronary artery based on a consensus read of the interventionalist and the CMR reader taking the respective coronary dominance type into account. Patients without WMAs during DS-CMR and exclusion of CAD by coronary angiography were defined as normal and served as control. The remaining segments in patients with significant CAD were considered as remote.

CMR image acquisition and analysis

CMR was performed using a conventional 1.5 T magnetic resonance system (Achieva, Philips, Best, The Netherlands) and a 5 array cardiac surface coil. During image acquisition ECG and breathing motion were detected continuously. Cine imaging was performed using balanced SSFP and retrospective gating (repetition time, 3.4 ms; echo time, 1.7 ms; flip angle, 60, in-plane spatial resolution was 1.8 × 1.8 mm with a slice thickness of 8 mm). Patients were instructed to stop beta-blocker medication at least 24 hours before DS-CMR.

All patients underwent a standardized DS-CMR described elsewhere [9]. Standard LGE imaging was performed 10 minutes after the termination of dobutamine infusion. For LGE an intravenous bolus of 0.2 mmol/kg gadolinium-diethylenetriamine-pentaacetic acid (Magnevist, Bayer, Berlin, Germany) was administered.

For CMR image analyses of left ventricular ejection fraction (LVEF), left ventricular end-diastolic volume (LVEDV), and left ventricular end-systolic volume (LVESV) the custom software package (Philips, MR WorkSpace 2.6.3.3) was used. Volumetric analysis of the LV was performed using Simpson's method. For WMA analysis 2 observers performed a consensus segmental analysis. Both were blinded to the patients' identities and results of the coronary angiography.

Feature tracking

Cine balanced SSFP (bSSFP) SAX images (basal, medial and apical) were used for the Ecc analysis with FT. The bSSFP cine images were stored as Digital Imaging and Communication in Medicine (DICOM) and analysed using the CMR FT software (TomTec Imaging Systems, Munich, Germany). Endocardial contours were drawn manually at end-diastole. The software tracks different features and generates information about myocardial deformation throughout the cardiac cycle [4]. In case of unsatisfactory detection of the endocardial border the contour was modified until a satisfying tracing resulted.

One operator, who was blinded to the results of the DS-CMR and coronary angiogram, drew the contours at rest, low- (10 μg), intermediate (20 μg)- and high-dose (40 μg) dobutamine. Additional to comparing segments defined by coronary angiography into normal, stenotic and remote we specifically analyzed those that developed a WMA during DS-CMR. Time to peak Ecc was compared between segments with WMA and remote segments. In order to assess interobserver variability a random subset of rest and stress images were re-analysed in 9 subjects (144 segments) by a second operator.

Statistical analysis

Statistical analysis was performed using SPSS 18.0 for Windows (SPSS Inc.) and MedCalc. All parameters were given as mean ± standard deviation (SD). Segmental based data were compared using a one-way ANOVA followed by the Scheffé's post-hoc analysis or in case of not normal distribution with Tamhane's post-hoc analysis. T-tests were performed for analysis of low-dose and intermediate dose Ecc values. For testing differences of time to peak values the paired t-test was used. For assessment of the interobserver variability the intraclass correlation coefficient and Bland-Altman analysis was used.

Results

DS-CMR

In all patients the target heart rate was achieved. All patients tolerated the protocol and no premature termination was necessary. Overall no severe adverse events were observed. Fifteen patients developed a WMA (34 segments) during DS-CMR, in 10 patients no WMA (160 segments) was detectable. All patients showed a normal LVEF. Remaining CMR results and hemodynamic data are reported in Table 1.

Coronary angiography

All patients underwent coronary angiography. Significant CAD was diagnosed in 15 patients. The remaining 10 patients had no significant CAD and were defined as normal. Based on coronary angiogram 64 segments were defined as stenotic (≥70% stenosis), 176 as remote (no significant stenosis in patients with CAD) and 160 as normal (Figure 1).

Feature tracking

At rest no differences in Ecc were observed between the different groups (normal: −28.1 ± 8.9%; stenotic: −25.9 ± 10.7%; remote: −27.5 ± 11.6% and WMA: −24.8 ± 12.9%; p = 0.62 for normal vs. stenotic, p = 0.66 for nomal vs. WMAs, p = 0.97 for normal vs. remote and p = 0.79 for

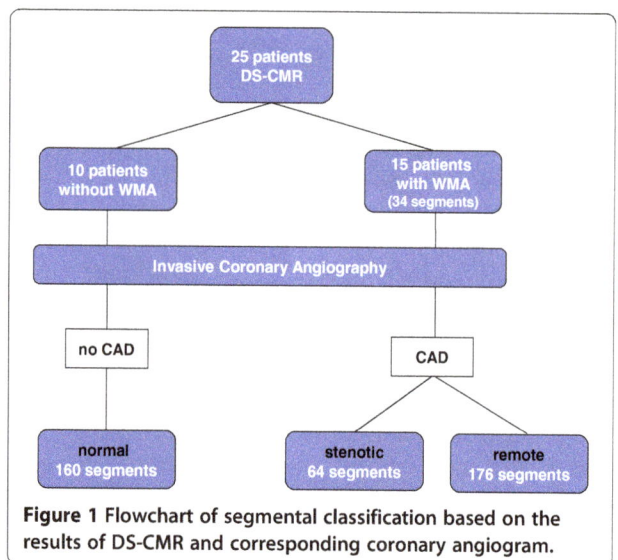

Figure 1 Flowchart of segmental classification based on the results of DS-CMR and corresponding coronary angiogram.

remote vs. stenotic segments). Ecc analysis at high-dose dobutamine stress showed highly significant differences between normal and stenotic segments (normal: –39.3 ± 11.3%; stenotic: –23.8 ± 15.9%, p < 0.001, representative imaging examples are given in Figures 2A, 2B and 2C) as well as between normal segments and segments which developed WMAs (–19.2 ± 19.1%, p < 0.001). Furthermore, Ecc

differed significantly between normal and remote segments (remote: –33.9 ± 15.1%, p = 0.002), while no difference was observed between segments with WMAs and stenotic segments (p = 0.79). The difference between remote segments and stenotic segments was highly significant (p < 0.001).

Similar results were seen when comparing the absolute change (Δ) of Ecc between rest and stress for normal vs.

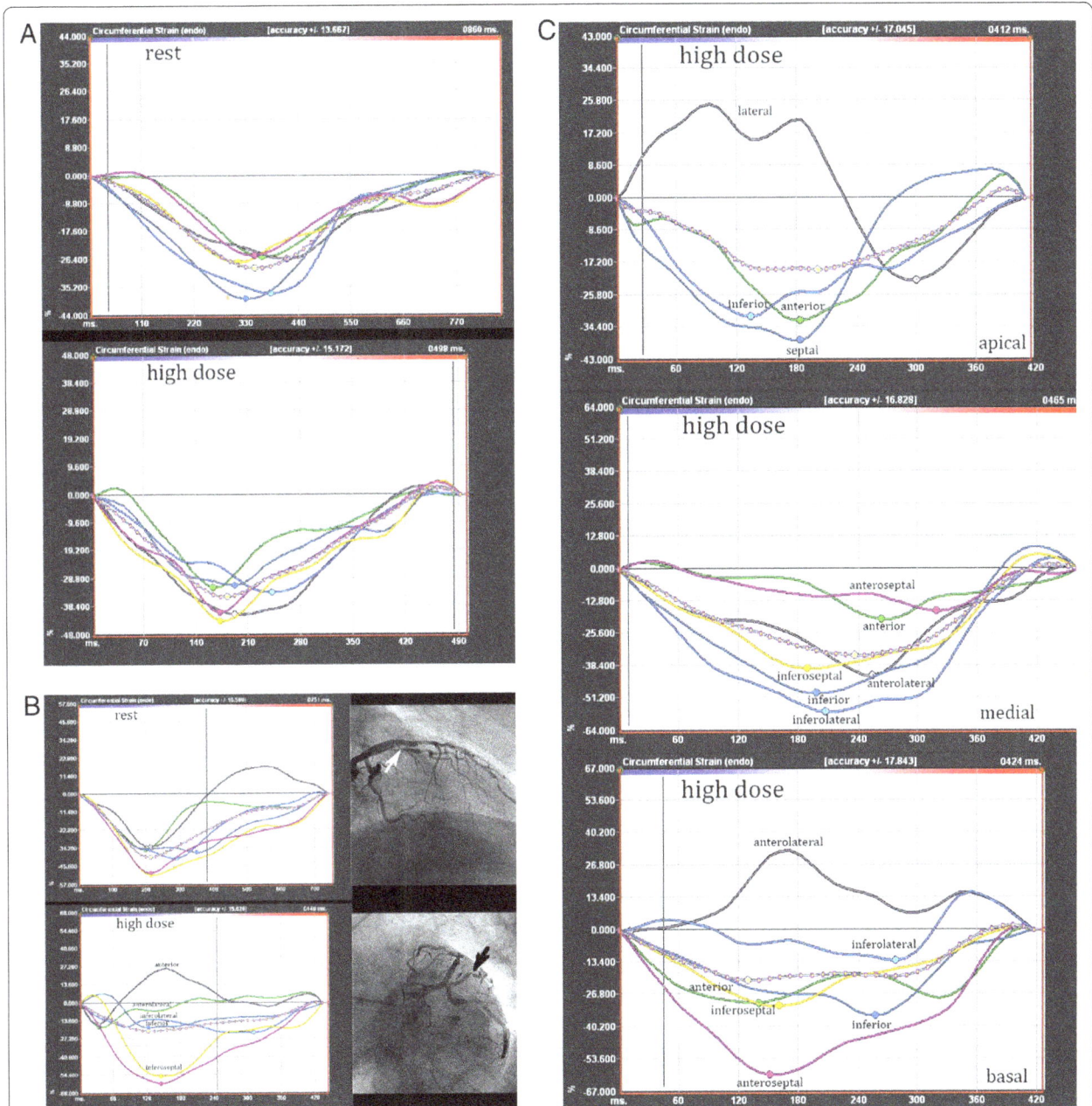

Figure 2 Segmental strain analysis. A: Segmental based circumferential strain analysis at rest and during high-dose dobutamine in a patient without WMA and normal coronary angiogram. **B:** Segmental strain analysis in a patient, who developed a WMA of the anterolateral segment. The Ecc of the neighbouring anterior and inferolateral segments was also impaired. The coronary angiogram showed a corresponding high-grade stenosis of the first diagonal branch. **C:** Ecc analysis of basal, medial and apical SAX under high-dose dobutamine stress. The depicted strain curves originate from three different patients, who all developed a WMA. Angiography showed high grade stenosis of the left circumflex artery in the patient at the bottom (basal SAX). Both patients in the middle and at the top had stenoses of the left anterior descending artery.

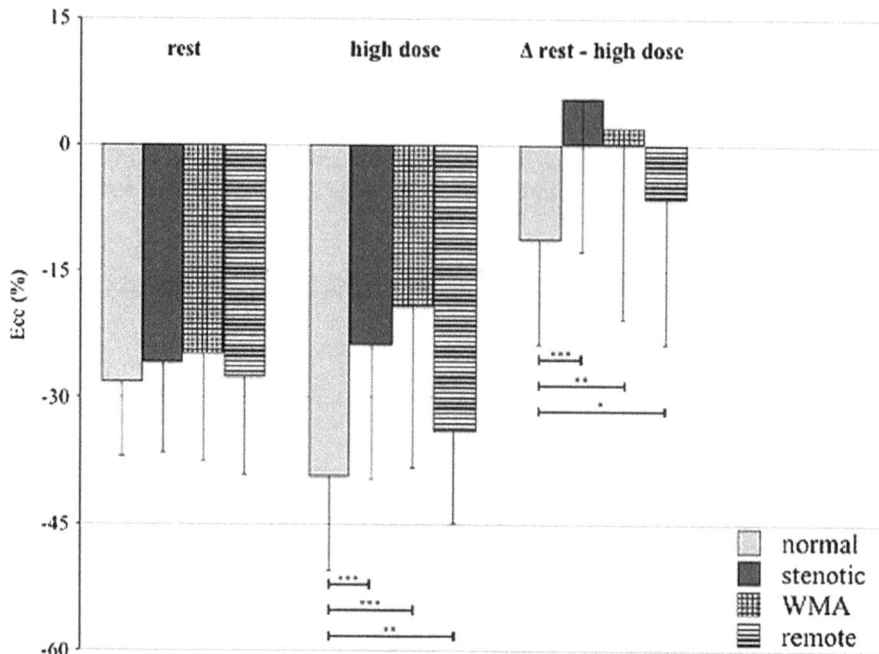

Figure 3 Bar graphs displaying the circumferential strain values at rest and high-dose dobutamine stress as well as the absolute change (Δ) of Ecc. Significant differences were observed between normal segments and the remaining segments.

stenotic segments (Δ normal: −11.2 ± 12.6%, Δ stenotic: 2.1 ± 18.4%; p < 0.001) and vs. segments with WMAs (Δ WMA: 5.6 ± 22.9%; p = 0.001), as well as between normal and remote segments (Δ remote: −6.5 ± 17.2%; p = 0.023). Furthermore, the difference between remote and stenotic segments was significant (p = 0.01) and no difference was detected between segments with WMAs and stenotic segments (p = 0.97).

Results of the Ecc analysis are summarized in Figure 3. ROC analysis for Ecc during high-dose DS-CMR differentiated normal from stenotic segments with a sensitivity of 75% and specificity of 67% using a cut-off of −33.2%

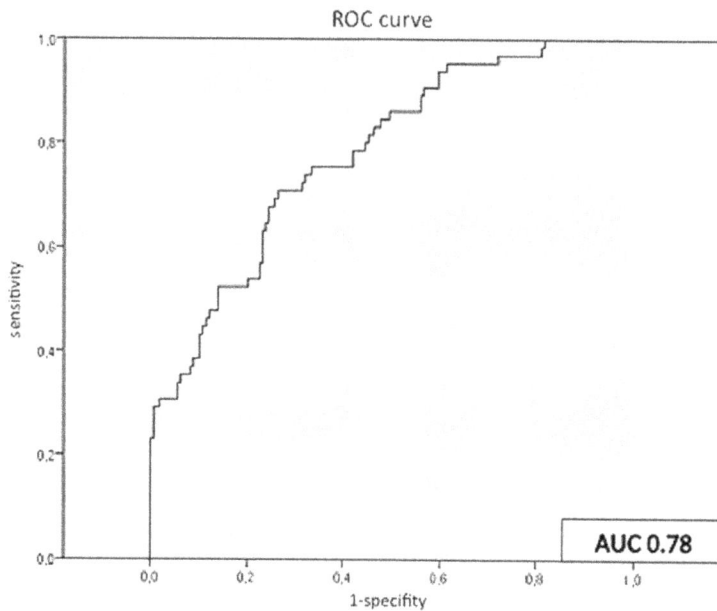

Figure 4 ROC analysis for Ecc during maximum DS-CMR. At a cutoff of -33.2% sensitivity and specificity to differentiate between normal and stenotic segments was 75% and 67%, respectively.

with an area under the curve of 0.78 (95% CI 0.72-0.85) (Figure 4). Due to the observed significant differences between normal and stenotic segments, we performed additional analyses for Ecc at low- and intermediate dobutamine stress. At low-dose dobutamine there was no difference between normal and stenotic segments (−32.9 ± 11%; −30.1 ± 9.6%; p = 0.08) However, at intermediate-dose dobutamine stress normal and stenotic segments differed significantly (−39.5 ± 10.4%; −33.9 ± 13.2%; p = 0.001). In regard to the absolute change (Δ normal: 11.4 ± 11.5%; Δ stenotic: 8.5 ± 14.9%) the difference was not statistically significant (p = 0.18).

In segments with WMA time to peak Ecc was longer than in remote segments (203.4 ± 56.8 ms vs. 163.7 ± 41.4 ms, p = 0.007).

Interobserver agreement

The intraclass correlation coefficients (ICC) indicated a strong agreement for Ecc at rest (0.7) and very high agreement at high-dose dobutamine stress (0.85). The Bland-Altman analyses showed reasonable agreement at rest as well as during high-dose dobutamine stress, but lack of consistent agreement for Ecc values less than −20% at rest and stress. Variability above −20% for rest as well as stress was mainly within 50% difference levels and nearly half of all values were within the 15% difference level (Figure 5A and B).

Discussion

The aim of this work was to evaluate the ability of FT derived Ecc to detect stress-inducible myocardial ischemia during high-dose DS-CMR. FT is a new method for assessing myocardial strain based on the analysis of cine images. There is growing interest in this method as reflected by a number of recently published studies that compared FT to other strain analysis tools such as myocardial tagging [4] and speckle tracking [10]. Until now the utility of FT for DS-CMR has only been demonstrated using low-dose

regimen in healthy volunteers [5] and patients with ischemic cardiomyopathy [6]. The application of FT during low-dose dobutamine or in patients with decreased LV function may be somewhat easier. Due to the increasing myocardial contractility and consecutive partial obliteration of the LV cavity during high-dose dobutamine, discrimination of the endocardial border using FT becomes more challenging. Our study demonstrated that FT was feasible and allowed to distinguish between stenotic, remote and normal segments. The Ecc values from our study at rest were within the range of previously published data [5]. Furthermore, FT demonstrated quantitative changes of Ecc during DS-CMR in segments that developed WMAs based on conventional visual analysis. The significant differences of Ecc in segments with WMA were accompanied by higher time to peak values thus indicating that peak Ecc is not only decreased but also delayed in segments with WMA.

Overall 64 segments were defined as stenotic, while only in 34 segments a WMA was visually detected. Ecc did not show differences between stenotic segments and segments, which developed WMAs. This indicates that Ecc may detect more ischemic segments as compared to the visual analysis of wall motion. Physiologically a perfusion deficit appears as the earliest sign of myocardial ischemia followed by metabolic alterations. With continuation of ischemia these effects become more pronounced and induce diastolic and systolic dysfunction before finally leading to myocardial infarction. Based on this, inducible WMAs during high-dose DS-CMR appear relatively late in the ischemic cascade.

Interestingly, we could show a difference of Ecc between normal and remote segments during high-dose dobutamine stress. Deterioration of strain in stenotic segments may not only be limited to the segment itself and will consequently affect neighbouring segments. Thus, these findings could be an expression of generalized changes of strain in the presence of only a regional coronary narrowing.

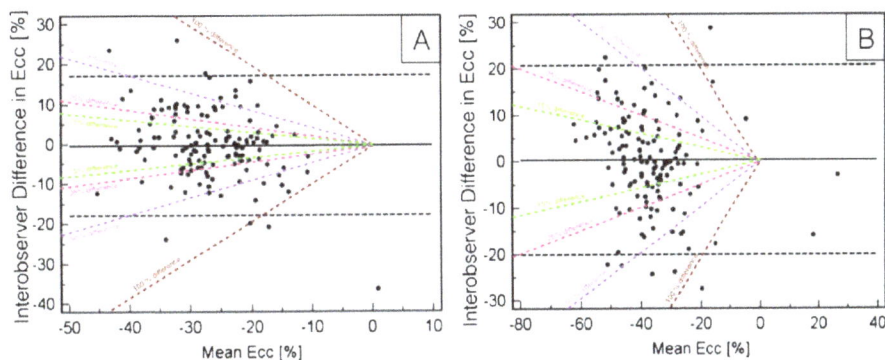

Figure 5 A and B: Bland Altman plots with bias (solid black line) and limits of agreement (dotted black line) for interobserver agreement at rest (A) and high-dose dobutamine stress (B). Values are expressed as %. The oblique dashed lines demonstrate 15, 25, 50 and 100% difference levels.

Our study demonstrated that the earliest sign of ischaemia detectable by Ecc using FT occurred during intermediate dose dobutamine stress. Differences in Ecc between stenotic and normal segments became even more pronounced at high-dose dobutamine stress. Furthermore, in normal segments strain did not increase further between intermediate and high-dose dobutamine stress. These findings are in line with a previous study that used direct color-coded visualization of myocardial strain with Strain-Encoded MR (SENC) [11]. The implementation of FT in clinical routine may help in earlier detection of ischaemia during intermediate stages, thereby increasing patient safety during pharmacologic stress testing.

Overall the analysis of myocardial strain during high-dose DS-CMR has been limited to a few studies using tagging [3,7,12] and SENC [8]. These studies have shown promising results to improve the accuracy for the detection of myocardial ischemia. However, most data were assessed only visually and quantitative data are only available for the apical SAX [7]. The limited amount of studies using tagging is most likely related to the necessity of acquiring additional sequences and the time-consuming post processing to assess strain values. In contrast, FT can process conventional cine images thus being potentially more time efficient. Previous studies demonstrated that Ecc seems to be the most robust and reproducible strain parameter [13]. For the interobserver agreement we noted a strong agreement for Ecc at rest (0.7) and very high agreement at high-dose dobutamine stress (0.85) when using ICC. Additional analysis with Bland Altman plots showed a reasonable agreement for Ecc values at rest and high-dose and are comparable to published data [5,6]. In our study half of the inter-observer measurements were within the 15% difference level, which implies that FT Ecc analysis on a segmental level becomes challenging at rest, but does not become worse during dobutamine stress.

Conclusion

The results of FT in DS-CMR seem to be promising and may improve the diagnostic accuracy of DS-CMR for the detection of ischemia. Further studies are necessary to evaluate FT in intermediate and high-dose DS-CMR and to determine whether a robust threshold for discriminating ischemic from non-ischemic segments can be given.

Limitations

Our study has important limitations. Conventional coronary angiography with visual assessment of severity of stenoses was used rather than fractional flow reserve (FFR) or quantitative coronary angiography (QCA) to distinguish between stenotic, remote and normal segments. The discrepancies between the anatomical and physiological approach are well known which may have introduced a bias to our

study. Also, we included patients with relatively good image quality only. Furthermore, patients with previous myocardial infarction were excluded; hence our results may not be applicable to patients with known myocardial infarction and pre-existing WMAs. The results of this study were based on the circumferential strain of the short axis geometry as it seems to be the most reliable and reproducible parameter [14].

Abbreviations

DS-CMR: Dobutamine stress cardiovascular magnetic resonance; CAD: Coronary artery disease; FT: Feature tracking; Ecc: Circumferential strain; SAX: Short axis; WMA: Wall motion abnormality; SSFP: Steady state free precession; bSSFP: Balanced SSFP; LVEF: Left ventricular ejection fraction; LVEDV: Left ventricular end-diastolic volume; LVESV: Left ventricular end-systolic volume; LGE: Late gadolinium enhancement; CMR: Cardiovascular magnetic resonance; SD: Standard deviation; SENC: Strain-encoded MR; FFR: Fractional flow reserve.

Competing interests

The authors declare that they have no competing interests.

Authors' contribution

RG, EF and CS were responsible for the conception and the design of the study. CS drafted the manuscript. RG and CS interpreted and analysed the data. AB, SK and CS were involved in CMR acquisition of data. EF and RG performed the coronary angiographies, RG and CS performed the consensus read of angiographic and CMR results. BS was responsible for the physical setup and helped to improve our image quality by his knowledge. JQ performed the FT analysis, CS the interobserver FT analysis. All authors were involved in reading and revising the manuscript carefully for important intellectual content and improvement. All authors have given their agreement for this manuscript to be published. All authors read and approved the final manuscript.

Author details

[1]Department of Internal Medicine/Cardiology, German Heart Institute Berlin, Augustenburger Platz 1, 13353 Berlin, Germany. [2]Department of Radiology, Peking University First Hospital, Beijing, China. [3]Philips Research Hamburg, Hamburg, Germany.

References

1. Nagel E, Lehmkuhl HB, Bocksch W, Klein C, Vogel U, Frantz E, Ellmer A, Dreysse S, Fleck E. Noninvasive diagnosis of ischemia-induced wall motion abnormalities with the use of high-dose dobutamine stress MRI: comparison with dobutamine stress echocardiography. Circulation. 1999; 99:763–70.
2. Flamm SD. High-dose dobutamine stress cardiac magnetic resonance imaging–has its time come? Eur Heart J. 2004; 25:1183–84.
3. Kuijpers D. Dobutamine cardiovascular magnetic resonance for the detection of myocardial ischemia with the use of myocardial tagging. Circulation. 2003; 107:1592–97.
4. Hor KN, Gottliebson WM, Carson C, Wash E, Cnota J, Fleck R, Wansapura J, Klimeczek P, Al-Khalidi HR, Chung ES, Benson DW, Mazur W. Comparison of magnetic resonance feature tracking for strain calculation with harmonic phase imaging analysis. JCMG. 2010; 3:144–51.
5. Schuster A, Kutty S, Padiyath A, Parish V, Gribben P, Danford DA, Makowski MR, Bigalke B, Beerbaum P, Nagel E. Cardiovascular magnetic resonance myocardialfeature tracking detects quantitative wall motionduring dobutamine stress. J Cardiovasc Magn Reson. 2011; 13:58.
6. Schuster A, Paul M, Bettencourt N, Morton G, Chiribiri A, Ishida M, Hussain S, Jogiya R, Kutty S, Bigalke B, Perera D, Nagel E. Cardiovascular magnetic resonance myocardial feature tracking for quantitative viability assessment in ischemic cardiomyopathy. Int J Cardiol. 2011; doi:10.1016/j.ijcard.2011.10.137.
7. Paetsch I. Magnetic resonance stress tagging in ischemic heart disease. AJP. 2005; 288:H2708–14.

8. Korosoglou G, Futterer S, Humpert PM, Riedle N, Lossnitzer D, Hoerig B, Steen H, Giannitsis E, Osman NF, Katus HA. Strain-encoded cardiac MR during high-dose dobutamine stress testing: comparison to cine imaging and to myocardial tagging. *J Magn Reson Imaging.* 2009; **29**:1053–61.
9. Gebker R, Frick M, Jahnke C, Berger A, Schneeweis C, Manka R, Kelle S, Klein C, Schnackenburg B, Fleck E, Paetsch I. Value of additional myocardial perfusion imaging during dobutamine stress magnetic resonance for the assessment of intermediate coronary artery disease. *Int J Cardiovasc Imaging.* 2010; **28**:89–97.
10. Onishi T, Saha SK, Ludwig DR, Onishi T, Marek JJ, Cavalcante JOL, Schelbert EB, Schwartzman D, Gorcsan J III. Feature tracking measurement of dyssynchrony from cardiovascular magnetic resonance cine acquisitions: comparison with echocardiographic speckle tracking. *J Cardiovasc Magn Reson.* 2013; **15**:1–1.
11. Korosoglou G, Lehrke S, Wochele A, Hoerig B, Lossnitzer D, Steen H, Giannitsis E, Osman NF, Katus HA. Strain-encoded CMR for the detection of inducible ischemia during intermediate stress. *JCMG.* 2010; **3**:361–71.
12. Thomas D, Meyer C, Strach K, Naehle CP, Mazraeh J, Gampert T, Schild HH, Sommer T. Dobutamine stress tagging and gradient-echo imaging for detection of coronary heart disease at 3 T. *Br J Radiol.* 2010; **84**:44–50.
13. Augustine D, Lewandowski AJ, Lazdam M, Rai A, Francis J, Myerson S, Noble A, Becher H, Neubauer S, Petersen SE, Leeson P. Global and regional left ventricular myocardial deformation measures by magnetic resonance feature tracking in healthy volunteers: comparison with tagging and relevance of gender. *J Cardiovasc Magn Reson.* 2013; **15** IS:8–8.
14. Morton G, Schuster A, Jogiya R, Kutty S, Beerbaum P, Nagel E. Inter-study reproducibility of cardiovascular magnetic resonance myocardial feature tracking. *J Cardiovasc Magn Reson.* 2012; **14** IS:43–43.

8

Cardiovascular magnetic resonance imaging of myocardial oedema following acute myocardial infarction: Is whole heart coverage necessary?

Stephen Hamshere[1*], Daniel A. Jones[1,2], Cyril Pellaton[1], Danielle Longchamp[1], Tom Burchell[1], Saidi Mohiddin[1], James C. Moon[1], Jens Kastrup[4], Didier Locca[1,3], Steffen E. Petersen[1,2], Mark Westwood[1] and Anthony Mathur[1,2]

Abstract

Background: AAR measurement is useful when assessing the efficacy of reperfusion therapy and novel cardioprotective agents after myocardial infarction. Multi-slice (Typically 10-12) T2-STIR has been used widely for its measurement, typically with a short axis stack (SAX) covering the entire left ventricle, which can result in long acquisition times and multiple breath holds. This study sought to compare 3-slice T2-short-tau inversion recovery (T2- STIR) technique against conventional multi-slice T2-STIR technique for the assessment of area at risk (AAR).

Methods: CMR imaging was performed on 167 patients after successful primary percutaneous coronary intervention. 82 patients underwent a novel 3-slice SAX protocol and 85 patients underwent standard 10-slice SAX protocol. AAR was obtained by manual endocardial and epicardial contour mapping followed by a semi-automated selection of normal myocardium; the volume was expressed as mass (%) by two independent observers.

Results: 85 patients underwent both 10-slice and 3-slice imaging assessment showing a significant and strong correlation (intraclass correlation coefficient = 0.92; $p < 0.0001$) and a low Bland-Altman limit (mean difference -0.03 ± 3.21 %, 95 % limit of agreement,- 6.3 to 6.3) between the 2 analysis techniques. A further 82 patients underwent 3-slice imaging alone, both the 3-slice and the 10-slice techniques showed statistically significant correlations with angiographic risk scores (3-slice to BARI $r = 0.36$, 3-slice to APPROACH $r = 0.42$, 10-slice to BARI $r = 0.27$, 10-slice to APPROACH $r = 0.46$). There was low inter-observer variability demonstrated in the 3-slice technique, which was comparable to the 10-slice method ($z = 1.035$, $p = 0.15$). Acquisition and analysis times were quicker in the 3-slice compared to the 10-slice method (3-slice median time: 100 seconds (IQR: 65-171 s) vs (10-slice time: 355 seconds (IQR: 275-603 s); $p < 0.0001$.

Conclusions: AAR measured using 3-slice T2-STIR technique correlates well with standard 10-slice techniques, with no significant bias demonstrated in assessing the AAR. The 3-slice technique requires less time to perform and analyse and is therefore advantageous for both patients and clinicians.

* Correspondence: stephenmark.hamshere@bartshealth.nhs.uk
[1]Department of Cardiology, Barts Heart Centre, St Bartholomews Hospital, Barts Health NHS Trust, London EC1A 7BE, UK
Full list of author information is available at the end of the article

Background

Cardiac magnetic resonance (CMR) imaging has become the reference standard in the quantification of ventricular volumes, function and tissue characterisation [1]. T2 weighted imaging has been widely used in the assessment of myocardial oedema and area at risk (AAR) following an acute myocardial infarction (AMI) and has been hailed as a potential 'gold standard' [2]. The AAR is defined as the area of ischaemic myocardium that occurs distally to a coronary artery occlusion and its quantification has become crucial in assessing the efficacy of reperfusion therapy and novel cardioprotective agents. Additionally the AAR acts as a prognostic factor in patients following AMI and can play a role in decision-making regarding myocardial revascularization helping distinguish between necrosed and viable myocardium [3, 4].

Currently methods for assessing AAR require coverage of the whole left ventricle with the acquisition of 10–12 continuous myocardial short axis slices, with each slice acquired with a single breath hold of 10–15 seconds. This lengthens the overall duration of a CMR scan in patients early after a myocardial infarction and therefore techniques that shorten examination times may be advantageous to improve patient compliance. Furthermore, despite advances in semi-automated software, post processing and analysis of these images requires time-consuming manual analysis.

Our goal was to assess the AAR using 3 non-contiguous slices in comparison to conventional multi-slice contiguous slices in patients following successful primary percutaneous coronary intervention (PPCI) for acute myocardial infarction.

Methods

Between April 2008 and November 2012, 167 patients with ST-segment elevation MI successfully reperfused through primary percutaneous coronary intervention (PPCI) and undergoing CMR within the first week after reperfusion were studied. All of these patients had been consented into interventional clinical trials including stem cell trial and pharmacological intervention trials (REGENERATE-AMI (NCT00765453), NITRITE-AMI (NCT01584453) and myocardial oedema in acute myocardial infarction (NCT00987259)) [5, 6]. These studies were approved by local ethics committee. Patients underwent either 3 or 10-slice T2 weighted imaging for the assessment of the AAR.

CMR Protocol

Cardiac magnetic resonance (CMR) imaging was performed on a 1·5 T Philips Achieva scanner with a cardiac 32-channel phased array coil. Balanced steady-state free precession cine imaging was used to acquire 10–12 short axis slices (8 mm slice thickness, 2 mm gap) with one slice per breath-hold. Sequence parameters were 1.5 ms echo time (TE), 3.1 ms repetition time (TR), and acquired voxel size was 1.8×1.86 mm with a typical FOV of 360 mm in the phase encoding direction. We acquired 45 phases with 25 % phase sharing. Parallel imaging (SENSE) was used with an acceleration factor of 2.0.

Myocardial oedema was assessed using fat suppressed T2-weighted triple inversion turbo spin echo STIR (Short tau inversion recovery) imaging (TE 80 ms, TR 2 heart beats, TSE factor 31, voxel size 1.8×1.8 mm). Either 10-slices (8 mm per slice, 2 mm gap matched to LGE/cine slices) or 3-slices (8 mm per slice, 19 mm gap with basal, midventricular and apical slices) with one slice per breath-hold (Fig. 1). This sequence has previously been used and validated for assessment of myocardial oedema and myocardial salvage index (MSI) [7–10].

Late gadolinium enhancement (LGE) images were acquired ten minutes after injection of a dose of 0·2 mmol/kg of gadoterate meglumine (Dotarem). A T1-weighted segmented inversion-recovery gradient echo pulse sequence (TR 3.9 ms TE 1.9 ms, flip angle 15°, voxel size of 2×2 mm, typical FOV 360 mm) was used to obtain 10–12 short axis slices (matched with the short-axis cine images) with one slice per breath-hold. The inversion time was adjusted individually according to a T1 scout sequence (Look-Locker). Images were acquired every other heart beat with 2 signal averages.

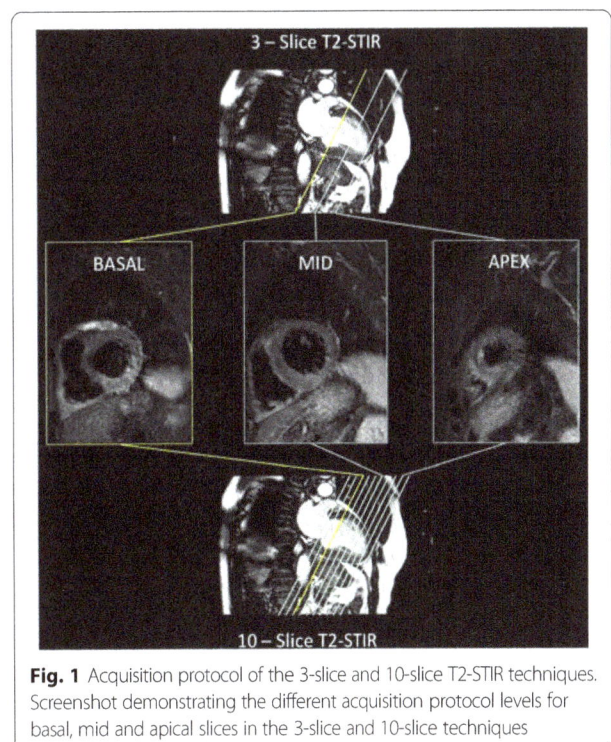

Fig. 1 Acquisition protocol of the 3-slice and 10-slice T2-STIR techniques. Screenshot demonstrating the different acquisition protocol levels for basal, mid and apical slices in the 3-slice and 10-slice techniques

Coronary angiography

All patients underwent coronary angiography according to local cardiac catheterisation laboratory protocols and standard primary percutaneous coronary intervention (PCI) with insertion of at least one stent after admission with a an acute STEMI with an ECG showing ST-segment elevation of 0.1 mV in two or more limb leads or 0.2 mV in two or more contiguous precordial leads, or presumed new left bundle branch block. Flow of the infarct related artery prior to PCI was characterized using the TIMI system (Thrombolysis in Myocardial Infarction) [11]. The AAR was established using angiographic risk scores (BARI and modified APPROACH scores [12, 13].

Image analysis

All analysis was performed using a dedicated software reporting system (CVI[42], Circle Cardiovascular Imaging Inc, Calgary, Alberta, Canada). All images were anonymised, batched and analysed in a blinded fashion by two experienced CMR operators. Manual endocardial and epicardial contours were drawn to calculate myocardial mass (MM), followed by semi-automated selection of normal myocardium with the oedema volumes being expressed as a mass (%). Area at risk (myocardial oedema) was described as >2SD in signal intensity from remote normal myocardium [14]. If present, a central core of hypointense signal within the area of increased signal intensity (hemorrhagic infarction) was included in the AAR [15]. Increased signal intensity from the blood pool adjacent to the endocardium due to slow flow was excluded. Infarct size was calculated using the full-width half maximum method as previously described [16–18]. Infarct and oedema endocardial surface area (ESA) was the percentage of the endocardial enhancement against the total endocardial area. In case of discordance between operators, blinded review by a level III certified CMR reader was performed. If myocardial haemorrhage was present within the area of increased signal intensity it was included in assessment area [15].

Angiographic risk scores

The angiographic area at risk was assessed by the Modified Bypass Angioplasty Revascularisation Investigation [12] and the modified Alberta Provincial Project for Outcome Assessment in Coronary Heart Disease [APPROACH] [13] jeopardy scores). Coronary angiograms were reviewed by two experienced observers blinded to CMR scan and clinical data.

Interobserver variability

Each AAR calculation method was assessed with the evaluator blinded to the results of other techniques. All studies, both angiographic and CMR, were evaluated separately by 2 cardiologists specialized in cardiac imaging and 2 interventional cardiologists to obtain the interobserver variability of each AAR estimation method.

Statistical analysis

Baseline demographics and continuous variables are summarized for 3-slice and 10-slice groups. Continuous variables are presented as a mean ± SD and categorical variables are presented as a percentage. 95 % confidence intervals (CI) are given. Intra-observer variability and correlation between methods was calculated using the coefficient of intraclass correlation coefficient (ICC). All p-values are 2-sided and a value of <0.05 was considered to indicate statistical significance. The comparison of the different correlation coefficients was performed using a 2-tailed Fisher's z-transformation statistical analysis. Data plotting used in analyzing the agreement between the different methods was made with Bland-Altman analysis [19]. All statistical analyses were performed using SPSS version 19 (IBM Corp. Armonk, NY, USA) and graphs produced using Graphpad Prism version 5.0 (GraphPad Software, San Diego, CA).

Results

167 patients presenting with AMI undergoing PPCI at 3 European cardiac intervention centre {Barts Heart Centre, UK; Centre Hospitalier Universitaire, Switzerland; Rigshospitalet, Denmark), were included in the analysis. The mean ages of patient was 56.2 ± 10·2 years and 88 % were male. Clinical, CMR and angiographic characteristics of the population are shown in Table 1. Patients underwent either 10-slice ($n = 85$) or 3-slice ($n = 82$) T2-STIR imaging for AAR assessment as previously described (Additional file 1: Figure S1). The 2 groups were similar with regards to age, sex, LVEF and medical therapy, due to the inclusion criteria of the individual clinical studies there were a greater number of left anterior descending artery (LAD) occlusions in the 3 slice group. CMR was performed at a median of 3 days (range: 2–3 days) after PPCI. In all cases, increased signal intensity was detected in T2-STIR as well as in late gadolinium enhancement sequences.

Comparison of 3-slice and 10-slice AAR in the 10-slice cohort

The 10-Slice AAR group underwent both 10-slice and 3-slice analysis to directly compare the 2 techniques. When assessing the 3-slice acquisition in the 10-slice cohort, all scans had the same level basal, mid and apical slice assessed (defined as 2nd basal slice after the aortic valve, 2nd slice with presence of papillary muscles defined as the mid ventricle and penultimate slice within the apex). Within the 10-slice AAR group the AAR ranged from 11.5 % of the myocardium to 46.8 % (mean

Table 1 Baseline characteristics

	3-slice	10-slice	
	($n = 82$)	($n = 85$)	P value
Age (yr)	57.0 ± 10.5	55.9 ± 11.4	0.6202
Sex (M/F)	71/11	75/12	0.3037
BMI (kg/m^2)	27.0 ± 3.8	27.4 ± 3.9	0.5277
Ethnicity (Caucasian) (No. (%))	66 (80 %)	71 (83.5 %)	0.6113
Medical History:			
Hypertension (No. (%))	30 (36.5 %)	28 (32.9 %)	0.6235
Hypercholesterolemia (No. (%))	24 (29.3 %)	31 (26.4 %)	0.3251
Diabetes mellitus (No. (%))	10 (12.2 %)	9 (11.6 %)	0.5766
Active smoker (No. (%))	42 (51.2 %)	47 (55.3 %)	0.6004
Previous MI (No. (%))	1 (1.2 %)	2 (2.4 %)	0.5841
Previous PCI (No. (%))	1 (1.2 %)	3 (3.5 %)	0.3320
Family history (No. (%))	25 (30.5 %)	19 (22.4 %)	0.2354
Culprit Vessel:			<0.0001
LAD (No. (%))	82 (100 %)	23 (27 %)	
LCx (No. (%))	0 (0 %)	11 (13 %)	
RCA (No. (%))	0 (0 %)	51 (60 %)	
Timings:			
Chest Pain to PCI (min)	194.5 ± 25.4	201.0 ± 32.2	0.8459
Infarct Size (%)	17.01 ± 8.88	18.02 ± 8.82	0.4543
AAR (%)	27.9 ± 8.3	27.27 ± 7.3	0.9800

Plus-minus values are mean ± SEM. No denotes number

BMI body mass index, *AAR* area at risk, *LAD* left anterior descending artery, *LCx* circumflex artery, *RCA* right coronary artery

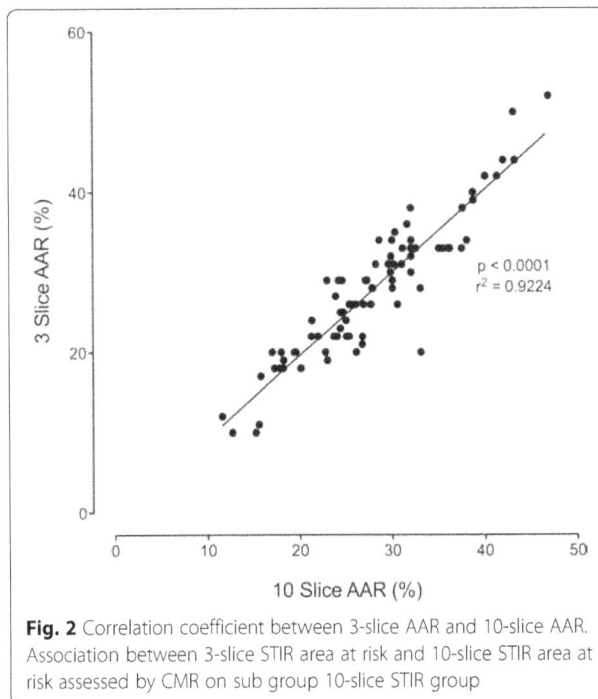

Fig. 2 Correlation coefficient between 3-slice AAR and 10-slice AAR. Association between 3-slice STIR area at risk and 10-slice STIR area at risk assessed by CMR on sub group 10-slice STIR group

27.8 ± 7.3) and the 3-slice AAR assessment of the same patients showed similar values ranging from 10.0 to 52.0 % (mean 27.9 ± 8.3) ($p = 0.9800$). There were strong correlations between 3-slice AAR and 10-slice AAR in this patient group ($r = 0.92$, $p < 0.0001$) (Fig. 2). Bland-Atman assessment of the two assessment groups shows a low limit of agreement (mean difference -0.03 ± 3.21 %, 95 % limit of agreement, -6.3 to 6.3, containing 95.3 % (81/85) of the difference scores). In addition there was a strong correlation between 3-slice MM and 10-slice MM ($r = 0.90$, $p < 0.0001$) (Additional file 2: Figure S2).

Comparison of CMR assessed AAR size and angiographic AAR

Angiographic risk assessment was performed for all patients in this study. In the 10-slice AAR group the BARI angiographic risk score ranged from 10.5 % to 47.4 % (mean 26.6 ± 10.1), and the APPROACH angiographic risk score ranged from 6.5 % to 47.8 % (mean 29.2 ± 9.0 %) of the left ventricle (LV) myocardium. There was good correlation between the 2 angiographic risk scores ($r = 0.85$, $p < 0.0001$). There was a statistically significant correlation with discrepant strength between the 10-slice AAR and the APPROACH angiographic risk score ($r = 0.46$, $p < 0.0001$)

with a weaker correlation seen between the 10-slice AAR and BARI angiographic risk score ($r = 0.27$, $p = 0.0124$) (Fig. 3). For the 10-slice AAR group infarct and oedema ESA was assessed for all patients, with Infarct ESA ranging from 0 to 45 % (mean 17.3 ± 9.8 %) and oedema ESA ranging from 10 to 44 % (mean 27.2 ± 7.8 %). There was a strong correlation between 10-slice AAR and oedema EAS ($r = 0.79$, $p < 0.0001$), there was a low correlation between 10-slice AAR and infarct EAS ($r = 0.42$, $p < 0.0001$).

In all 3-slice AAR studies the BARI angiographic risk score ranged from 10.5 to 47.4 % (mean 30.9 ± 10.5) and the APPROACH angiographic risk score ranging from 6.5 to 47.8 % (mean 33.4 ± 9.3 %) of the LV myocardium. As was seen within the 10-slice group there was a good correlation between the 2 angiographic risk scores ($r = 0.88$ $p < 0.0001$). Within the 3-slice AAR group the AAR ranged from 3 to 56 % (mean 30.1 ± 9.8). The 3-slice AAR assessment was correlated with both angiographic risk scores (BARI: $r = 0.36$, p <0.0001, APPROACH; $r = 0.42$, $p < 0.0001$) (Fig. 4) (Table 2). For the 3-slice AAR group infarct and oedema ESA was assessed, with infarct ESA ranging from 1 to 57 % (mean 17.3 ± 9.7 %) and oedema ESA ranging from 2 to 59 % (mean 29.1 ± 9.9 %). There was a strong correlation between 3-slice AAR and oedema EAS ($r = 0.89$, $p < 0.0001$), there was a low correlation between 3-slice AAR and infarct EAS ($r = 0.45$, $p < 0.0001$).

Comparison between infarct size and myocardial AAR Scores

Infarct size as measured by CMR ranged from 1.0 % to 44.0 % of the LV myocardium (mean 18.0 ± 8.8 %). There

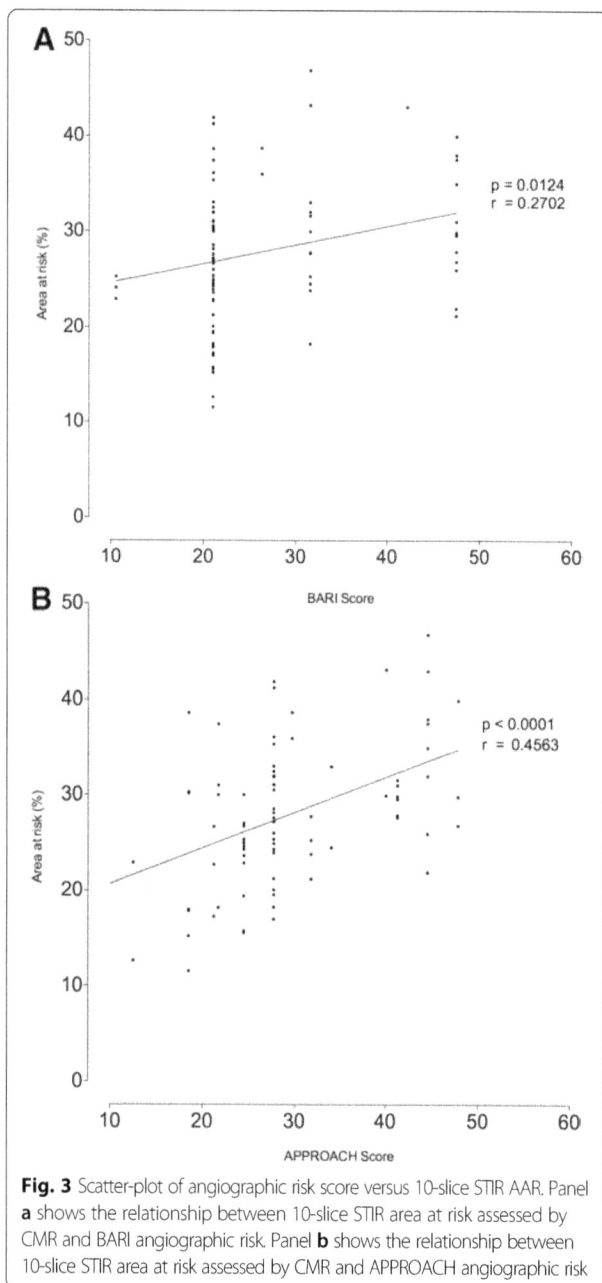

Fig. 3 Scatter-plot of angiographic risk score versus 10-slice STIR AAR. Panel **a** shows the relationship between 10-slice STIR area at risk assessed by CMR and BARI angiographic risk. Panel **b** shows the relationship between 10-slice STIR area at risk assessed by CMR and APPROACH angiographic risk

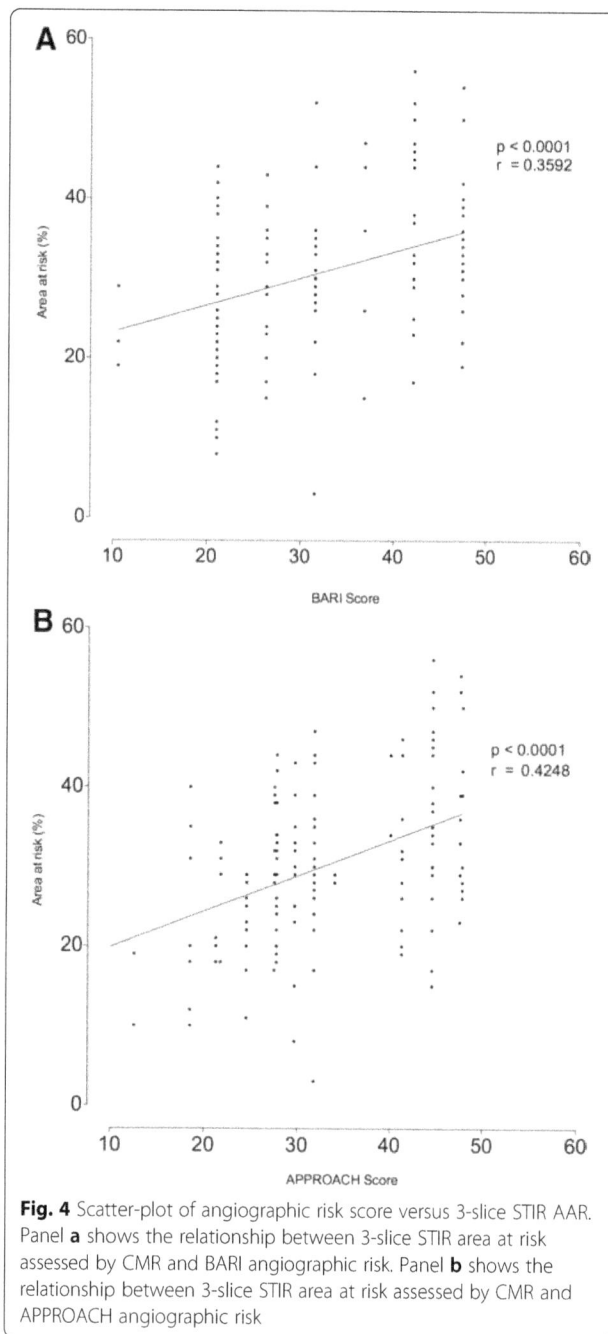

Fig. 4 Scatter-plot of angiographic risk score versus 3-slice STIR AAR. Panel **a** shows the relationship between 3-slice STIR area at risk assessed by CMR and BARI angiographic risk. Panel **b** shows the relationship between 3-slice STIR area at risk assessed by CMR and APPROACH angiographic risk

was a significant correlation between infarct size and 10-slice AAR ($r = 0.73$, $p < 0.0001$), with a lower correlation seen between infarct size and 3-slice AAR studies ($r = 0.48$ $p < 0.0001$) (Fig. 5). Myocardial salvage was calculated for both 3-slice and 10-slice assessments with no significant difference between the two imaging modalities (41.30 % ± 22.41 % in the 3-slice group vs. 39.39 % ± 21.59 % in the 10-slice group; $p = 0.5712$) (Fig. 6).

Timing for acquisition and analysis of 3-slice versus 10-slice AAR

The time taken for the acquisition of the T2-STIR sequences was assessed from the initiation of the scan to the start of the next imaging sequence. The 3-slice group had a median acquisition time of 100 seconds (range: 65–171 seconds) and the 10-slice group had a median acquisition time of 355 seconds (range: 275–603 seconds), with a significant difference seen between the two groups ($p < 0.0001$) (Fig. 7a).

For analysis the 3-slice group had a median time of 43 seconds (IQR: 36–56 seconds) and 10-slice group had a median time of 137 seconds (IQR: 133–144 seconds), with a significant difference seen between the two groups ($p < 0.0001$). The inter-observer timing variability

Table 2 Intraclass correlation coefficients between angiographic and cardiovascular magnetic resonance methods of 3-slice and 10-slice oedema CMR (T2-STIR) imaging techniques

3-slice Assessment	T2 STIR	APPROACH	BARI
Infarct ESA	0.50 (0.30–0.66)***	0.27 (0.12–0.41)**	0.19 (0.05–0.34)**
Oedema ESA	0.91 (0.86–0.95)***	0.36 (0.22–0.49)**	0.27 (0.12–0.41)*
Infarct %	0.47 (0.26–0.64)***	0.28 (0.13–0.41)**	0.20 (0.05–0.35)*
BARI	0.35 (0.21–0.49)***	0.88 (0.85–0.91)***	
APPROACH	0.42 (0.29–0.55)***		
10-slice Assessment	T2 STIR	APPROACH	BARI
Infarct ESA	0.64 (0.50–0.75)***	0.44 (0.25–0.60)***	0.28 (0.07–0.47)**
Oedema ESA	0.89 (0.84–0.93)***	0.40 (0.20–0.56)***	0.17 (−0.05–0.37)
Infarct %	0.73 (0.61–0.82)***	0.50 (0.32–0.64)***	0.33 (0.13–0.51)**
BARI	0.27 (0.06–0.46)***	0.85 (0.78–0.90)***	
APPROACH	0.46 (0.27–0.61)***		

Data are expressed intraclass correlation coefficients (confidence interval). *p* value <0.05 = *, <0.01 = **, <0.001 = ***. *APPROACH* Alberta provincial project for outcome assessment in coronary heart disease, *BARI* bypass angioplasty revascularization investigation myocardial jeopardy index, *ESA* endocardial surface area, *STIR T2*, short tau inversion recovery, *LAD* left anterior descending artery

correlated well between analysers; 3-slice $r = 0.96$ $p < 0.0001$, 10-slice $r = 0.93$ $p < 0.0001$ (Fig. 7b).

Combined acquisition and analysis time showed a significant difference between the two groups ($p < 0.0001$). The median time of 143 seconds (IQR: 131–171 seconds) in the 3-slice group was on average 5 minutes quicker than the 10-slice group (median time of 492 seconds (IQR: 472–565 seconds).

Overall scan time was taken from initiation of first scouting image to the end of the final image. Within the 3-slice group there was a median time of 2163 seconds (IQR: 1740–2520 seconds) and 10-slice group had a median time of 2448 seconds (IQR: 1986–2835 seconds), with a significant difference seen between the two groups ($p = 0.0057$).

Inter-observer variability
3-slice STIR imaging showed low inter-observer variability. For the Bland-Altman plot, the 95 % limits of agreement (−5.3 %, 3.6 %) contained 95.1 % (78/82) of the difference scores. The mean bias of the measurements between observers was 0.08 %, and the maximum and minimum difference was 8.0 % and −7.0 % respectively (Fig. 8). The 10-slice STIR imaging showed similar inter-observer variability ($z = 1.035$, $p = 0.15$). For the Bland-Altman plot, the 95 % limits of agreement (−4.68 %, 4.04 %) contained 94.1 % (80/85) of the difference scores. The mean bias of the measurements between observers was −0.32 %, and the maximum and minimum difference was 5.0 % and −5.6 % respectively.

Discussion
Oedema CMR imaging using T2-STIR remains an important technique to quantify the AAR. The aim of this study was to validate a 3-slice oedema CMR quantification of

the myocardial AAR following PPCI for STEMI. We demonstrated that 3-slice quantification remains accurate for the detection of myocardial oedema after an AMI when compared to the conventional 10-slice technique with no significant bias demonstrated in assessing the AAR. The 3-slice technique also requires less time to acquire and analyse compared to the conventional 10-slice approach.

Oedema CMR using T2-STIR imaging remains popular for assessing myocardial oedema [20] and the AAR after AMI, with studies showing the superiority of the clinical use of oedema CMR imaging in both AMI and chronic heart disease [4, 21]. The benefit of oedema CMR assessment over previous AAR assessment such as single-photon emission computed tomography (SPECT) is the lack of ionising radiation or the need for tracer administration. Although the benefit of SPECT imaging processes removes the issues of claustrophobia that is found in CMR imaging. The majority of these studies have used 10–12 slice oedema CMR covering the whole left ventricle, however due to the need for adequate breath holding techniques and the possibility of artefact the overall image acquisition time is long for the 10-slice STIR imaging technique.

Previous studies have demonstrated the suitability of 3-slice imaging in the assessment of myocardial scar as well as LV volumes [22]. However this is the first study to assess whether or not the AAR can also be assessed using a 3-slice technique, demonstrating the technique is comparable to the conventional 10-slice approach. The main benefit of the 3-slice oedema CMR in comparison to 10-slice oedema CMR is a quicker acquisition and analysis time. The overall scan time was nearly 5 minutes shorter with the 3-slice oedema sequence compared to the longer 10-slice sequences. The difference of over 5 minutes due to a shorter acquisition time and

A

B

Fig. 5 Correlation coefficient between infarct size and AAR. Panel **a** shows the association between 3-slice STIR area at risk assessed by CMR and infarct size. Panel **b** shows the association between 10-slice STIR area at risk assessed by CMR and infarct size

Fig. 6 Myocardial salvage assessment between 3-Slice and 10-Slice technique. Panel **a** shows the relationship between 3-slice STIR area at risk assessed by CMR and infarct size. Panel **b** shows the relationship between 10-slice STIR area at risk assessed by CMR and infarct size

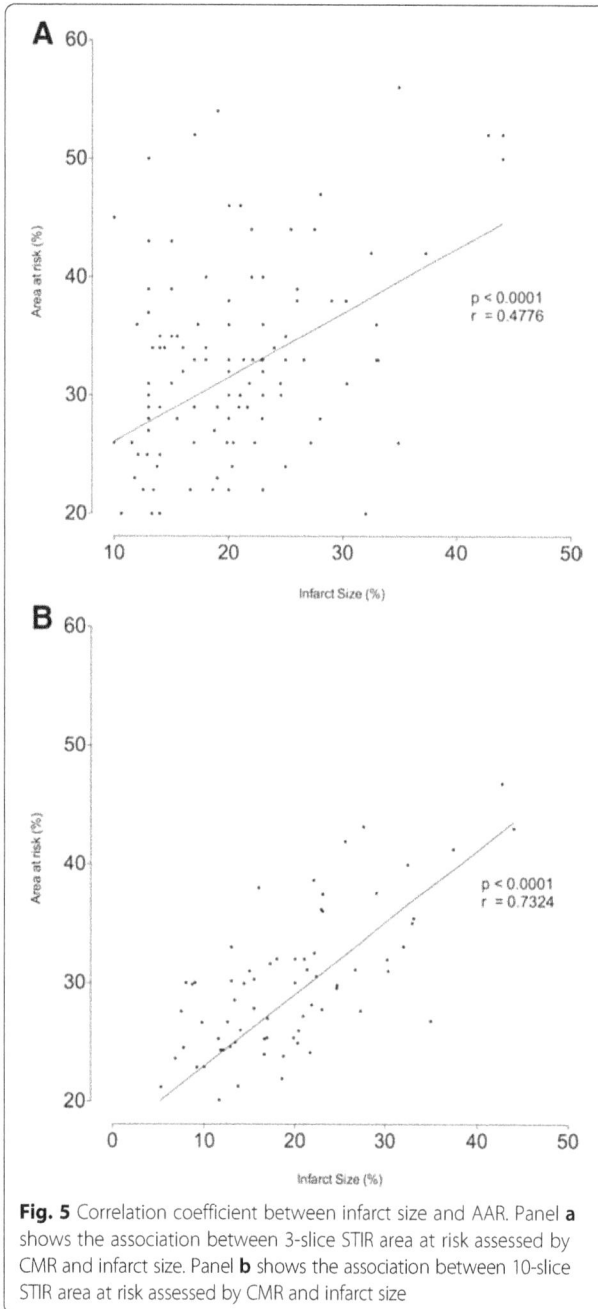

analysis time would have clinical benefit. The use for only 3 breath holds in comparison to the 10 or 12 without loss of required clinical information is of benefit especially in patients who have issues including claustrophobia or who are unable to lie flat for extended periods. These are common factors in patients 3 days post primary PCI for AMI. The benefit that could be applied to patients could also be seen finically by performing 3-slice AAR in the clinical setting. In a busy CMR centre where multiple clinical scans are performed each day the reduction of acquisition time could result in additional scans being performed and improved financial incentive. In addition the timing for

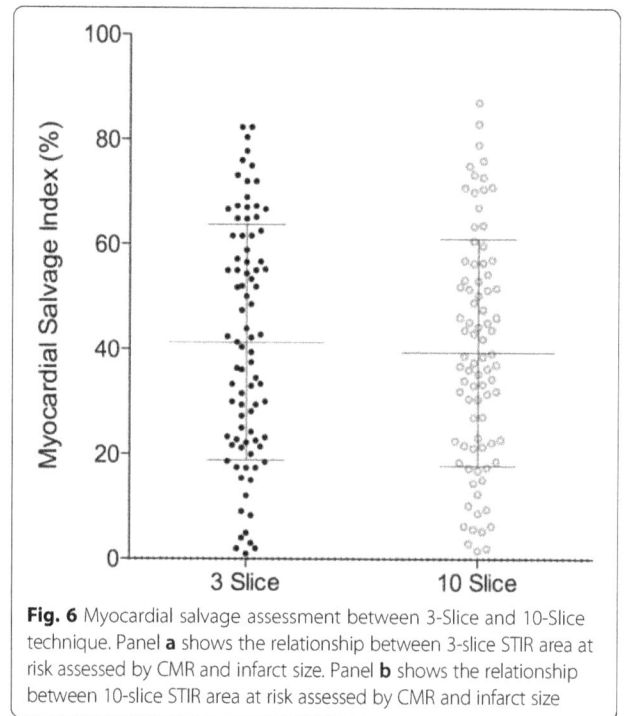

analysis was significantly shorter within the 3-slice approach without the loss of significant clinical information, which may be of benefit when multiple analysis are required thus reducing analysis times in large quantity analysis.

The assessment of AAR has become increasingly important when testing potentially cardioprotective therapies. Conventional imaging techniques in such trials tend to assess changes in left ventricular ejection fraction for their surrogate endpoint that require multiple visits. The use of a single AAR image acquisition at an early time point could possibly reduce the need for multiple scans and give early results without the need for protracted follow up. Although more information maybe required in the research setting the shorter image analysis times could have be an important factor when assessing multiple images within a study.

One particular issue with T2-STIR imaging is the false signal that occurs in area of blood pooling especially in patients with poor LV function [23]. In the apical segments of the LV there is increased blood pooling causing greater sub-endocardial bright artefact during myocardial quantification. The imaging technique for 10-slice acquisition takes single contiguous 1 cm slices from mid atria to true apex, whereas the 3-slice acquisition takes a slice in the basal, mid and apical segment of the LV therefore reducing true apical blood pooling (Additional file 3: Figure S3). The observer variability was similar in the 3 slice and 10-slice acquisition groups. This implies that the use of 3-slice acquisition imaging may not result in the loss of important

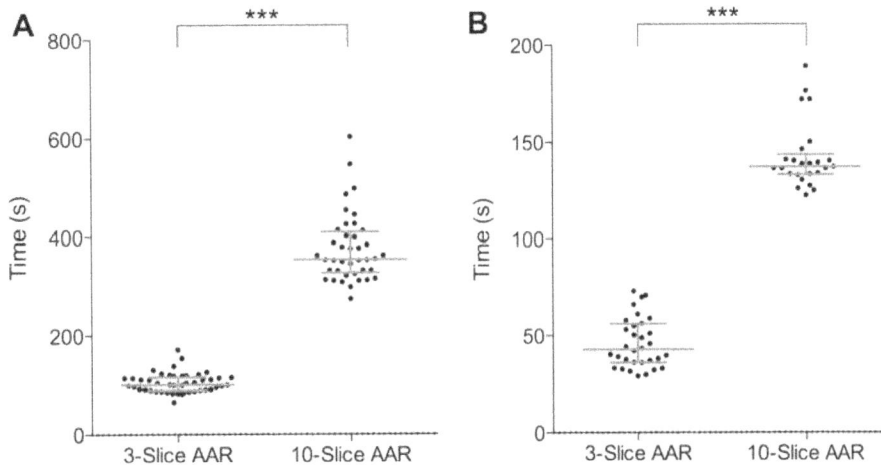

Fig. 7 Comparison of acquisition **a** and analysis **b** time between 3-slice and 10-slice imaging technique. Panel **a** shows the relationship between 3-slice STIR area at risk assessed by CMR and infarct size. Panel **b** shows the relationship between 10-slice STIR area at risk assessed by CMR and infarct size

clinical information and may reduce the issue of increased signal from pooled blood in comparison to 10-slice acquisition. Although T2-STIR imaging has been used widely other methods or programming techniques are available to reduce acquisition time such as navigator gated imaging technique and the use of early gadolinium enhancement that could be beneficial in the clinical setting.

In summary the advantages of 3-slice oedema CMR imaging over 10-slice imaging in assessing myocardial AAR are: 1) equal clinical information; 2) reduced imaging protocol time; 3) reduced breath holding time; and 4) reduced combined acquisition and analysis time.

Study limitations
The present study was performed on a small limited patient population in patients who after suffered a STEMI

and underwent successful PPCI with the majority of patients receiving a novel cardioprotective intervention at the time prior to undergoing CMR imaging within 3 days. One of the studies included in the analysis recruited only patients with anterior infarcts due to occlusions of the LAD which may have lead to bias in the results.

Conclusions
This study was able to validate 3-slice oedema CMR quantification of AAR showing good correlations with current full coverage imaging techniques. The quicker and easier analysis method is advantageous for both patients and clinicians and could shorten acquisition time in patients who are either claustrophobic or have difficulty with breath holding technique.

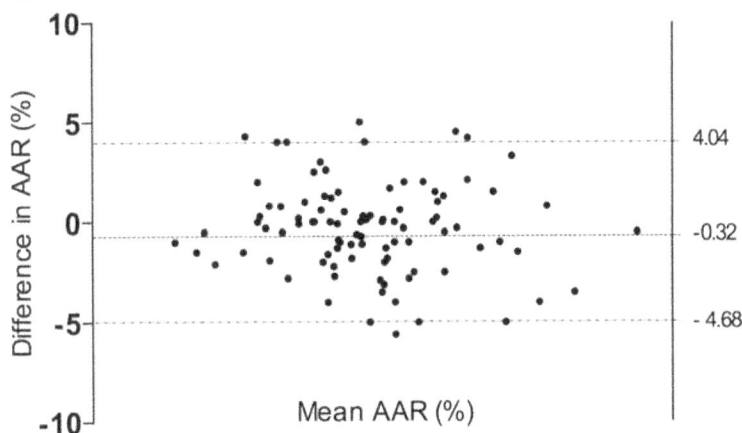

Fig. 8 Bland-Altman plot for the inter-observer variability of the 3-slice STIR AAR assessment

Additional files

Additional file 1: Figure S1. Consort diagram. Flow chart of study design summarizing flow of patients through study.

Additional file 2: Figure S2. Correlation coefficient between 3-slice MM and 10-slice MM. Association between 3-slice MM quantification and 10-slice MM quantification assessed by CMR.

Additional file 3: Figure S3. Difference between T2-STIR distributions after myocardial infarction. Screenshot demonstrating the increased signal seen in the basal, mid and apical slices in a T2-STIR imaging technique after a ST elevation myocardial infarction involving each of the major epicardial coronary arteries.

Competing interests
The authors declare that they have no competing interests.

Authors' contributions
SH carried out recruitment, procedures, data collection, data analysis, statistical analysis, writing of publication. DJ carried out data analysis, statistical analysis, co-writing of publication. CP carried out data analysis. DL carried out data analysis. TB carried out recruitment, CMR protocol. SM carried out CMR protocol and CMR imaging. JM carried out CMR imaging. JK carried out recruitment, procedures, data collection. DL carried out recruitment, procedures. SP carried out CMR protocol and CMR imaging. MW carried out CMR protocol and CMR imaging. AM carried out trial design, procedures, overall lead of project and co-writing of publication. All authors read and approved the final manuscript.

Acknowledgements
We would like to thank the support of all the staff at the Barts Heart Centre, Centre Hospitalier Universitaire Vaudois, Rigshospitalet, The Heart Cell Foundation, Barts and the London Charity, The UK Stem Cell Foundation and the support of the National Institute for Health Research Cardiovascular Biomedical Research Unit.

Funding
No funding for this study to declare

Author details
[1]Department of Cardiology, Barts Heart Centre, St Bartholomews Hospital, Barts Health NHS Trust, London EC1A 7BE, UK. [2]William Harvey Research Institute, NIHR Cardiovascular Biomedical Research Unit at Barts, Queen Mary University of London, Charterhouse Square, London EC1M 6BQ, UK. [3]Service de Cardiologie et Département de Médecine Interne, Centre Hospitalier Universitaire, Vaudois, Lausanne, Switzerland. [4]Department of Cardiology, Rigshopitale, University of Copenhagen, Copenhagen, Denmark.

References
1. Lorenz CH, Walker ES, Morgan VL, Klein SS, Graham Jr TP. Normal human right and left ventricular mass, systolic function, and gender differences by cine magnetic resonance imaging. J Cardiovasc Magn Reson. 1999;1:7–21.
2. McAlindon E, Pufulete M, Lawton C, Angelini GD, Bucciarelli-Ducci C. Quantification of infarct size and myocardium at risk: evaluation of different techniques and its implications. Eur Heart Cardiovasc Imag. 2015;16:738–46.
3. Monmeneu JV, Bodi V, Sanchis J, Lopez-Lereu MP, Mainar L, Nunez J et al. Cardiac magnetic resonance evaluation of edema after ST-elevation acute myocardial infarction. Rev Esp Cardiol. 2009;62:858–66.
4. Friedrich MG, Abdel-Aty H, Taylor A, Schulz-Menger J, Messroghli D, Dietz R. The salvaged area at risk in reperfused acute myocardial infarction as visualized by cardiovascular magnetic resonance. J Am Coll Cardiol. 2008;51:1581–7.
5. Hamshere S, Choudhury T, Jones DA, Locca D, Mills P, Rothman M, et al. A randomised double-blind control study of early intracoronary autologous bone marrow cell infusion in acute myocardial infarction (REGENERATE-AMI). BMJ Open. 2014;4, e004258.
6. Jones DA, Andiapen M, Van-Eijl TJ, Webb AJ, Antoniou S, Schilling RJ, et al. The safety and efficacy of intracoronary nitrite infusion during acute myocardial

infarction (NITRITE-AMI): study protocol of a randomised controlled trial. BMJ Open. 2013;3.
7. Fuernau G, Eitel I, Franke V, Hildebrandt L, Meissner J, de Waha S, et al. Myocardium at risk in ST-segment elevation myocardial infarction comparison of T2-weighted edema imaging with the MR-assessed endocardial surface area and validation against angiographic scoring. J Am Coll Cardiol Img. 2011;4:967–76.
8. Hadamitzky M, Langhans B, Hausleiter J, Sonne C, Kastrati A, Martinoff S, et al. The assessment of area at risk and myocardial salvage after coronary revascularization in acute myocardial infarction: comparison between CMR and SPECT. J Am Coll Cardiol Img. 2013;6:358–69.
9. Botker HE, Kaltoft AK, Pedersen SF, Kim WY. Measuring myocardial salvage. Cardiovasc Res. 2012;94:266–75.
10. Oh-I D, Ridgway JP, Kuehne T, Berger F, Plein S, Sivananthan M, et al. Cardiovascular magnetic resonance of myocardial edema using a short inversion time inversion recovery (STIR) black-blood technique: diagnostic accuracy of visual and semi-quantitative assessment. J Cardiovasc Imag Magn Reson. 2012;14:22.
11. Chesebro JH, Knatterud G, Roberts R, Borer J, Cohen LS, Dalen J, et al. Thrombolysis in Myocardial Infarction (TIMI) Trial, Phase I: A comparison between intravenous tissue plasminogen activator and intravenous streptokinase. Clinical findings through hospital discharge. Circulation. 1987; 76:142–54.
12. Alderman EL, Kip KE, Whitlow PL, Bashore T, Fortin D, Bourassa MG, et al. Native coronary disease progression exceeds failed revascularization as cause of angina after five years in the Bypass Angioplasty Revascularization Investigation (BARI). J Am Coll Cardiol. 2004;44:766–74.
13. Ghali WA, Knudtson ML. Overview of the Alberta Provincial Project for Outcome Assessment in Coronary Heart Disease. On behalf of the APPROACH investigators. Can J Cardiol. 2000;16:1225–30.
14. Wright J, Adriaenssens T, Dymarkowski S, Desmet W, Bogaert J. Quantification of myocardial area at risk with T2-weighted CMR: comparison with contrast-enhanced CMR and coronary angiography. J Am Coll Cardiol Img. 2009;2:825–31.
15. Lotan CS, Bouchard A, Cranney GB, Bishop SP, Pohost GM. Assessment of postreperfusion myocardial hemorrhage using proton NMR imaging at 1. 5 T. Circulation. 1992;86:1018–25.
16. Rajchl M, Stirrat J, Goubran M, Yu J, Scholl D, Peters TM, et al. Comparison of semi-automated scar quantification techniques using high-resolution, 3-dimensional late-gadolinium-enhancement magnetic resonance imaging. Int J Cardiovasc Imaging. 2014.
17. Khan JN, Nazir SA, Horsfield MA, Singh A, Kanagala P, Greenwood JP, et al. Comparison of semi-automated methods to quantify infarct size and area at risk by cardiovascular magnetic resonance imaging at 1.5T and 3.0T field strengths. BMC Res Notes. 2015;8:52.
18. Bulluck H, White SK, Rosmini S, Bhuva A, Treibel TA, Fontana M, et al. T1 mapping and T2 mapping at 3 T for quantifying the area-at-risk in reperfused STEMI patients. J Cardiovasc Magn Reson. 2015;17:73.
19. Bland JM, Altman DG. Statistical methods for assessing agreement between two methods of clinical measurement. Lancet. 1986;1:307–10.
20. h-Ici D, Ridgway J, Kuehne T, Berger F, Plein S, Sivananthan M, et al. Cardiovascular magnetic resonance of myocardial edema using a short inversion time inversion recovery (STIR) black-blood technique: Diagnostic accuracy of visual and semi-quantitative assessment. J Cardiovasc Magn Reson. 2012;14:22.
21. Abdel-Aty H, Cocker M, Meek C, Tyberg JV, Friedrich MG. Edema as a very early marker for acute myocardial ischemia: a cardiovascular magnetic resonance study. J Am Coll Cardiol. 2009;53:1194–201.
22. Kuoy E, Nguyen C, Dissanayake S, Nelson K, Abbona P, Krishnam M. Quantitative assessment of LV function and volumes with 3-slice segmentation of cine SSFP short axis images: our experience. J Cardiovasc Magn Reson. 2014;16:P384.
23. Higgins CB, Lanzer P, Stark D, Botvinick E, Schiller NB, Crooks L, et al. Imaging by nuclear magnetic resonance in patients with chronic ischemic heart disease. Circulation. 1984;69:523–31.

9

4D MUSIC CMR: value-based imaging of neonates and infants with congenital heart disease

Kim-Lien Nguyen[1,2], Fei Han[1,3,7], Ziwu Zhou[1,3,7], Daniel Z. Brunengraber[1,7], Ihab Ayad[4], Daniel S. Levi[5], Gary M. Satou[5], Brian L. Reemtsen[6], Peng Hu[1,3,7] and J. Paul Finn[1,3,7]*

Abstract

Background: 4D Multiphase Steady State Imaging with Contrast (MUSIC) acquires high-resolution volumetric images of the beating heart during uninterrupted ventilation. We aim to evaluate the diagnostic performance and clinical impact of 4D MUSIC in a cohort of neonates and infants with congenital heart disease (CHD).

Methods: Forty consecutive neonates and infants with CHD (age range 2 days to 2 years, weight 1 to 13 kg) underwent 3.0 T CMR with ferumoxytol enhancement (FE) at a single institution. Independently, two readers graded the diagnostic image quality of intra-cardiac structures and related vascular segments on FE-MUSIC and breath held FE-CMRA images using a four-point scale. Correlation of the CMR findings with surgery and other imaging modalities was performed in all patients. Clinical impact was evaluated in consensus with referring surgeons and cardiologists. One point was given for each of five key outcome measures: 1) change in overall management, 2) change in surgical approach, 3) reduction in the need for diagnostic catheterization, 4) improved assessment of risk-to-benefit for planned intervention and discussion with parents, 5) accurate pre-procedural roadmap.

Results: All FE-CMR studies were completed successfully, safely and without adverse events. On a four-point scale, the average FE-MUSIC image quality scores were >3.5 for intra-cardiac structures and >3.0 for coronary arteries. Intra-cardiac morphology and vascular anatomy were well visualized with good interobserver agreement ($r = 0.46$). Correspondence between the findings on MUSIC, surgery, correlative imaging and autopsy was excellent. The average clinical impact score was 4.2 ± 0.9. In five patients with discordant findings on echo/MUSIC ($n = 5$) and catheter angiography/MUSIC ($n = 1$), findings on FE-MUSIC were shown to be accurate at autopsy ($n = 1$) and surgery ($n = 4$). The decision to undertake biventricular vs univentricular repair was amended in 2 patients based on FE-MUSIC findings. Plans for surgical approaches which would have involved circulatory arrest were amended in two of 28 surgical cases. In all 28 cases requiring procedural intervention, FE-MUSIC provided accurate dynamic 3D roadmaps and more confident risk-to-benefit assessments for proposed interventions.

Conclusions: FE-MUSIC CMR has high clinical impact by providing accurate, high quality, simple and safe dynamic 3D imaging of cardiac and vascular anatomy in neonates and infants with CHD. The findings influenced patient management in a positive manner.

Keywords: Congenital heart disease, Magnetic resonance angiography, Cardiovascular magnetic resonance, Ferumoxytol, 4-D imaging

Journal Subject Codes: Magnetic resonance angiography, Neonates, Infants, Congenital heart disease, Ferumoxytol, 4D

* Correspondence: pfinn@mednet.ucla.edu
[1]Diagnostic Cardiovascular Imaging Laboratory, Department of Radiological Sciences, David Geffen School of Medicine at UCLA, Los Angeles, CA, USA
[3]Department of Biomedical Physics, University of California, Los Angeles, CA, USA
Full list of author information is available at the end of the article

Background

Within the past decade, advances in cardiovascular imaging and therapeutic interventions have improved the care of newborns with congenital heart disease (CHD). Severe congenital anomalies are nowadays often detected with fetal echocardiography during gestation such that elective deliveries can be planned at centers of excellence. While echocardiography is clearly the first line of imaging in neonates, even in the best of hands there may remain unanswered questions. In these cases, cardiovascular magnetic resonance (CMR) has emerged as a second line technique that does not involve ionizing radiation. Further, in small children with complex CHD and multisystem involvement, CMR holds promise for comprehensive pre-surgical evaluation with catheter angiography reserved for select indications and image-guided interventions.

CMR in pediatric CHD however, is highly specialized and individualized as almost all sequences require adaptation for body size, heart rate and specific clinical questions. Compared to older children, the requirement for spatial resolution is more stringent. Further, CMR exams in this population should be brief due to the high acuity of many cases and to minimize time outside of the neonatal intensive care unit (NICU). Conventional CMR techniques for pediatric CHD typically involve a timed bolus of a gadolinium based contrast agent (GBCA) for 3D vascular evaluation, in addition to multiple 2D breath hold cine acquisitions in customized orientations. A 4D imaging approach can potentially combine the best of both worlds, providing high resolution 3D anatomy and an unlimited number of 2D cine planes for reconstruction in arbitrary orientations.

Recently, a 4D Multiphase Steady-state Imaging with Contrast (MUSIC) CMR technique was introduced, which generates sub-millimeter, isotropic 3D voxels over multiple phases of the cardiac cycle [1]. MUSIC data are acquired without breath holding during continuous positive pressure ventilation, and the airway pressure signal is used for respiratory gating. Cardiac gating is implemented using the ECG and a stable blood pool signal is assured by imaging during the steady state distribution of ferumoxytol (Feraheme®, AMAG, Lexington, MA). With a total scan time of 7–10 minutes, MUSIC offers the potential for rapid, simple, safe and versatile mapping of complex cardiovascular anatomy with dynamic resolution previously not available.

In this study, we aim to evaluate the diagnostic quality and performance of ferumoxytol (FE) enhanced MUSIC CMR in a cohort of neonates and infants with CHD and to assess its impact on patient management.

Methods

This prospective study was approved by our Institutional Review Board and was compliant with the Health Insurance Portability and Accountability Act. Written informed consent was obtained from legal guardians of all subjects. Forty consecutive neonates and infants with CHD (age range 2 days to 2 years; 21 females; weight range 1 to 13 kg) undergoing an FE-CMR from 2013 to 2016 were enrolled, including two recent subjects enrolled under IND #129441 (Clinicaltrials.gov NCT02752191). No patients were excluded. Primary study indications were: 1) assessment of vascular anatomy ($n = 20$), 2) intra-cardiac anatomy ($n = 17$), 3) pre-interventional or surgical planning ($n = 16$). Primary diagnoses are outlined in Additional file 1: Table S1.

In patients whose blood gas status was felt sufficiently stable for safe breath holding by attending neonatologists or anesthesiologists, breath-held 3D FE-CMRA (cardiovascular magnetic resonance angiography) was performed as a standard of care reference for comparison of image quality with MUSIC.

MR Acquisition

All neonates and infants were examined during continuous positive pressure ventilation as is standard at our institution and at many centers performing neonatal CMR [2, 3]. Patients were transported directly to the CMR suites, already intubated and sedated. Sedation management and physiologic monitoring have been described previously [4] and typically included IV fentanyl and rocuronium. Continuous monitoring of heart rate, blood pressure, pulse oximetry, and end-tidal CO_2 was performed and recorded in all cases.

All studies were performed on a clinical 32-channel 3.0 T system (Magnetom TIM Trio, Siemens Medical Solutions). Phased-array multi-element coils were used for signal reception, in configurations based on body size. For children weighing less than 2 kg, a 16-channel adult extremity (knee) coil was employed. For children weighing 2 kg or more, a combination of head-neck (posterior elements) and small flex coil (anterior elements) was used. Imaging parameters for breath-held FE-CMRA were: repetition time/echo time (TR/TE) 2.9/0.9 ms; flip angle 15-17°; in-plane resolution 0.9–1.2 mm; slice thickness 0.9–1.1 mm; GRAPPA acceleration 3×–4×; 75% partial Fourier acquisition in both phase encoding directions. FE-MUSIC was acquired during continuous ventilation using the airway pressure signal for respiratory gating [1]. No adjustments were made to the ventilatory frequency, amplitude or waveform to maximize gating efficiency and the default settings were employed.

Technical parameters for FE-MUSIC were: TR/TE 2.9/0.9 ms; flip angle, 25°; 3D isotropic (non-interpolated) resolution 0.6–0.9 mm; GRAPPA 2×–3×; 75% partial Fourier in both phase encoding and partition encoding directions. The pressure waveform from the endotracheal tube was input into the physiological monitoring unit of the CMR scanner and served as a surrogate respiratory gating signal. An empiric respiratory gate time delay of three cardiac segments (~200 msec) was used to account for the temporal phase lag between the upper airway pressure wave and resulting diaphragmatic movement. A 50% threshold of the pressure peak defined the acceptance range for the respiratory gating.

A total of 4 mg/kg (elemental iron per kg of body weight) of the stock ferumoxytol formulation was diluted with normal saline by 8×–10× based on patient size [4]. For first pass imaging ($n = 15$), half of the diluted ferumoxytol solution (2 mg/kg) was infused over 15 s [5]. The injection duration was 75% of the acquisition time window [4]. Subsequently, the remaining half of the diluted ferumoxytol was administered over 30 s to provide a total dose of 4 mg/kg for steady state imaging. To comply with a warning issued by U.S. Food and Drug Administration (FDA) in March 2015 [6], our protocol was amended to give ferumoxytol only by slow infusion at a rate of 0.8 mg/kg/min. Therefore, in 25 of 40 subjects who received ferumoxytol, only steady state imaging was performed.

Image analysis

Two experienced CMR readers independently scored the images. FE-MUSIC images were reviewed using 'multiplanar reconstruction (MPR) cine mode' on a Mac-OsiriX workstation (OsiriX MD version 6.5, Pixmeo, Switzerland), which enables interactive dynamic, multiphase interrogation of arbitrary imaging planes until the optimal plane for visualization is chosen. For comparison with the single phase, breath-held FE-CMRA images, each reader was free to choose a preferred single 3D phase of the FE-MUSIC images for each of the intra-cardiac structures (valves, cardiac chambers), ventricular outflow tracts, and named vascular segments, including the proximal coronary arteries, using a four-point scale [7] (Additional file 1: Table S1). For coronary artery visualization, the optimal cardiac phase and plane for coronary visualization was interrogated. Based on border definition, image contrast, and presence of artifacts, scores of 1 or 2 were considered non-diagnostic whereas scores of 3 or 4 were considered diagnostic. MUSIC findings were correlated with surgical reports ($n = 28$), catheterization data ($n = 14$), cardiac CT data ($n = 4$), and autopsy findings ($n = 1$). The signal-to-noise ratio (SNR) was calculated as the ratio of the mean luminal signal intensity (SI) divided by the standard deviation of noise and was further divided by 1.53 to adjust for Rayleigh noise distribution [8]. The contrast-to-noise ratio (CNR) was calculated as the difference between the SNR of the lumen and SNR of nearby muscle tissue. Noise was defined by the standard deviation in regions of interest of air within the imaging field of view.

Clinical impact

The impact of FE-MUSIC on overall diagnosis and patient management for each case was scored in consensus with collaborating surgeons and cardiologists. Five key measures of added value were assessed: 1) change in overall surgical management, 2) change in surgical approach, 3) reduction in the need for diagnostic catheterization, 4) improved assessment of risk-to-benefit for planned intervention and discussion with parents, 5) accurate pre-procedural roadmap.

Statistical analysis

Statistical analysis was performed using MedCalc 12.0.1.0 (Mariakerke, Belgium). Continuous data were summarized as mean ± standard deviation or as mean and interquartile. Categorical data were summarized as absolute values and frequencies. The Wilcoxon rank sum test was used to compare the image quality scores between breath-held FE-CMRA and FE-MUSIC. Pearson's correlation coefficient was used to determine inter-observer correlation. Analysis of variance (ANOVA) for repeated measurements was used to determine the statistical significance of temporal changes in mean heart rate, blood pressure, pulse oximetry (SpO_2), and end-tidal CO_2. A p value < 0.05 is considered significant.

Results

All 40 patients (neonates [$n = 20$, 2 to 25 days, 1–4 kg]; infants [$n = 20$, 1.2 months to 2 years, 2–13 kg]) underwent the ferumoxytol-enhanced exam safely and without any adverse events, including those who had bolus injection of ferumoxytol for breath held FE-CMRA. Total image acquisition time for FE-MUSIC ranged from 7 to 10 mins. The SNR and CNR of the FE-MUSIC images were 54 ± 21 and 38 ± 15, respectively. Clinical complexity and diagnoses of the patient cases are outlined in Additional file 1: Table S2. Heart rate, blood pressure, blood oxygenation and end tidal CO_2 remained stable throughout the procedure and variations were not statistically significant ($p > 0.05$) (Additional file 1: Table S3).

Image quality

Image quality scores are reported in Table 1. Respiratory gating efficiency for the MUSIC acquisition ranged from 45 to 58%. Of the 13 intra-cardiac structures and

Table 1 Image quality score of FE-CMRA and FE-MUSIC

	FE-CMRA (n = 15)	FE-MUSIC (n = 40)	P value*
Right atrium	1.9 ± 0.4	3.7 ± 0.5	p < 0.001
Left atrium	2.0 ± 0.4	3.8 ± 0.4	p < 0.001
Right ventricle	2.0 ± 0.4	3.6 ± 0.5	p < 0.001
Left ventricle	2.0 ± 0.4	3.7 ± 0.5	p < 0.001
Interatrial septum	1.5 ± 0.6	3.8 ± 0.4	p < 0.001
Interventricular septum	2.2 ± 0.7	3.8 ± 0.4	p < 0.001
Tricuspid valve	1.4 ± 0.5	3.6 ± 0.5	p < 0.001
Mitral valve	1.4 ± 0.5	3.7 ± 0.4	p < 0.001
LVOT, aortic valve, and aortic root	2.0 ± 0.7	3.7 ± 0.5	p < 0.001
RVOT, pulmonary valve	1.9 ± 0.7	3.6 ± 0.5	p < 0.001
Main pulmonary artery and second order branches	2.7 ± 0.6	3.6 ± 0.6	p < 0.001
Proximal ascending aorta	2.8 ± 0.6	3.7 ± 0.6	p < 0.001
Coronaries	1.2 ± 0.5	3.3 ± 1.0	p < 0.001

LVOT left ventricular outflow tract, PV pulmonic valve, RVOT right ventricular outflow tract
*P values reflect comparisons between average image quality scores for FE-CMRA and FE-MUSIC using the Wilcoxon rank sum test

vascular segments evaluated, FE-MUSIC had an average image quality score greater than 3.5 in 12 structures and 3.3 for the coronary arteries. Based on a four-point scoring system, scores of 3 or greater indicate that all relevant cardiac and vascular structures within the imaged field of view were confidently evaluable on FE-MUSIC images. Inter-reader correlation of FE-MUSIC scores was higher ($r = 0.46$, 95% CI 0.37 to 0.55, $p < 0.01$) compared to FE-CMRA ($r = 0.41$, 95% CI 0.30 to 0.58, $p < 0.01$). In the subset of babies ($n = 15$) with both FE-CMRA and FE-MUSIC, FE-MUSIC images provided superior visualization of intra-cardiac anatomy and superior vascular definition ($p < 0.001$). For FE-CMRA images, the average image quality scores were <2.5 for all intra-cardiac structures, outflow tracts, and coronary arteries.

Figures 1 and 2 and Additional file 2: Figure S1 provide a range of comparative examples of FE-CMRA and FE-MUSIC image quality. Videos are provided as online files to highlight the incremental benefit of dynamic multiphase display. The online videos illustrate clear definition of valve leaflets and the dynamic relationship of great vessels to intracardiac structures over multiple phases of the cardiac cycle. Using the interactive cine mode of multiplanar reformats, arbitrary planes of the beating heart could be interrogated. This latter feature facilitated more confident visualization of cardiac chambers and coronary anatomy, provided a roadmap for surgical planning, and enabled more confident risk-to-benefit assessment. The quality of FE-MUSIC is exemplified by illustrative examples of coronary anatomy in neonates and infants whose heart rate are physiologically tachycardic and clear visualization requires high spatial resolution (Additional file 2: Figure S1, Fig. 2c-d, Fig. 4b-c, Fig. 6,

Additional file 3: online video 6a). In an unstable 1.1 kg patient with a tiny 700 micron patent ductus arteriosus (PDA), acidosis, and a heart rate of 160–180 bpm (Fig. 1), multi-planar thin slice (0.8 mm) cine reconstruction of the FE-MUSIC data showed the origin, nature and extent of thrombus from an infected umbilical vein catheter to the right atrium. Successful and complete surgical thrombectomy was performed without further imaging.

Correlation of MUSIC Findings with other Modalities
MUSIC findings correlated well with angiographic data ($n = 14$), cardiac CT ($n = 4$), and surgical reports ($n = 28$). Autopsy findings were available for one neonate (Fig. 2). In five patients with discordant findings (echo and MUSIC [$n = 5$]; catheter angiography and MUSIC [$n = 1$]), the findings on FE-MUSIC were shown to be accurate at autopsy ($n = 1$) or surgery ($n = 4$). Images in Fig. 2 are of a premature neonate weighing 1.5 kg who underwent CMR following echo and angiography to further clarify vascular and intra-cardiac anatomy. The patient had a heart rate of 160–170 beats per minute (bpm). FE-MUSIC showed a dysplastic pulmonic valve with right ventricular enlargement, an aneurysmal pulmonary artery and severe pulmonary regurgitation. An anomalous right coronary artery was incidentally noted on FE-MUSIC (Fig. 2d), which had not been evident on echo or catheterization nor well-visualized on FE-CMRA (Fig. 2c). Comparative breath-held FE-CMRA produced poor definition of intra-cardiac (Fig. 2a) and coronary anatomy (Fig. 2c). Autopsy examination confirmed the aforementioned findings from FE-MUSIC, in addition to a small PDA. Because of the neonate's poor renal function and critically ill status, very little iodinated contrast could be used during catheterization.

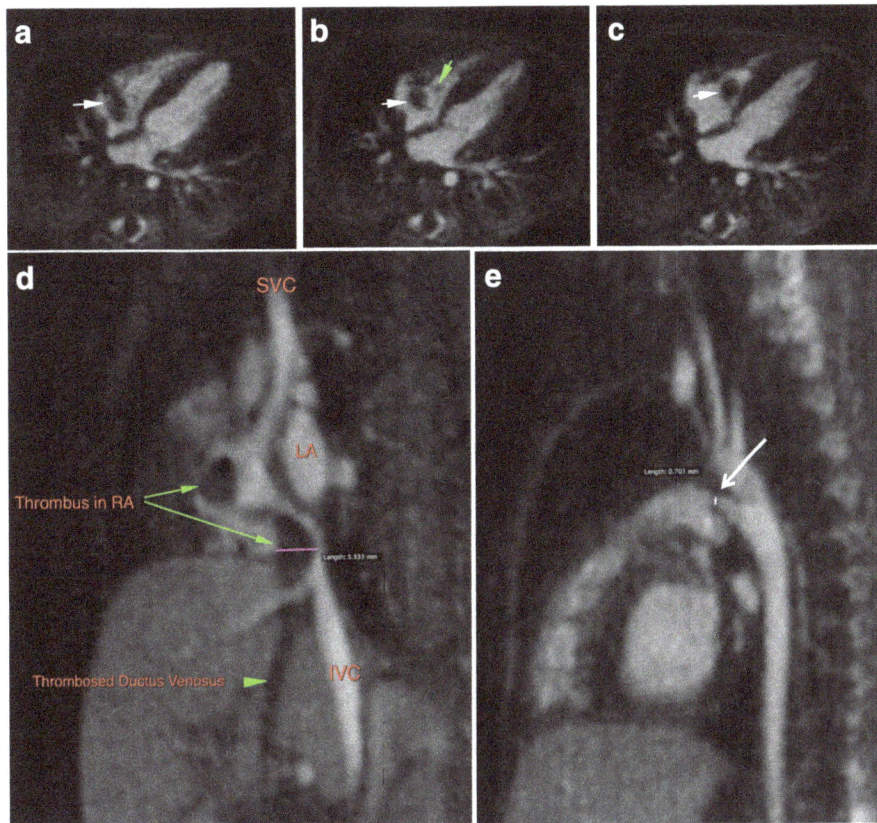

Fig. 1 FE-MUSIC images of a twenty-one-day old boy (1.1 kg) with a patent ductus arteriosus (**a-e**). A mobile right atrial mass of uncertain etiology was noted on echocardiography after birth. Three of 8 frames from FE-MUSIC show a large mobile mass (*white arrow*) in the right atrium (RA) abutting the tricuspid annulus and valve leaflets (*green arrow*). The mass has to-and-fro motion and connects via a thin stalk to thrombus (**d**, Additional file 3: online video 1a) in the inferior vena cava, which in turn, is continuous with thrombus in the ductus venosus originating from an infected umbilical vein catheter. A patent ductus arteriosus measuring 700 microns at its waist is shown bridging the pulmonary artery and descending aorta in the FE-MUSIC image (**e**, Additional file 3: online video 1b)

Thus, there was poor contrast opacification of the high capacity right ventricular outflow tract, where suboptimal visualization suggested an aortopulmonary window versus a large PDA. FE-MUSIC clarified and reconciled the findings between echo and catheterization, and definitively depicted the vascular and intra-cardiac anatomy.

Impact of FE-MUSIC on Patient Management

In all cases, FE-MUSIC satisfactorily answered all clinical questions requested by referring surgeons or cardiologists and in many cases provided additional insight, which impacted the overall patient care plan. Table 2 provides sample cases highlighting the clinical impact of the FE-MUSIC findings on patient management. On a five-point scale (with one point for each key clinical outcome measure), the average clinical impact score was 4.2 ± 0.9. In all cases, results from FE-MUSIC informed the overall management of the patient and informed the risk-to-benefit evaluation for discussion with the patient's parents regarding the treatment plan (Figs. 3, 4, 5 and 6). Of the 28 cases where management may have needed

additional assessment by catheterization, further diagnostic evaluation was avoided in 13 patients because relationships between vascular anatomy and its relationship to intracardiac morphology were well visualized on FE-MUSIC imaging. Supplemental information regarding flow patterns and volume was available as a part of the entire clinical CMR exam (Fig. 3, Additional file 3: online video 3b; Fig. 5, Additional file 3: online video 5b and 5c). One diagnostic cath was performed at an outside facility prior to CMR. Of the remaining 14 cases that had catheterization, three patients had necessary pre-Glenn angiograms and 11 underwent catheterization for therapeutic purposes (four of which were transcatheter interventions that were in lieu of high risk surgery). Sixty-eight percent of patients ($n = 16$ neonates; $n = 12$ infants) had successful surgical correction or palliation of congenital anomalies. Circulatory arrest was avoided in 2 surgical cases. In all cases requiring intervention, multiphase assessment of vessel size and dynamic 3D imaging of intra- and extra-cardiac structures facilitated procedural planning by decreasing projected operative time as well as informing more confident assessment of the true

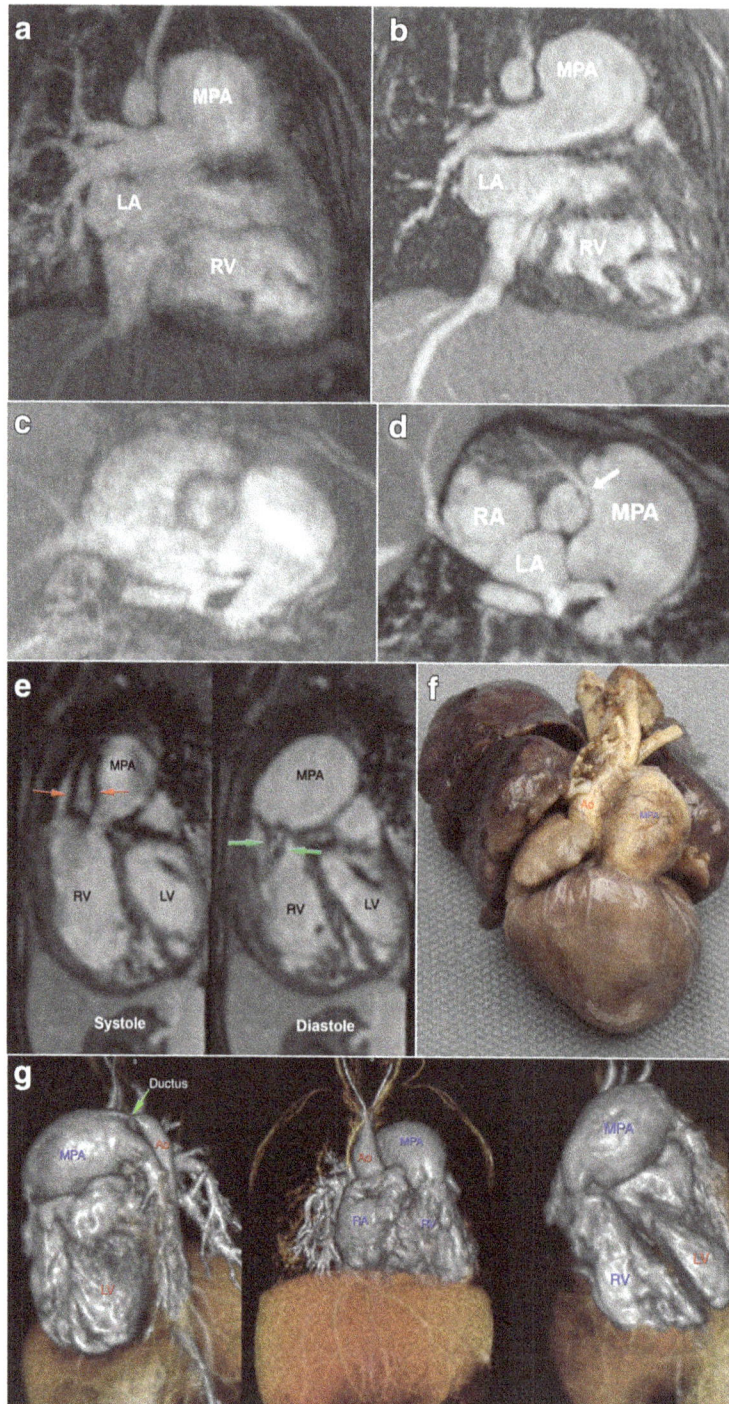

Fig. 2 Correlative FE-MUSIC and autopsy findings of a premature newborn girl (1.6 kg) with severe pulmonary regurgitation, dilated main pulmonary artery, right ventricular hypertrophy, and anomalous right coronary artery are shown. Breath held FE-CMRA (**a**, **c**) shows blurred cardiac borders, poor definition of RV trabeculae (scored 1) and mild blurring of the severely dilated main pulmonary artery (scored 3). FE-MUSIC (**b**, **d**) shows defined cardiac chambers with hypertrophied and trabeculated right ventricle (RV, scored 4) and interatrial septum (scored 4). The right coronary artery has an anomalous origin from the left coronary cusp and an inter-arterial course (*white arrow* in **d**, scored 3). An ejection flow jet (*red arrows*) and a regurgitant flow jet (*green arrows*) are visualized in systolic and diastolic FE-MUSIC frames (**e**) respectively. Autopsy findings (**f**) show full agreement with volume-rendered FE-MUSIC images (**g**). Ao, aorta; MPA, main pulmonary artery; RA, right atrium; RV, right ventricle

Table 2 Case examples highlighting the clinical impact of FE-MUSIC CMR on the management of neonates and infants with congenital heart disease

Pt	Weight (kg)	Pre-MUSIC diagnosis	Post-MUSIC diagnosis	Management and impact on patient care
1	2.2[d]	TOF-PA, discontinuous PAs	TOF-PA, right-sided aortic arch with diminutive MPA (1.3 mm) and branch PAs, MAPCAs arising from LSCA & DAo	Balloon angioplasty of PAs, BT shunt deferred until patient is ~3 kg
2	2.6	TOF-PA, ?discontinuous PAs	TOF-PA with discontinuous PAs, MAPCAs supplied RPA, ductus/APCs from distal abdominal aorta supplies LPA	Unifocalization of PAs, patch angioplasty at small MPA/RPA juncture, and modified left BT shunt
3	3.3	D-TGA with VSD, double aortic arch, sub-PS/PS	D-TGA, VSD, double aortic arch with tracheo-esophageal compression, sub-PS/PS. Incomplete tracheal rings.	Underwent balloon atrial septostomy; subsequent staged surgery with modified right BT shunt, division of DAA
4	2.5[ac]	Hypoplastic aortic arch; VSD	Severe aortic arch hypoplasia, near IAA, VSD, normal LV volume/size	VSD closure and aortic arch augmentation
5	3.5	TOF-PS	TOF-PS, hypoplastic MPA continuing as RPA. No APCs. LPA comes from transverse aorta. LCA originates from LCC and courses between RPA and aorta without compression	Staged unifocalization of LPA aided by visualization of unconventional coronary course
6	1.5[ab]	PV dysplasia, moderate PR, bicuspid AV, severe RVH, ?AP window	PV dysplasia, severe PR, anomalous RCA from LCC with acute anterior angulation, severe RVH. Left-sided aortic arch. No AP window seen	Unsuccessful PDA closure. Patient expired prior to surgery. Autopsy confirmed MUSIC findings.
7	3.6	HLHS;?pulmonary vein stenosis	HLHS, large PAs, no pulmonary vein stenosis. Preserved ventricular function. Large APC from DAo	Occlusion of APC and ductal stenting prior to hybrid Norwood with bilateral banding of PAs
8	2.8[d]	SV/heterotaxy with PA, ?APCs, PAPVR vs TAPVR	SV/heterotaxy with PA, hypoplastic PAs with MAPCAs	Ductal stenting; No surgery
9	1.5	Parachute MV, bicuspid AV with AS, aortic coarctation	Parachute MV, hypoplastic LV, bicuspid AV with severe AS, hypoplastic aortic arch	ABVP and BAS, Subsequent aortic arch repair
10	2.6	TOF-PA	TOF-PA, confluent branch pulmonary arteries. No MAPCAs.	BT shunt, ductal ligation
11	2.4[d]	TOF-PA, Unclear PAs anatomy	TOF-PA, absent MPA, tortuous L/RPA, MAPCAs from proximal left vertebral artery to LPA, MAPCAs from RSCA to RPA. Severe RPA hypoplasia (1.7 mm)	Left subclavian collateral stenting. Small PAs size led to stenting and deferring unifocalization
12	4.2[a]	VSD, aortic arch and branching not well seen	VSD, vascular ring with right aortic arch and aberrant left brachiocephalic artery coursing posteriorly, inferiorly behind esophagus and trachea. No tracheal compression.	VSD closure, division of vascular ring. Extracardiac characterization of vascular ring's unusual course facilitated surgical planning; surgery occurred earlier because of VSD
13	3.2a	Double aortic arch, large VSD	IAA with LPA & LSCA arising from left branch of hypoplastic AA, large VSD	VSD closure, IAA repair, LPA reimplantation rather than ring division
14	2.3	PAPVR, aortic arch hypoplasia	Scimitar syndrome with right-sided pulmonary sequestration; aortic arch hypoplasia	Occlusion of APCs, Surgical aortic arch repair
15	3.1	TOF-PA, LPA not well seen	TOF-PA, confluent branch PAs with discrete LPA stenosis, no MAPCAs	Surgery rather than watchful waiting. BT shunt with plasty of PAs rather than shunt only.
16	2.6	TOF-PA, LPA not well seen, ?APCs	TOF-PA, severe LPA stenosis, no MAPCAs	BT shunt with LPA plasty rather than watchful waiting
17	3.5[a]	Hypoplastic aortic arch	Double aortic arch forming complete vascular ring without tracheal or esophageal compression	Division of vascular ring rather than coarctation repair

Table 2 Case examples highlighting the clinical impact of FE-MUSIC CMR on the management of neonates and infants with congenital heart disease *(Continued)*

Pt	Weight (kg)	Pre-MUSIC diagnosis	Post-MUSIC diagnosis	Management and impact on patient care
18	2.1[c]	IAA/VSD, large PDA, hypoplastic bicuspid AV	IAA/VSD, large PDA, hypoplastic bicuspid AV; predominant flow thru VSD determined final surgical decision	Rastelli-type VSD closure with RV- PA conduit, Damus-Kaye-Stansel arch reconstruction
19	12.7	TOF/PA s/p repair (RV-PA conduit, VSD closure), MAPCAs s/p coil occlusion, RPA stenting	TOF/PA s/p unifocalization. No significant APCs. Findings of markedly diminished perfusion and arterial vascularity in the left lung base along with diminutive and pruned PAs to the LLL as well as dynamic compression of the LIPV determined surgical course	RV to pulmonary artery conduit replacement, aortic homograft, RPA stent removal, LPA repair
20	7.7	TOF/PS, double aortic arch with vascular ring, PAPVR	TOF/PS, double aortic arch with vascular ring. No compression of airways. 3D visualization of the PAPVR (left superior vertical vein joining the LSPV to the left innominate vein/subclavian vein junction) facilitated surgical approach and planning.	TOF repair, division of vascular ring, ligation of levoatrial cardinal vein

[a]Discordant echo/MUSIC findings (*n* = 5)
[b]Discordant catheterization/MUSIC findings (*n* = 1)
[c]Change from single ventricle to biventricular repair or vice-versa (*n* = 2)
[d]Percutaneous transcatheter intervention in lieu of immediate high risk cardiothoracic surgery (*n* = 3)

AA ascending aorta, *ABVP* aortic balloon valvuloplasty, *ASD* atrial septal defect, *AV* aortic valve, *BAS* balloon atrial septostomy, *BT* blalock-taussig, *DAo* descending aorta, *IAA* interrupted aortic arch, *LCA* left coronary artery, *L (R) PA* left (right) pulmonary artery, *L (R) (I) (S) PV* left (right) (inferior) (superior) pulmonary vein, *L (R) SCA* left (right) subclavian artery, *LV* left ventricle, *MAPCAs* major aortopulmonary collateral arteries, *MPA* main pulmonary artery, *MV* mitral valve, *NA* not applicable, *PA* pulmonary atresia, *PAs* pulmonary arteries, *PDA* patent ductus arteriosus, *PFO* patent foramen ovale, *PH* pulmonary hypertension, *PV* pulmonic valve, *RCA* right coronary artery, *RV* right ventricle, *SV* single ventricle, *TAPVR* total anomalous pulmonary venous return, *TGA* transposition of the great arteries, *TOF* tetralogy of fallot, *VSD* ventricular septal defect

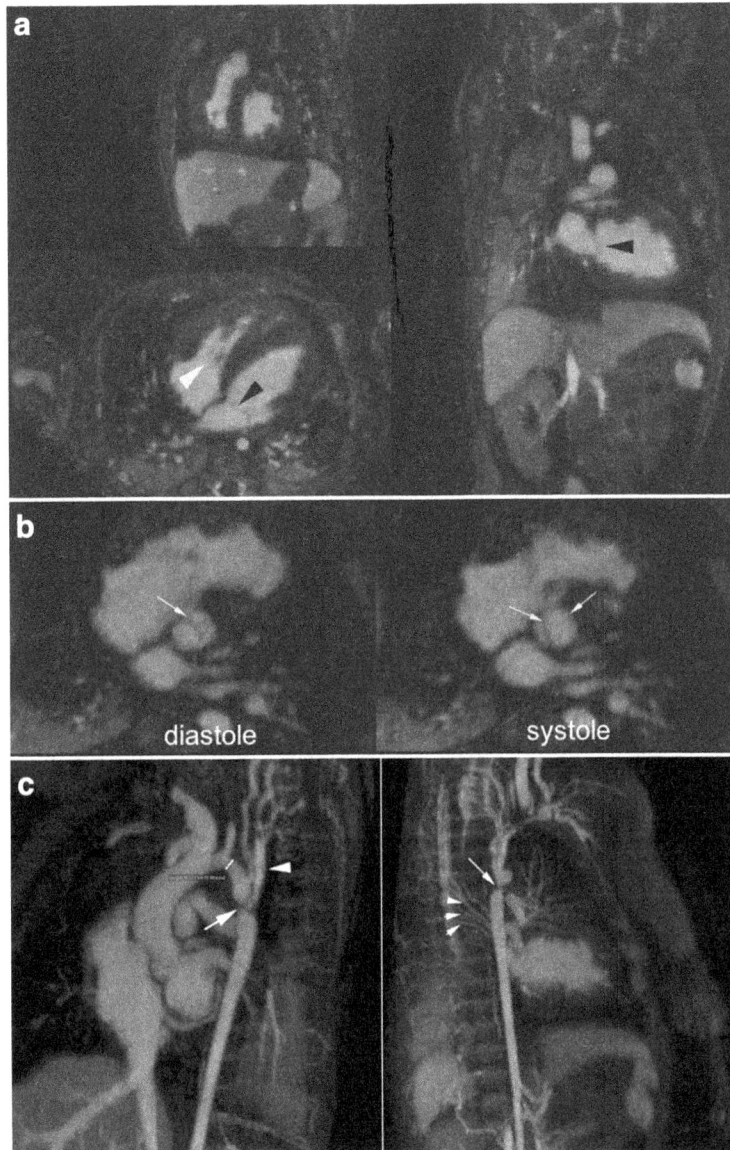

Fig. 3 Multiplanar reformat MUSIC images of a 1-month old boy infant (4.4 kg) with biventricular hypertrophy (**a**), bicuspid aortic valve (**b**), and critical aortic coarctation (**c**) are shown. *Black arrowheads* (**a**) point to thin mitral valve leaflets. Tricuspid valve leaflets and chordae are well characterized (**a**, *white arrowhead*). Bicuspid aortic valve leaflets (**b**, *white arrows*) demonstrate good excursion throughout the cardiac cycle. The transverse aortic arch (**c**, *white line*) is hypoplastic (0.32 cm). Critical aortic coarctation (**c**, *white arrow*) along with collaterals (**c**, *white arrowheads*) and their dynamic relationship to intracardiac anatomy are well characterized (Additional file 3: Online video 3b). Vessels and intracardiac borders are sharp. There is moderately reduced left ventricular systolic function (Additional file 3: Online video 3b). Turbulent flow through the bicuspid valve and minimal flow through the coarctation are demonstrated in Additional file 3: Online video 3b. FE-MUSIC CMR was ordered to define vascular structures prior to surgery and to delineate the etiology for reduced left ventricular systolic function. Because of the severe coarctation, arch hypoplasia, and reduced left ventricular systolic function, the patient underwent repair of the coarctation and arch augmentation. The global LV hypokinesis and systolic function improved after surgical intervention. The arch anatomy was unclear on echo and the FE-MUSIC findings changed the surgical plan as well as facilitated discussion with parents regarding the overall management plan

risks and benefits of the proposed procedure. For example, in the case involving a 10-day neonate with hypoplastic left heart syndrome (Fig. 4, Additional file 3: online video 4a-4b), identification of large aortopulmonary collaterals from the abdominal aorta altered the course of management and surgical approach. In another patient,

clarification of the complex anatomy with 3D volumetric reconstructions (Fig. 6) and 3D printing of FE-MUSIC images (Fig. 6d, Additional file 3: online video 6b-6c) helped cardiologists to communicate with parents and allowed surgeons to visually describe the operative plan to them. Prior knowledge of potential procedural risks was felt to

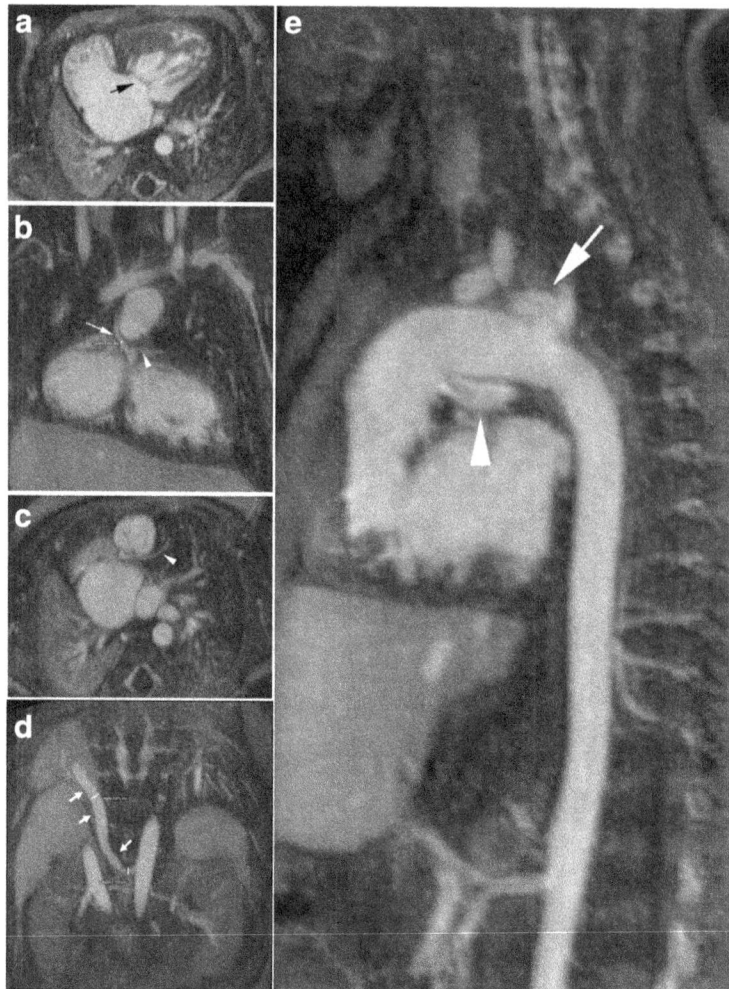

Fig. 4 A 10-day old neonate (3.6 kg) with hypoplastic left heart syndrome (HLHS) who was referred for FE-MUSIC CMR to assess pulmonary vein stenosis and to delineate intra-cardiac and extracardiac vascular anatomy prior to defining a surgical approach. His heart rate ranged from 126 to 140 beats per minute. HLHS with predominant right heart anatomy (**a**, multiplanar reformat) and common atrioventricular valve (*black arrow*) were confirmed. There were large pulmonary arteries and a diminutive aortic root (**b**, *white arrow*; aortic annulus 2.5 mm, sinotubular junction 1.2 mm) with the left main coronary artery (white arrowhead) coming off the aortic sinus. The left anterior descending artery courses between the RVOT and ventricle (**c**, white arrowhead). Large APCs (**d** and Additional file 3: Online video 4a-4b, *white arrows*) from the abdominal aorta were seen. The ductal arch (**e**) is continuous with the descending aorta. *White* arrow points to the innominate artery and *white arrowhead* points to the left pulmonary artery. No pulmonary vein stenosis. Based on the findings, the patient underwent occlusion of APCs and ductal stenting prior to proceeding with a hybrid Norwood and bilateral banding of the pulmonary arteries. Because MUSIC images provided a clear roadmap for surgery planning, our surgeons and cardiologists had a better sense of the child's higher risk profile. MUSIC enhanced the risk discussion with the child's parents. As a result, the decision was to palliate rather than pursue a staged operation

be of significant value when discussing treatment options with parents or guardians. Of those undergoing surgery, decisions about the optimal surgical approach were informed by visualization of dynamic cardiac anatomy shown with FE-MUSIC (Figs. 3, 4, 5 and 6).

Discussion

Our results affirm that FE-MUSIC provided detailed and reliable multiphase 3D visualization of intra-cardiac and extra-cardiac vascular anatomy in small babies. We also demonstrate that findings on MUSIC images had high

clinical impact on the care of neonates and infants with CHD. FE-MUSIC represents a promising step towards practical and simplified image acquisition for combined assessment of dynamic cardiac and vascular anatomy in this complex patient group. Once the imaging volume is prescribed, no further interaction is required of the machine operator. FE-MUSIC images were immediately available for interrogation by interpreting physicians without additional post-processing. All relevant analyses and desired reconstructions were performed using a commercially available software with 4D capability. FE-MUSIC

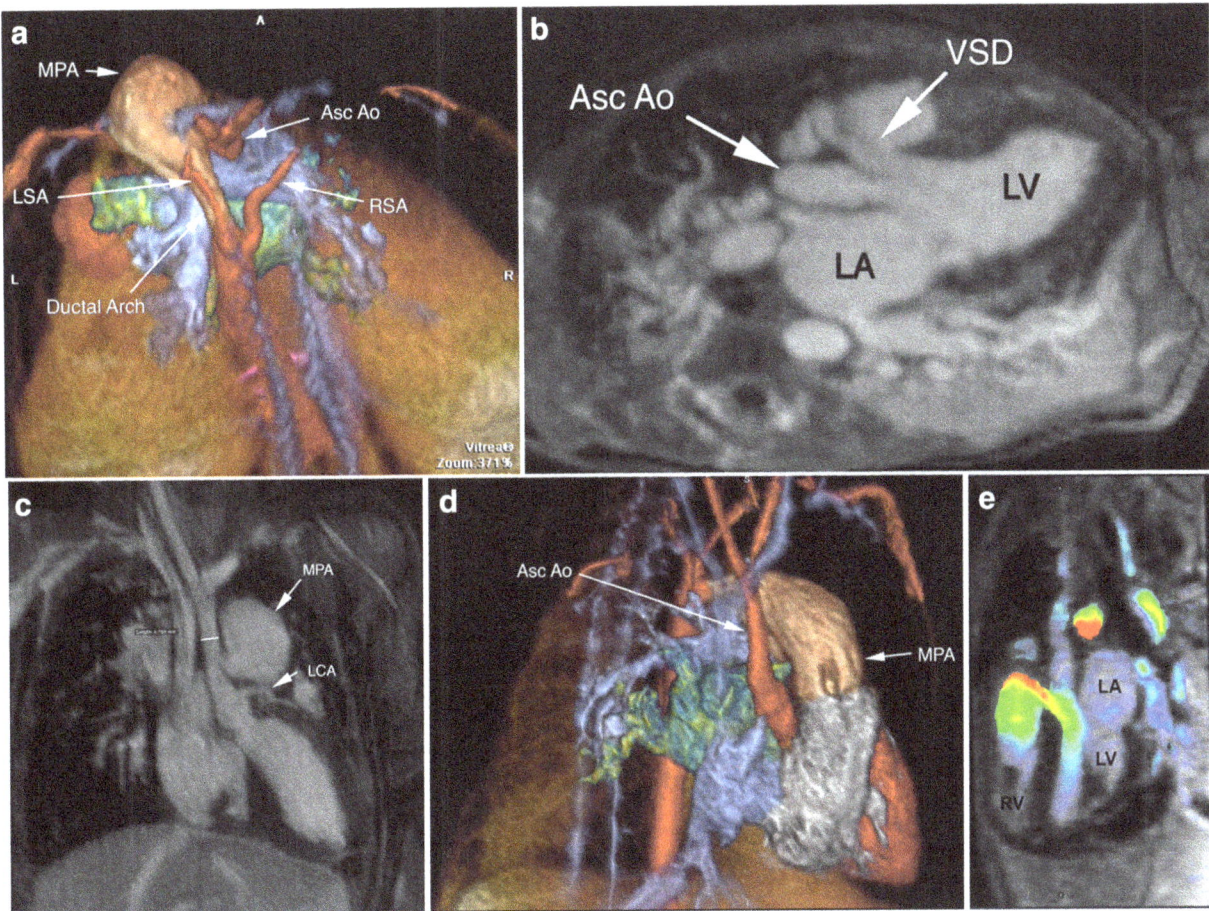

Fig. 5 3D multiplanar reformat and color volume rendered MUSIC images of a 20-day old neonate (2.1 kg) with interrupted ascending aorta (**a**, bird's eye view, Asc Ao) and ventricular septal defect (VSD, **b**) are shown. 4D color volume rendered MUSIC images are available as Additional file 3: Online video 5a. Relationships between the large main pulmonary artery (MPA), hypoplastic ascending aorta (3.8 mm), ductal arch, and intracardiac structures are depicted in **c** and **d**. Their 4D dynamic relationships are exemplified in Additional file 3: Online video 5a. The proximal course of the left coronary artery (LCA) is well visualized (**c**). FE-MUSIC CMR was obtained to clarify extra-cardiac vessels and intra-cardiac anatomy. Her heart rate ranged between 137 and 184 beats per minute. Clear definition of intra-cardiac anatomy along with findings of predominant flow through the VSD (**e**, Additional file 3: Online video 5b-c) resulted in the patient undergoing biventricular rather than single ventricle repair. LA, left atrium; LSA, left subclavian artery; LV, left ventricle; RSA, right subclavian artery

added clinical value by defining relevant dynamic anatomy clearly, providing detailed diagnostic data and procedural roadmaps, which informed decision-making, procedural planning and assessment of risks and benefits. Because no ionizing radiation is involved, CMR aligns well with the Image Gently® campaign to explore radiation-free imaging alternatives in children [9].

FE-MUSIC leverages reliable cardio-respiratory gating and ferumoxytol enhancement at 3.0 T to generate 4D images of the beating heart with true isotropic voxel dimensions of 0.6–0.9 mm [1]. This was accomplished by exploiting the high relaxivity and stable blood-pool concentration of ferumoxytol for steady state imaging, combined with regular airway pressure and ECG signals for optimal cardio-respiratory gating. Together, these strategies mitigate both respiratory and cardiac motion artifact

and enable permanent and retrospective interrogation of cine images in any plane. Moreover, insofar as the respiratory waveform and heart rate remain regular and the blood concentration of ferumoxytol remains stable, FE-MUSIC can in principle expand to a high limit in both spatial and temporal resolution, overcoming many of the inherent challenges associated with CMR in pediatric CHD. These inherent challenges include small body size, high heart rates, immature renal function, need for repeated apnea, prolonged examination time, and dedicated physician supervision.

Several possible approaches exist for CMR in small children. Breath held, cardiac gated 3D contrast enhanced CMRA with gadolinium is an option [10, 11], but image acquisition is limited to one or two cardiac phases. Further, the limited time window for breath holding sets a

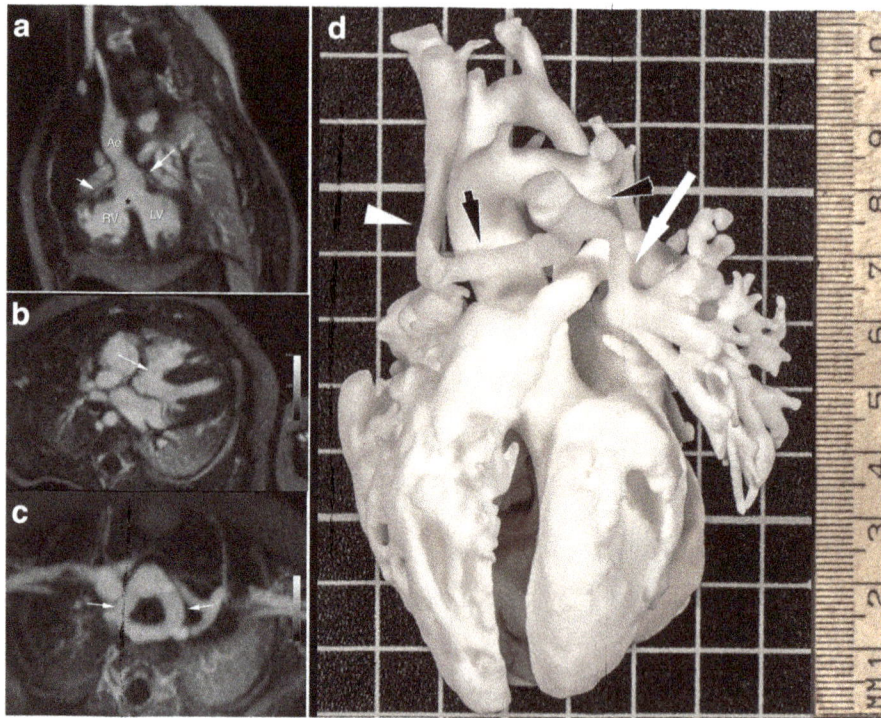

Fig. 6 Multiplanar reformats of FE-MUSIC in a 3-month old girl (7.7 kg) with Tetralogy of Fallot (ToF) and a double aortic arch. Characteristic features of ToF (**a**, Additional file 3: Online video 6a) including right ventricular (RV) hypertrophy with dynamic RV outflow tract obstruction, an overriding aorta, and a perimembranous ventricular septal defect (*black asterisk*) are clearly visualized on dynamic review. Both proximal courses of the left and right coronary arteries (**a**, *white arrow*; Additional file 3: Online video 6a) are also well visualized; the distal right coronary artery can be seen coursing along the right ventricle. Additional file 3: Online video 6a exemplifies the value of dynamic, multiphase imaging in the setting of coronary visualization. The large ventricular septal defect (**a**, *black asterisk*; **b**, *white arrow*) and the complete vascular ring from a double aortic arch (**c**, *white arrows*) are clearly delineated. There is no dynamic compression of the trachea. Colorized volume rendered cine MUSIC images (Additional file 3: Online video 6b) illustrate the dynamic complex extra-cardiac vascular anatomy and its relationship to intra-cardiac structures, which can be used to provide a more concrete image of the anatomic problem and explain a clearly complex case to parents and guardians (**d**, Additional file 3: Online video 6c). There is anomalous pulmonary venous drainage with the left innominate vein (*black arrow*, **d**) dipping inferiorly before joining the right innominate vein (*white arrowhead*, **d**) to form a right-sided superior vena cava. The left superior vertical vein (*black arrowhead*, **d**) joins the low bridging left innominate vein (*black arrow*, **d**) and the left superior pulmonary vein (*white arrow*, **d**), which forms the confluence of the superior pulmonary venous trunk (Additional file 3: Online video 6b, left panel). There is also a double aortic arch, which forms a complete vascular ring without tracheal compression (Additional file 3: Online video 6b, right panel). The FE-MUSIC data were further processed for 3D printing (photographed in **d**, Additional file 3: Online video 6c). The patient subsequently underwent successful surgical repair

limit on spatial resolution, temporal resolution and SNR. With FE-MUSIC, spatial resolution, temporal resolution and SNR have a high upper bound because breath holding is not necessary and image acquisition spans several minutes. SNR is likely higher for MUSIC at 3.0 T than at 1.5 T, although a comparison has not yet been performed in practice.

Others have described the use of 3D bSSFP [12–14] without contrast at 1.5 T. However, the requirement for high spatial resolution in small patients mandates a longer minimum TR per line for bSSFP which, when combined with the fast blood flow in neonates, predisposes to troublesome off-resonance artifact [15]. At 3.0 T, this phenomenon becomes even more problematic. On the other hand, the spoiled gradient echo acquisition in FE-

MUSIC is insensitive to off-resonance effects at both field strengths and pulsatility artifacts are mitigated through gated, multiphase acquisitions. Although 3D respiratory navigator-gated and ECG-triggered IR-FLASH (inversion recovery - fast low-angle shot) with gadofosveset trisodium (Ablavar®, Lantheus Medical Imaging, MA) [16] has been described in CHD imaging, this technique produces only a single cardiac phase. FE-MUSIC provides a permanent 4D archive for reconstruction of cardiac-phase resolved images into any imaging plane, such that the requirement to acquire customized or unusual planes at the time of the study is obviated.

4D flow techniques represent another approach to image acquisition [17–19] in CHD and supplemental information on blood flow can be very helpful. However, with current 4D flow acquisitions, the requisite scan time needed to achieve the same spatial and temporal resolution as 4D MUSIC is greater by a factor of six or more, such that spatial and temporal resolution is usually dialed back with 4D flow [17]. Strategies for accelerated image acquisition are constantly in evolution and these will no doubt improve the performance of 4D flow techniques. Similar acceleration approaches can also be applied to 4D MUSIC such that it will likely remain proportionately faster than 4D flow. In practice, both techniques are complementary and it should not be necessary to choose one over the other. Ferumoxytol supports higher CNR for 4D flow as it does for 4D MUSIC and it seems logical to acquire both sets of data sequentially and to overlay the 4D velocity fields onto the high resolution dynamic anatomy of 4D MUSIC. While evaluation of 4D flow was not the focus of this current work, our referring surgeons and cardiologists had access to 4D flow images in the course of clinical decision making. Systematic evaluation of accelerated, ferumoxytol-enhanced 4D MUSIC and 4D flow as a single comprehensive technique for imaging of CHD is the subject of ongoing work in our laboratory and others.

With modern CT technology, it has become possible to generate 4D datasets at increasingly lower radiation doses. However, the radiation dose with multi-phase CT is proportionately greater than with single phase and raises concerns in young children, especially those who will likely require follow up studies. Nonetheless, clinical decisions are best made for individual patients depending on the required information and where ultrafast, low dose CT scanning is available, this may prove adequate and appropriate for assessment of static anatomy such as the site and size of aorto-pulmonary collateral vessels.

Although no ionizing radiation is involved with CMR, repeated imaging of babies with traditional approaches poses lifelong gadolinium exposure risks. In this regard, ferumoxytol offers an attractive alternative to GBCAs. Moreover, with the recent discontinuation of gadofosveset trisodium (Ablavar®), no blood pool CMR contrast agent is available clinically. Although ferumoxytol is approved by the FDA for treatment of iron deficiency anemia in adults with chronic kidney disease [20], as a theranostic agent, ferumoxytol also has potential for high fidelity steady state blood pool imaging because of its long intravascular half-life and high r_1 relaxivity [5, 21–26]. Following US FDA approval in 2009, ferumoxytol has been used off-label [21, 22] as an alternative to GBCAs in patients with renal impairment [5, 24, 25, 27, 28]. In addition to its unique properties, the elemental iron in ferumoxytol is incorporated into the hematopoietic pathway once the outer carbohydrate shell is degraded providing a therapeutic source of iron, unlike GBCAs which has been shown to accumulate in biologic tissue [29] after repeated exposure. In neonates and children, the therapeutic effects

of ferumoxytol may also be favorable as iron deficiency anemia is common in this population [30]. However, in light of a recent FDA warning regarding the rare potential for fatal hypersensitivity reactions, the benefit to risk ratios must be carefully weighed. To date, no major adverse events have been associated with the diagnostic use of ferumoxytol at our institution [31] and others [32, 33]. Moreover, in children, and particularly neonates, serious allergic reactions of any type tend to be less common than in adults (3–5.8% in children vs 6–10% in adults) [34] potentially because of a less developed immune system [35, 36].

While it is incumbent on caregivers to offer the best available options to patients and to inform management decisions thoughtfully, additional precautionary processes were implemented in our study. All of the patients had protected airways from the start of the procedure and hemodynamic monitoring was performed throughout the exam. While no adverse events occurred in our study, protocols were also in place to deal with them.

The focus on our current study is on the 4D MUSIC sequence in CHD for high resolution, dynamic imaging as opposed to the use of ferumoxytol as a contrast agent to replace gadolinium for all CMR applications. With this in mind, our study does have limitations. First, we did not directly compare GBCA-enhanced vs FE-CMRA in the same population for ethical and practical reasons. Second, we did not perform a systematic comparison between ferumoxytol and another blood pool contrast agent such as gadofosveset trisodium. Additionally, due to the retrospective and non-randomized nature of our study design, there is selection bias – the neonates and infants studied generally represent the most complex cases and frequently with the highest degree of acuity. Because our study is retrospective and the investigation was implemented as a pragmatic clinical study in the context of routine clinical care, the surgical team was not blinded to the FE-MUSIC findings and an independent panel was not formed beforehand to assess the degree of divergence in the surgical plan pre and post FE-MUSIC results. Although preliminary work supports good agreement in volumetry between MUSIC and conventional 2D multi-slice SSFP cine imaging [1], effort is currently underway to systematically evaluate precision and reproducibility of volumetric measurements from 4D MUSIC. Our sample size is also modest. However, a multi-center clinical study is underway to systematically evaluate FE-MUSIC in CHD imaging and to adequately address these concerns. In spite of these limitations, our work demonstrates promising clinical evidence for using FE-MUSIC in neonates and infants with a wide range of CHD. Our findings also support the need for continued work towards the development and validation of streamlined, comprehensive techniques for imaging CHD.

Conclusion

In neonates and infants with CHD, FE-MUSIC at 3.0 T depicts detailed, dynamic 4D anatomy reliably and with high clinical value, without the need for breath holding, contrast bolus timing or prescription of customized imaging planes. Further studies are warranted to assess the performance of FE-MUSIC across field strengths and imaging platforms.

Abbreviations

CHD: Congenital heart disease; CMR: Cardiovascular magnetic resonance; CMRA: Cardiovascular magnetic resonance angiography; FDA: Food and Drug Administration; FE: Ferumoxytol enhanced; GBCA (s): Gadolinium based contrast agent (s); MUSIC: Multiphase steady state imaging with contrast; NICU: Neonatal intensive care unit; SSFP: Steady state free precession

Acknowledgements

The authors would like to acknowledge Dr. Michael Fishbein (Professor of Medicine, Pathology, and Laboratory Medicine; David Geffen School of Medicine at UCLA) for his assistance with autopsy images and pathology results.

Funding

This work is supported by grant R01HL127153 from the National Heart, Lung, and Blood Institute.

Authors' contributions

BLR participated in its design, scored clinical outcomes, and revised the manuscript. DSL participated in its design, scored clinical outcomes, and revised the manuscript. DZG participated in the design, scored the studies, and revised the manuscript. FH participated in the design, facilitated image reconstruction, and revised the manuscript. GMS participated in its design, scored clinical outcomes, and revised the manuscript. IA provided anesthesia support and revised the manuscript. JPF conceived the study, participated in its design, performed the CMR studies, and revised the manuscript. KLN conceived the study, participated in its design, scored the studies, performed the statistical analysis, and drafted the manuscript. PH conceived the study, participated in its design, and revised the manuscript. ZZ facilitated the image reconstruction and revised the manuscript. All authors read and approved the final manuscript.

Competing interests

Dr. J. Paul Finn serves on the Scientific Advisory Board for AMAG, Bracco, and Bayer. The other authors declare they have no competing interests.

Author details

[1]Diagnostic Cardiovascular Imaging Laboratory, Department of Radiological Sciences, David Geffen School of Medicine at UCLA, Los Angeles, CA, USA. [2]Division of Cardiology, David Geffen School of Medicine at UCLA and VA Greater Los Angeles Healthcare System, Los Angeles, CA, USA. [3]Department of Biomedical Physics, University of California, Los Angeles, CA, USA. [4]Department of Anesthesiology, David Geffen School of Medicine at UCLA, Los Angeles, CA, USA. [5]Division of Pediatric Cardiology, David Geffen School of Medicine at UCLA, Los Angeles, CA, USA. [6]Division of Cardiothoracic Surgery, David Geffen School of Medicine at UCLA, Los Angeles, CA, USA. [7]Department of Radiological Sciences, University of California at Los Angeles, Peter V. Ueberroth Building Suite 3371, 10945 Le Conte Ave., Los Angeles, CA 90095-7206, USA.

References

1. Han F, Rapacchi S, Khan S, Ayad I, Salusky I, Gabriel S, Plotnik A, Finn JP, Hu P. Four-dimensional, multiphase, steady-state imaging with contrast enhancement (MUSIC) in the heart: A feasibility study in children. Magn Reson Med. 2015;74:1042–9.
2. Saleh RS, Patel S, Lee MH, Boechat MI, Ratib O, Saraiva CR, Finn JP. Contrast-enhanced MR angiography of the chest and abdomen with use of controlled apnea in children. Radiology. 2007;243:837–46.
3. Tsai-Goodman B, Geva T, Odegard KC, Sena LM, Powell AJ. Clinical role, accuracy, and technical aspects of cardiovascular magnetic resonance imaging in infants. Am J Cardiol. 2004;94:69–74.
4. Nguyen KL, Khan SN, Moriarty JM, Mohajer K, Renella P, Satou G, Ayad I, Patel S, Boechat MI, Finn JP. High-field MR imaging in pediatric congenital heart disease: Initial results. Pediatr Radiol. 2015;45:42–54.
5. Li W, Tutton S, Vu AT, Pierchala L, Li BS, Lewis JM, Prasad PV, Edelman RR. First-pass contrast-enhanced magnetic resonance angiography in humans using ferumoxytol, a novel ultrasmall superparamagnetic iron oxide (USPIO)-based blood pool agent. J Magn Reson Imaging. 2005;21:46–52.
6. US Food and Drug Administration. FDA Drug Safety Communication: FDA strengthens warnings and changes prescribing instructions to decrease the risk of serious allergic reactions with anemia drug Feraheme (ferumoxytol). 2015; Accessed 30 March 2015. http://www.fda.gov/Drugs/DrugSafety/ucm440138.htm.
7. Han F, Zhou Z, Han E, Gao Y, Nguyen KL, Finn JP, Hu P. Self-gated 4D multiphase, steady-state imaging with contrast enhancement (MUSIC) using rotating cartesian K-space (ROCK): Validation in children with congenital heart disease. Magn Reson Med. 2016. doi:10.1002/mrm.26376 [Epub ahead of print].
8. Dietrich O, Raya JG, Reeder SB, Reiser MF, Schoenberg SO. Measurement of signal-to-noise ratios in MR images: influence of multichannel coils, parallel imaging, and reconstruction filters. J Magn Reson Imaging. 2007;26:375–85.
9. Image Gently: The Alliance for Radiation Safety in Pediatric Imaging. Accessed 23 May 2016. http://www.imagegently.org/.
10. Arpasi PJ, Bis KG, Shetty AN, White RD, Simonetti OP. MR angiography of the thoracic aorta with an electrocardiographically triggered breath-hold contrast-enhanced sequence. Radiographics. 2000;20:107–20.
11. Groves EM, Bireley W, Dill K, Carroll TJ, Carr JC. Quantitative analysis of ECG-gated high-resolution contrast-enhanced MR angiography of the thoracic aorta. AJR Am J Roentgenol. 2007;188:522–8.
12. Sorensen TS, Korperich H, Greil GF, Eichhorn J, Barth P, Meyer H, Pedersen EM, Beerbaum P. Operator-independent isotropic three-dimensional magnetic resonance imaging for morphology in congenital heart disease: a validation study. Circulation. 2004;110:163–9.
13. Fenchel M, Greil GF, Martirosian P, Kramer U, Schick F, Claussen CD, Sieverding L, Miller S. Three-dimensional morphological magnetic resonance imaging in infants and children with congenital heart disease. Pediatr Radiol. 2006;36:1265–72.
14. Seeger A, Fenchel MC, Greil GF, Martirosian P, Kramer U, Bretschneider C, Doering J, Claussen CD, Sieverding L, Miller S. Three-dimensional cine MRI in free-breathing infants and children with congenital heart disease. Pediatr Radiol. 2009;39:1333–42.
15. Ferreira PF, Gatehouse PD, Mohiaddin RH, Firmin DN. Cardiovascular magnetic resonance artefacts. J Cardiovasc Magn Reson. 2013;15:41.
16. Febbo JA, Galizia MS, Murphy IG, Popescu A, Bi X, Turin A, Collins J, Markl M, Edelman RR, Carr JC. Congenital heart disease in adults: Quantitative and qualitative evaluation of IR FLASH and IR SSFP MRA techniques using a blood pool contrast agent in the steady state and comparison to first pass MRA. Eur J Radiol. 2015;84:1921–9.
17. Markl M, Kilner PJ, Ebbers T. Comprehensive 4D velocity mapping of the heart and great vessels by cardiovascular magnetic resonance. J Cardiovasc Magn Reson. 2011;13:7.
18. Cheng JY, Hanneman K, Zhang T, Alley MT, Lai P, Tamir JI, Uecker M, Pauly JM, Lustig M, Vasanawala SS. Comprehensive motion-compensated highly accelerated 4D flow MRI with ferumoxytol enhancement for pediatric congenital heart disease. J Magn Reson Imaging. 2016;43(6):1355–68.
19. Lai LM, Cheng JY, Alley MT, Zhang T, Lustig M and Vasanawala SS. Feasibility of ferumoxytol-enhanced neonatal and young infant cardiac MRI without general anesthesia. J Magn Reson Imaging. 2016 Sep 28. doi:10.1002/jmri.25482.
20. AMAG Pharmaceuticals. Feraheme Drug Label. 2014. (revised March 2015); April 2015.
21. Bashir MR, Bhatti L, Marin D, Nelson RC. Emerging applications for ferumoxytol as a contrast agent in MRI. J Magn Reson Imaging. 2015;41:884–98.

22. Finn JP, Nguyen KL, Han F, Zhou Z, Salusky I, Ayad I, Hu P. Cardiovascular MRI with ferumoxytol. Clin Radiol. 2016;71:796–806.
23. Bashir MR, Jaffe TA, Brennan TV, Patel UD, Ellis MJ. Renal transplant imaging using magnetic resonance angiography with a nonnephrotoxic contrast agent. Transplantation. 2013;96:91.
24. Prince MR, Zhang HL, Chabra SG, Jacobs P, Wang Y. A pilot investigation of new superparamagnetic iron oxide (ferumoxytol) as a contrast agent for cardiovascular MRI. J Xray Sci Technol. 2003;11:231–40.
25. Nayak AB, Luhar A, Hanudel M, Gales B, Hall TR, Finn JP, Salusky IB, Zaritsky J. High-resolution, whole-body vascular imaging with ferumoxytol as an alternative to gadolinium agents in a pediatric chronic kidney disease cohort. Pediatr Nephrol. 2015;30:515–21.
26. Neuwelt EA, Hamilton BE, Varallyay CG, Rooney WR, Edelman RD, Jacobs PM, Watnick SG. Ultrasmall superparamagnetic iron oxides (USPIOs): a future alternative magnetic resonance (MR) contrast agent for patients at risk for nephrogenic systemic fibrosis (NSF)? Kidney Int. 2009;75:465–74.
27. Bashir MR, Mody R, Neville A, Javan R, Seaman D, Kim CY, Gupta RT, Jaffe TA. Retrospective assessment of the utility of an iron-based agent for contrast-enhanced magnetic resonance venography in patients with endstage renal diseases. J Magn Reson Imaging. 2014;40:113–8.
28. Walker JP, Nosova E, Sigovan M, Rapp J, Grenon MS, Owens CD, Gasper WJ, Saloner DA. Ferumoxytol-Enhanced Magnetic Resonance Angiography is a Feasible Method for the Clinical Evaluation of Lower Extremity Arterial Disease. Ann Vasc Surg. 2015;29:63–8.
29. McDonald RJ, McDonald JS, Kallmes DF, Jentoft ME, Murray DL, Thielen KR, Williamson EE, Eckel LJ. Intracranial Gadolinium Deposition after Contrast-enhanced MR Imaging. Radiology. 2015;275:772–82.
30. Lopez A, Cacoub P, Macdougall IC, Peyrin-Biroulet L. Iron deficiency anaemia. Lancet. 2016;387:907–16.
31. Nguyen KL, Yoshida T, Han F, Ayad I, Reemtsen BL, Salusky IB, Satou GM, Hu P, Finn JP. MRI with Ferumoxytol: A Single Center Experience of Safety Across the Age Spectrum. J Magn Reson. 2017;45(3):804-812.
32. Ning P, Zucker EJ, Wong P, Vasanawala SS. Hemodynamic safety and efficacy of ferumoxytol as an intravenous contrast agents in pediatric patients and young adults. Magn Reson Imaging. 2016;34:152–8.
33. Muehe AM, Feng D, Von Eyben R, Luna-Fineman S, Link MP, Muthig T, Huddleston AE, Neuwelt EA, Daldrup-Link HE. Safety Report of Ferumoxytol for Magnetic Resonance Imaging in Children and Young Adults. Invest Radiol. 2016;51:221–7.
34. Elzouki AY HH, Nazer HM, Stapleton FB, Oh W, Whitley RJ. Textbook of Clinical Pediatrics. 2nd ed. New York: Springer; 2012.
35. Marodi L. Innate cellular immune responses in newborns. Clin Immunol. 2006;118:137–44.
36. Gervassi AL, Horton H. Is Infant Immunity Actively Suppressed or Immature? Virol. 2014;2014:1–9.

10

Quantification of myocardium at risk in ST-elevation myocardial infarction: a comparison of contrast-enhanced steady-state free precession cine cardiovascular magnetic resonance with coronary angiographic jeopardy scores

Rodney De Palma[*†], Peder Sörensson[†], Dinos Verouhis, John Pernow and Nawzad Saleh

Abstract

Background: Clinical outcome following acute myocardial infarction is predicted by final infarct size evaluated in relation to left ventricular myocardium at risk (MaR). Contrast-enhanced steady-state free precession (CE-SSFP) cardiovascular magnetic resonance imaging (CMR) is not widely used for assessing MaR. Evidence of its utility compared to traditional assessment methods and as a surrogate for clinical outcome is needed.

Methods: Retrospective analysis within a study evaluating post-conditioning during ST elevation myocardial infarction (STEMI) treated with coronary intervention ($n = 78$). CE-SSFP post-infarction was compared with angiographic jeopardy methods. Differences and variability between CMR and angiographic methods using Bland-Altman analyses were evaluated. Clinical outcomes were compared to MaR and extent of infarction.

Results: MaR showed correlation between CE-SSFP, and both BARI and APPROACH scores of 0.83 ($p < 0.0001$) and 0.84 ($p < 0.0001$) respectively. Bias between CE-SSFP and BARI was 1.1% (agreement limits -11.4 to +9.1). Bias between CE-SSFP and APPROACH was 1.2% (agreement limits -13 to +10.5). Inter-observer variability for the BARI score was 0.56 ± 2.9; 0.42 ± 2.1 for the APPROACH score; -1.4 ± 3.1% for CE-SSFP. Intra-observer variability was 0.15 ± 1.85 for the BARI score; for the APPROACH score 0.19 ± 1.6; and for CE-SSFP -0.58 ± 2.9%.

Conclusion: Quantification of MaR with CE-SSFP imaging following STEMI shows high correlation and low bias compared with angiographic scoring and supports its use as a reliable and practical method to determine myocardial salvage in this patient population.

Keywords: Myocardium, myocardial salvage, cardiovascular magnetic resonance imaging

* Correspondence: rodney_de_palma@icloud.com
[†]Equal contributors
Karolinska Institutet, Department of Medicine, Unit of Cardiology, Karolinska University Hospital, Stockholm, Sweden

Background

The clinical outcome following acute ST-segment elevation myocardial infarction (STEMI) is predicted by the final infarct size [1, 2]. This in turn is determined by a complex interplay between several factors including the duration of myocardial ischemia, the presence of collateral blood supply, reperfusion injury and left ventricular myocardium at risk (MaR). Therapies to restore myocardial perfusion and/or limit reperfusion injury, whether mechanical or pharmacological, are incompletely assessed by final absolute infarct size alone [3]. Evaluation of infarct size has to be performed in relation to the MaR. The myocardial salvage index, calculated as (MaR-final infarct size)/MaR, is a more robust surrogate for therapeutic efficacy. The reference technique for assessing the MaR is nuclear single photon emission computed tomography (SPECT) [4–6]. This imaging modality, however, is not practical in the clinical setting as it requires acute imaging when a patient may remain clinically unstable as well as two subsequent image acquisitions. Furthermore, it has relatively limited spatial resolution and involves exposure to ionizing radiation. It is therefore of interest that several studies have demonstrated that cardiovascular magnetic resonance imaging (CMR) is equivalent to SPECT at 7 days following STEMI for assessing MaR using contrast-enhanced steady-state free precession cardiac magnetic resonance (CE-SSFP), or T2-weighted sequences in a single examination [4, 7–9].

CE-SSFP is not yet widely used for the assessment of MaR but has been shown to be more robust than T2-weighted imaging in multi-center, multi-vendor studies [10, 11]. Given the potential advantage of combining CE-CMR with SSFP and LGE to evaluate both MaR and final infarct size in this setting further evidence of its utility as a surrogate for clinical outcome is needed. Angiographic assessment of myocardium at risk has been shown to predict clinical outcome following myocardial infarction [12, 13]. A comparison of CE-SSFP and such angiographic evaluation has not been undertaken previously.

Aim

The aim of the current investigation was therefore to evaluate the relationship between CE-SSFP and two validated angiographic scoring techniques for anatomical left ventricular myocardial area at risk: the BARI (Bypass Angioplasty Revascularization Investigation Myocardial Jeopardy index) score and the modified APPROACH (Alberta Provincial Project for Outcome Assessment in Coronary Heart Disease) score [12, 13]. Clinical outcome data were also evaluated in the context of MaR and extent of infarction.

The main hypothesis tested was that CE-SSFP provides a coherent determination of MaR, when compared with angiographic scoring techniques.

Methods

Consecutive patients from a randomized trial evaluating post-conditioning during STEMI were analyzed retrospectively. This study was a single-center single-blinded prospective clinical trial evaluating the benefit of intracoronary balloon–mediated ischemic post-conditioning on myocardial infarct size in patients presenting with STEMI the setting of a primary percutaneous coronary intervention service with study recruitment between 1st January 2009-31st December 2009 and has been described in detail previously [14]. In brief, eligibility consisted of a presentation within 6 h compatible with acute ischemia, ST elevation on a 12 lead electrocardiogram (>0.1 mV in two contiguous leads, >0.2 mV in V1-V3, or new left bundle branch block and Thrombolysis in Myocardial Infarction (TIMI) 0 flow in an identifiable infarct-related artery on invasive coronary angiography. Exclusion criteria consisted of: previous myocardial infarction including the presence of pathological Q waves on the resting electrocardiogram, surgical revascularization, cardiogenic shock, a presentation with cardiac arrest, treatment with metformin, absolute contraindication to CMR, atrial fibrillation and known renal impairment (defined as creatinine >150 micromol/l).

Invasive coronary angiography

Invasive coronary angiography was performed to confirm complete coronary occlusion in the infarct related artery and determine the BARI and Modified APPROACH scores. Percutaneous coronary intervention (PCI) was then performed according to local standard procedures at the discretion of the individual physician. The intervention was completed by a coronary angiographic acquisition to determine final TIMI grade flow.

Visual angiographic scoring, using the BARI and modified APPROACH systems, was carried out retrospectively using pre- and post-PCI images. Two experienced assessors, each with direct clinical experience of more than 2000 invasive procedures, and blinded to the CMR results scored the angiograms. The Rentrop scoring system was used to assess collateralization (Table 2).

Post-conditioning protocol

After invasive coronary angiography, patients were randomized to primary PCI only or primary PCI followed by post-conditioning. This was performed by intracoronary occlusion using the PCI balloon to a pressure of 2-4 atmospheres for four cycles of 60 s starting 60 s after the initial reperfusion [14].

Cardiovascular magnetic resonance imaging

A standard CMR was scheduled between 5-7 days after admission. These investigations were performed in the supine position with an eight-channel cardiac coil by means of a 1.5 Tesla system (Signa Excite TwinSpeed, General Electric Healthcare, Waukesha, Wisconsin, USA) during vector-ECG monitoring. Intravenous gadolinium-DTPA chelated contrast (0.2 mmol/kg; Omniscan, GE Healthcare) was administered before positioning the patient in the scanner. The image protocol included scout images, localization of the short axis and then covering the whole left ventricle (LV) with cine balanced steady-state free precession (SSFP) images retrospectively-gated. Baseline images were acquired 5 min after contrast administration. The following parameters were used; SSFP (echo time (TE) 1.58 milliseconds (ms), repetition time (TR) 3.61 ms, flip angle 60°, 25 phases, 8 millimetres (mm) slice, no inter-slice gap, matrix 226x226). Late gadolinium enhancement (LGE) images were acquired 15-20 min after contrast injection using an inversion recovery gradient echo sequence (TE 3.3 ms, TR 7.0 ms, inversion time 180-250 ms to null the myocardium, 8 mm slice, no inter-slice gap, matrix 256x192) and the same slice orientation as cine SSFP images [15, 16].

Cardiac triggering was set for diastole to reduce motion artifacts. Each slice was obtained during end-expiratory breath holding. Two-, three- and four-chamber views were also obtained to confirm the findings.

CMR images were analyzed off-line at a later session using freely available segmentation software (Segment V.1.8 R0857; http://segment.heiberg.se/) [17]. End-diastolic and end-systolic volumes, ejection fraction, stroke volume and left ventricular volume were calculated on cine SSFP sequences. Infarct size was quantified using an automated quantification method that has been validated ex vivo and in vivo in which account is made for partial volume effects [18, 19]. The extent of infarction is expressed both in absolute mass and as the percentage of MaR with LGE.

MaR determined from CE-SSFP was assessed according to previously described methodology [9]. Endo- and epicardial borders were manually traced in all short-axis slices in both end-diastole and end-systole followed by manual delineation of the hyper-intense regions in end-diastole and end-systole, by one experienced observer (level 2 CMR certified and with 12 years of CMR experience) blinded to the LGE images and angiographic scores (Fig. 1). A second experienced observer (level 3 CMR certified and with 20 years of CMR experience) evaluated twelve patients for intra-observer variability. Hypo-intense myocardium within the area of increased signal intensity was regarded as microvascular obstruction and was included in the MaR. The values of MaR in end-diastole and end-systole were averaged and expressed as a percentage of LV mass, (Fig. 1 and Additional file 1: movie1).

BARI score

Left ventricular MaR was calculated by grading all terminating arteries. All branches were scored as 3, 2, 1 or 0 points, corresponding to, large, medium, small or absent respectively. The ventricular base to apex distance, approximated from the coronary angiogram, provided the basis for assessing the relative distribution of coronary branches. Branches were considered large if their length exceeded two- thirds of the distance from base to apex, medium if one-third to two-thirds the distance, small if less than one-third of the distance and absent if less than one-fifth of the distance from base to apex [12]. The risk score was calculated as a percentage of the left ventricular myocardial volume; by dividing summed scores of a jeopardized territory by the total score of the entire left ventricle.

Modified APPROACH score

This score, which is based on pathological and necropsy studies [20, 21], is derived from a template that

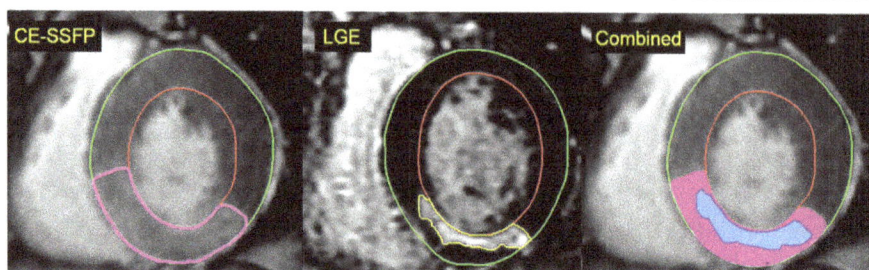

Fig. 1 Example of MaR and myocardial salvage index using contrast-enhanced SSFP magnetic resonance imaging. Corresponding left ventricular short axis views from a patient with an inferior STEMI caused by a right coronary artery occlusion. The epicardium is delineated by a *green* border, and the endocardium by a *red* border. The myocardium at risk (MaR) in the inferior segment is determined by area of early gadolinium enhancement on SSFP (delineated by a *pink* border in the *panel to the left*). The size of infarction in the inferior segment is determined by the area of late gadolinium enhancement delineated by a *yellow* border in the *middle panel*. Automatic computer-aided superimposition of the infarcted area and the MaR area can be used to calculate the myocardial salvage index (as a ratio of the two areas, 1-scar area/MaR), *panel to the right*. MaR = myocardium at risk; CE-SSFP = contrast-enhanced steady-state free precession; STEMI = ST-elevation myocardial infarction; LGE = late gadolinium enhancement

considers the culprit artery, dominance and lesion location (proximal or mid-vessel) together with the size (small, medium or large) of the remaining major non-culprit epicardial vessel [13]. The score in the template represents the percentage of LV MaR.

Statistical methods

Data management and analyses were performed using EXCEL version 14.4.3 (Microsoft Corporation, Redmond, Wisconsin, USA) and GraphPad Prism V.5.00 (GraphPad Software, San Diego, California, USA).

Continuous data are presented as means with standard deviations (SD). Categorical data are presented as frequencies with percentages or medians with interquartile ranges (IQR).

The endpoint was the mean bias between the angiographic scores and MaR derived from the CE-SSFP images using Bland-Altman plots and expressed as mean and limits of agreement (2 x SD).

Pearson's correlation coefficient was also used to evaluate the relationship between CE-SSFP and the angiographic risk scores.

Intra- and inter-observer variability was calculated as the SD of the difference between two calculations divided by the mean of the two observers and expressed as the mean+/- SD.

Statistical significance was accepted as $p < 0.05$.

Results

A total of 89 patients out of a screened cohort of 795 presented with acute STEMI and TIMI 0 flow in the infarct-related artery and were eligible. Those not fulfilling the inclusion criteria were excluded prior to randomization ($n = 706$). Eleven patients were excluded following randomization due to poor CMR image quality, not fulfilling the post-conditioning protocol, or in-hospital death prior to imaging.

Those finally selected comprised 78 patients who underwent CMR examination at a median of 7 days (IQR 6-9) following admission.

Baseline clinical characteristics show the group to be young and predominantly male. Smoking and hypertension were present in a substantial proportion of patients but diabetes mellitus and previous symptoms of ischemic heart disease were infrequent.

The absence of prior symptomatic ischemic heart disease is also reflected by the small proportion of patients on cardiovascular preventive therapies prior to admission (Table 1).

In 35% of patients the culprit artery was the left anterior descending artery, in 57% of patients it was the right coronary artery, and in 8% it was the circumflex artery. No patients presented with a left main occlusion. Collateral circulation was visible in 18% (Table 2).

Table 1 Clinical characteristics of the cohort

Variables	$N = 78$
On admission	
Age, years (SD)	62 ± 11
Male sex, n (%)	65 (83)
Body mass index, kg/m^2 (IQR)	27 (25-30)
Ischemia time, minutes (IQR)	173 (140-239)
Current smoker, n (%)	24 (31)
Hypertension, n (%)	18 (23)
Dyslipidemia, n (%)	6 (8)
Previous angina, n (%)	9 (12)
Previous known diabetes mellitus, n (%)	2 (3)
Treatment on admission	
Aspirin, n (%)	5 (6)
Beta-blocker, n (%)	6 (8)
ACE/ARB, n (%)	7 (9)
Statin	6 (8)
Treatment at discharge	
Aspirin, n (%)	77 (99)
Clopidogrel, n (%)	78 (100)
Beta-blocker, n (%)	77 (99)
ACE/ARB, n (%)	44 (56)
Statin, n (%)	76 (97)

Data are presented as number of patients and percentage in brackets for dichotomous variables or median and interquartile range. *ACE* angiotensin converting enzyme inhibitor, *ARB* angiotensin receptor blocker, *IQR* inter-quartile range

Table 2 Angiographic characteristics of the cohort

Variables	$N = 78$
Infarct related artery	
LAD	27 (35)
LCx	6 (8)
RCA	45 (57)
Disease pattern	
One-vessel disease	49 (63)
Two-vessel disease	22 (28)
Three-vessel disease	7 (9)
TIMI grade 3 flow after PCI	69 (88)
Collateral flow (Rentrop grade 0 or 1)	64 (82)
Collateral flow (Rentrop grade 2 or 3)	14 (18)

Data are presented as number of patients and percentage in brackets for dichotomous variables. *LAD* left anterior descending coronary artery, *RCA* right coronary artery, *LCx* left circumflex coronary artery, *TIMI* Thrombolysis In Myocardial Infarction, *PCI* percutaneous coronary intervention
Rentrop grade 0 = no filling of distal infarct vessel by collateral vessels
Rentrop grade 1 = filling of distal infarct vessel side branches only by collateral vessels
Rentrop grade 2 = partial filling of distal infarct main vessel by collateral vessels
Rentrop grade 3 = complete filling of distal infarct main vessel by collateral vessels

There were no significant differences in the percentage MaR based on culprit vessel or background coronary disease pattern between the methods (Table 3).

All patients had a sufficient number and quality of angiographic projections to determine the culprit and non-culprit coronary anatomy.

Relationship between CE-SSFP and angiographic scores

There was a good linear correlation between the BARI and modified APPROACH scores and that derived from CMR (0.83 $p < 0.0001$ and 0.84 respectively, $p < 0.0001$) (Figs. 2 and 3). Bland-Altman analysis demonstrated that there was good agreement of the size of the MaR between CE-SSFP and angiographic scores (mean of 1.1%+/-5.2 with limits of agreement -11.4 to +9.1, and 1.2%+/-6.0 with limits of agreement -13 to +10.5, for the BARI and Modified APPROACH scores respectively) (Figs. 2 and 3).

Reproducibility amongst observers

The angiographic and CMR estimated MaR did not differ between techniques (Table 3). The inter-observer variability showed a mean difference $0.56 \pm 2.9\%$ for the BARI score ($n = 12$, 95%CI = 0.84 to 0.28), $0.42 \pm 2.1\%$ for the Modified APPROACH score ($n = 12$, 95%CI = 0.70 to 0.14) and $-1.4 \pm 3.1\%$ for the CE-SSFP technique ($n = 12$, 95%Ci = -0.36 to -2.44)). The intra-observer variability showed a mean difference $0.15 \pm 1.85\%$ for the BARI score (95%CI = 0.35 to -0.20), $0.19 \pm 1.6\%$ for the

Table 3 Myocardium at risk by method used and angiographic characteristics

Variables	CMR	BARI	APPROACH
Total MaR	30 (7.7- 56.9)	28.5 (12-50)	28.0 (12-48)
Infarct related artery			
LAD	42 (32-49)	41 (33-46)	44 (30-47)
LCx	40 (35-46)	34 (32-37)	30 (28-40)
RCA	26 (22-32)	27 (22-29)	28 (24-28)
Disease pattern			
One-vessel disease	31 (25-44)	29 (27-40)	28 (27-44)
Two-vessel disease	31 (25-39)	30 (25-34)	28 (28-28)
Three-vessel disease	24 (22-32)	22 (22-26)	24 (22-28)
Collateral flow grade 0	31 (24-43)	30 (25-39)	28 (27-44)
Collateral flow grade 1	31 (27-39)	28 (27-36)	28 (27-29)
Collateral flow grade 2 or 3	21 (7-26)	27 (22-29)	28 (22-28)

Data on percentage myocardium at risk are presented as median and interquartile range (in brackets). There were no significant differences between the methods according to infarct-related artery or underlying coronary disease pattern. *LAD* left anterior descending coronary artery, *RCA* right coronary artery, *LCx* left circumflex coronary artery, *CMR* cardiac magnetic resonance, *MaR* myocardium at risk. There were no statistically significant differences between the MaR and collateralization for each of the angiographic techniques and CMR. Friedman test $p = 0.157$ and 0.06 respectively for collaterals 0 vs 2 and 3

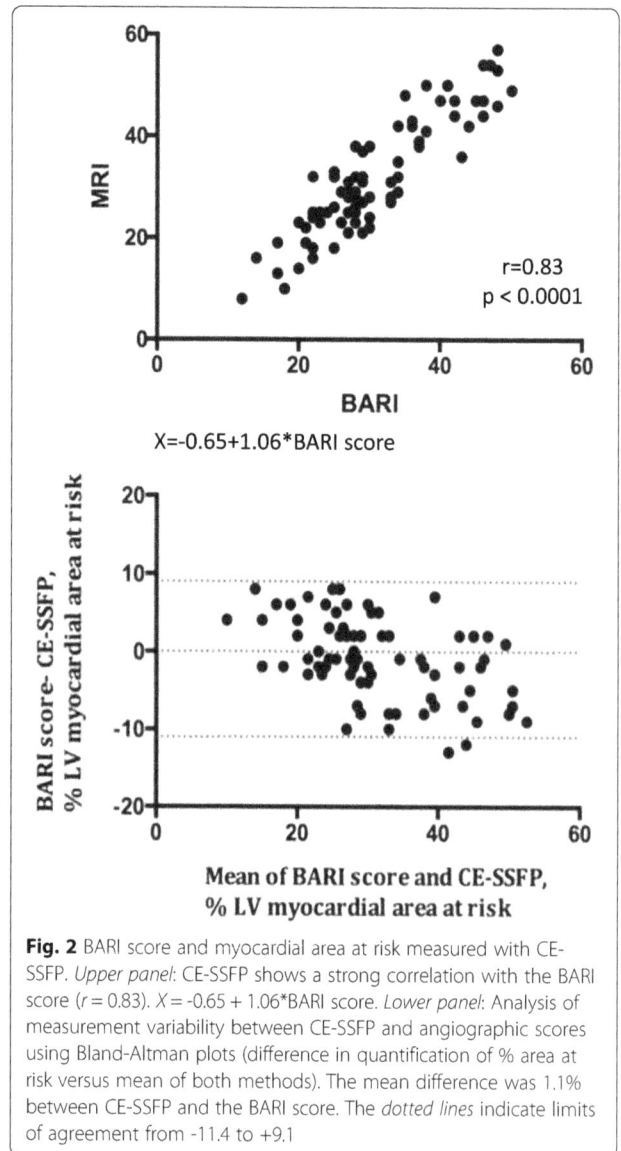

X=-0.65+1.06*BARI score

Fig. 2 BARI score and myocardial area at risk measured with CE-SSFP. *Upper panel*: CE-SSFP shows a strong correlation with the BARI score ($r = 0.83$). $X = -0.65 + 1.06*$BARI score. *Lower panel*: Analysis of measurement variability between CE-SSFP and angiographic scores using Bland-Altman plots (difference in quantification of % area at risk versus mean of both methods). The mean difference was 1.1% between CE-SSFP and the BARI score. The *dotted lines* indicate limits of agreement from -11.4 to +9.1

Modified APPROACH score (95%CI = 0.41 to -0.03) and for CE-SSFP $-0.58 \pm 2.9\%$ (95%CI = -0.04 to -1.12)

Discussion

The main finding is that contrast enhanced CE-SSFP CMR evaluation of MaR correlates well with angiographic jeopardy scores validated previously as surrogates for clinical outcome [22]. The bias was small with very mild overestimation, 1.1 and 1.2% for the BARI and Modified APPROACH scores respectively. The limits of agreement between the CMR and angiographic measurements were -11.4 to +9.1, and -13 to +10.5 for the BARI and Modified APPROACH scores respectively. There was consistent variability across the range of MaR measured.

Final infarct size in acute STEMI is a key determinant for clinical outcome and has to be determined in relation to MaR [1, 2]. Due to the large variability in

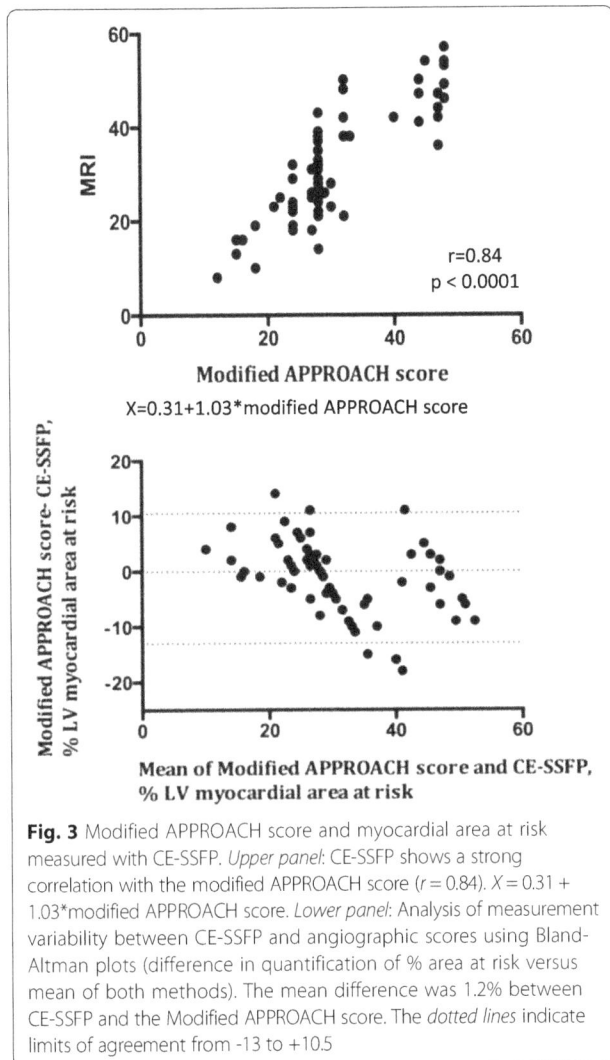

Fig. 3 Modified APPROACH score and myocardial area at risk measured with CE-SSFP. *Upper panel*: CE-SSFP shows a strong correlation with the modified APPROACH score ($r = 0.84$). $X = 0.31 + 1.03*$modified APPROACH score. *Lower panel*: Analysis of measurement variability between CE-SSFP and angiographic scores using Bland-Altman plots (difference in quantification of % area at risk versus mean of both methods). The mean difference was 1.2% between CE-SSFP and the Modified APPROACH score. The *dotted lines* indicate limits of agreement from -13 to +10.5

absolute infarct size, very large study groups are needed to achieve adequate power in clinical studies having infarct size as an end-point. Myocardial salvage is a pragmatic surrogate measurement for therapeutic efficacy of interventions aiming at limiting infarct size since it normalizes the infarct size to MaR. Thus, the use of CMR and myocardial salvage index (rather than myocardial infarction size alone) substantially reduces the study group sizes needed to evaluate efficacy in clinical trials [23]. It is therefore of utmost importance to develop feasible methods that accurately determine MaR in the clinical setting. Furthermore, the evaluation of the peri-infarct zone, which is also a feature of CMR evaluation, can add incremental prognostic value [24].

Cardiovascular magnetic resonance evaluation of myocardium at risk

CMR is increasingly recognized as equivalent to nuclear-based techniques for determining the MaR whilst also having inherent practical advantages. Several CMR sequences have been evaluated in this context including CE-SSFP [9, 11, 25, 26]. In 2012, Moral et al, compared BARI and APPROACH scores with T2-STIR and infarct endocardial surface area methods. They reported a good correlation between the different angiographic scores and their CMR-sequence [27]. The data presented here, as far as we are aware, represent the first comparison of CE-SSFP and angiographic jeopardy scores in the literature.

The advantage of this method is that it can be easily added to current standard clinical protocols, in scanners from all major vendors, simply by administering a single dose of gadolinium contrast agent before acquiring short-axis cine images. This shortens the CMR protocol in the scanner and the evaluation time after the examination since the same images can be used both for MaR determination and the evaluation of functional parameters. Unstable patients may also benefit from shorter CMR protocols.

Bright-blood T2-weighted sequences have been developed to increase the diagnostic accuracy of T2 CMR for depicting edema [28, 29]. One such sequence (ACUT2E) was more accurate for the determination of MaR and myocardial salvage than was dark-blood T2-weighted sequences, which results in underestimation of MaR [30]. Thus, CE-SSFP might be more accurate than dark-blood T2 since CE-SSFP showed larger MaR in a study by Ubachs et al [8]. Several limitations of different T2-weighted imaging protocols include a lack of consensus on the optimal quantification method, signal intensity variability within each slice and susceptibility to motion artefacts [7, 31, 32]. Newly developed T1- or T2-mapping techniques may improve accuracy considerably on these limitations when using motion correction and an absolute threshold for edema, [33–35] but further standardization and validation are still needed.

In patients, therefore, where there is no contraindication to gadolinium, the CE-SSFP may nevertheless still remain a more practical method to apply, particularly in time-constrained contemporary clinical working environments. Furthermore, the multi-phase acquisition of SSFP throughout the cardiac cycle allows for more robust delineation of endocardial and epicardial borders, less image artefacts, better spatial resolution, and as a consequence better inclusion rates of patients in clinical studies.

The mechanism for contrast-enhancement of the MaR during SSFP cannot be explained fully. The contrast in SSFP images is dependent on the sequence T2/T1 ratio. T2 relaxation times are based on the increase in tissue water content and mobility, which is a characteristic of MaR [36]. When using a gadolinium-based contrast agent, the T1 for the surrounding tissue is shortened. This is also the rationale for infarct visualization in T1-weighted inversion-recovery LGE imaging since the contrast agent distributes to the extracellular space. Here the concentration of an extracellular gadolinium-based contrast agent is increased due to an increased distribution volume in myocardium injured by ischemia [37–40]. It has been shown that even reversibly injured myocardium within the MaR has an increased distribution volume in the acute phase after an ischemic episode [41, 42]. The T2/T1 ratio in the entire MaR, including both reversible and irreversibly injured myocardium, is affected by the presence of gadolinium. This might therefore explain the increased signal intensity in the MaR seen by CE-SSFP.

There is an ongoing scientific discourse regarding the conditioning treatments of reperfusion injury and their effect on myocardial edema. Two recent studies [43, 44] have shown reduced MaR in the active group (local post-conditioning and remote pre-conditioning) of patients compared to controls, but the protocols and sequences used were not the same as the one used in our study. In addition, these studies used T2-STIR and T2-mapping respectively. The post-conditioning protocol in theory could have influenced the MaR calculated by CE-SSFP in the present study. The final infarct size and MaR, however, as judged by the extent of CE-SSFP and LGE was similar in both the control arm and post-conditioning arm. Furthermore, there were no differences in clinical outcomes between the groups. These observations suggest that any contribution of the treatment protocol to the MaR was minimal.

Collateral supply to an infarcted territory could also influence the final infarct size and MaR. Although there was no statistically significant difference between each of the angiographic quantification methods and the MaR for the extent of collateralization, there was a trend to significance with CE-SSFP evaluation ($p = 0.157$ and 0.06 respectively for Rentrop collaterals 0 vs a composite of Rentrop 2 and 3). This points to the intuitive consideration that CE-SSFP may have an added benefit as it takes the collateral supply into account whereas the rigid angiographic scoring techniques do not.

Angiographic evaluation of myocardium at risk

The modified–APPROACH score is based on pathological and necropsy studies and is derived from a template that considers the culprit artery, dominance and lesion location (proximal or mid-vessel) together with the size (small, medium or large) of the remaining major non-culprit epicardial vessel. The score in the template represents the percentage of left ventricle at risk.

The BARI score bases the anatomical area at risk and the length and caliber of the epicardial coronaries and has been validated against post-mortem histological studies [21].

Both scores have been validated with respect to adverse clinical outcome in a large population-based cohort (20,067 patients) undergoing PCI with similar c-statistics for predicting one-year mortality, when added to simple baseline characteristics, of 0.85 and 0.84 for the APPROACH and BARI scores respectively [22]. For both these angiographic scores their validity is based predominantly on left anterior descending and right coronary artery infarctions. Challenges in the electrocardiographic diagnosis of circumflex occlusion leads to under-representation of this category of infarction [45].

The BARI score is more precise than the modified APPROACH score but is also more time-consuming. The modified APPROACH score on the other hand is subject to more observer variability. This study also reflects the broader variability of the latter compared to the former on Bland-Altman analysis. Whilst the BARI score takes into consideration stenotic lesions >50% and the Modified APPROACH score considers a lesion >70% as being significant, in the context of acute STEMI this difference in scoring is not manifest as the culprit vessel is occluded. The Modified APPROACH score is based on fixed assumptions of the myocardium at risk subtended by the location of a lesion in the coronary artery and hence clustering of high, intermediate and lower values can be seen when compared with CE-SSFP. There was no difference, however, in clinical outcomes and the absolute extent of infarction or in relation to MaR as estimated by either angiographic score or CE-SSFP. In addition, there was no difference in extent of infarction when adjusted for angiographically-evident collateralization. These data thus indicate that despite the precision of the BARI score, both angiographic techniques for estimating the size of MaR appeared to be clinically equivalent in this study.

Angiographic risk scores have been used to validate single-photon emission computed tomography as well as T2 weighted CMR [7, 46].

This study was not able to disprove the hypothesis that there was no difference between angiographic scoring and CE-SSFP for the assessment of MaR, hence validating its use for this purpose. The close correlation between the angiographic and CE-SSFP measurements of myocardial area at risk adds further support that CE-SSFP may be a useful tool in studies investigating interventional, pharmacological and cardioprotective therapies in STEMI. These data and the practicality of adding early contrast enhancement to standard SSFP protocols, makes this a widely applicable method.

Limitations

The study was a single center retrospective analysis and thus subject to selection bias that may limit its external validity. The study was a post-hoc analysis from a parent study that was powered for clinical endpoints and so the analysis presented here is open to type 2 error. The results may have been influenced by the post-conditioning protocol and presence of collateral blood supply. The post-conditioning protocol, however, did not affect the overall infarct size. Furthermore, as infarct size was similar, an analysis on the differential predictive capacity for the techniques and infarct size based on therapy could not be performed

The angiographic jeopardy scores are based on anatomical assumptions and the relationships between these and other scoring systems in predicting clinical outcome is unclear.

No semi-quantitative method was used to determine MaR with the CE-SSFP sequence since the signal intensity difference between remote myocardium and MaR is small and makes it difficult to choose a fixed threshold value. Nevertheless, the inter-observer variability was excellent between the image readers. However, a new freely available semi-automatic software for estimating MaR using CE-SSFP has recently been validated and published [19]. This program can be used in all major vendors and can further decrease variability as well as increase the accuracy in estimating MaR for future reperfusion studies.

Conclusion

Quantification of MaR with contrast-enhanced SSFP imaging following acute STEMI shows high correlation and low bias compared with angiographic scoring and further supports its use as a reliable and practical method to determine myocardial salvage in this patient population.

Abbreviations

ACE: angiotensin converting enzyme inhibitor; APPROACH: Alberta Provincial Project for Outcome Assessment in Coronary Heart Disease; ARB: angiotensin receptor blocker; BARI: Bypass Angioplasty Revascularization Investigation Myocardial Jeopardy index; CE-SSFP: contrast-enhanced steady-state free precession; CI: confidence interval; CMR: cardiovascular magnetic resonance imaging; IQR: interquartile ranges; LAD: left anterior descending coronary artery; LCx: left circumflex coronary artery; LGE: late gadolinium enhancement; LV: left ventricle; MACCE: major adverse cardiovascular and cerebral events; MaR: myocardium at risk; PCI: percutaneous coronary intervention; RCA: right coronary artery; SD: standard deviation; SPECT: nuclear single photon emission computed tomography; STEMI: ST elevation myocardial infarction; TE: echo time; TIMI: Thrombolysis in Myocardial Infarction; TR: repetition time

Acknowledgements
Not applicable.

Funding
Not applicable for this study. The parent trial was funded originally by the Swedish Heart-Lung Foundation, Swedish Research Council of Medicine (10857, 14231), Stockholm County Council.

Authors' contributions
RDP data collection, data analysis and interpretation, drafting the article, critical revision of the article, final approval of the version to be published. PS data analysis and interpretation, drafting the article, critical revision of the article, final approval of the version to be published. DV critical revision of the article, final approval of the version to be published. JP Conception and design of the work, data analysis and interpretation, drafting the article, critical revision of the article, final approval of the version to be published. NS and design of the work, data collection,data analysis and interpretation, drafting the article, critical revision of the article, final approval of the version to be published.

Authors' information
Not applicable.

Competing interests
The authors declare that they have no competing interests.

References
1. Braunwald E. Myocardial reperfusion, limitation of infarct size, reduction of left ventricular dysfunction, and improved survival. Should the paradigm be expanded? Circulation. 1989;79:441–4.
2. Fibrinolytic Therapy Trialists' (FTT) Collaborative Group. Indications for fibrinolytic therapy in suspected acute myocardial infarction: collaborative overview of early mortality and major morbidity results from all randomised trials of more than 1000 patients. Lancet. 1994;343:311–22.
3. Wang QD, Pernow J, Sjoquist PO, Ryden L. Pharmacological possibilities for protection against myocardial reperfusion injury. Cardiovasc Res. 2002;55:25–37.
4. Gibbons RJ, Verani MS, Behrenbeck T, Pellikka PA, O'Connor MK, Mahmarian JJ, Chesebro JH, Wackers FJ. Feasibility of tomographic 99mTc-hexakis-2-methoxy-2-methylpropyl-isonitrile imaging for the assessment of myocardial area at risk and the effect of treatment in acute myocardial infarction. Circulation. 1989;80:1277–86.
5. De Coster PM, Wijns W, Cauwe F, Robert A, Beckers C, Melin JA. Area-at-risk determination by technetium-99 m-hexakis-2-methoxyisobutyl isonitrile in experimental reperfused myocardial infarction. Circulation. 1990;82:2152–62.
6. Sinusas AJ, Trautman KA, Bergin JD, Watson DD, Ruiz M, Smith WH, Beller GA. Quantification of area at risk during coronary occlusion and degree of myocardial salvage after reperfusion with technetium-99 m methoxyisobutyl isonitrile. Circulation. 1990;82:1424–37.
7. Fuernau G, Eitel I, Franke V, Hildebrandt L, Meissner J, de Waha S, Lurz P, Gutberlet M, Desch S, Schuler G, Thiele H. Myocardium at risk in ST-segment elevation myocardial infarction comparison of T2-weighted edema imaging with the MR-assessed endocardial surface area and validation against angiographic scoring. JACC Cardiovasc Imaging. 2011;4:967–76.
8. Ubachs JF, Sörensson P, Engblom H, Carlsson M, Jovinge S, Pernow J, Arheden H. Myocardium at risk by magnetic resonance imaging: head-to-head comparison of T2-weighted imaging and contrast-enhanced steady-state free precession. Eur Heart J Cardiovasc Imaging. 2012;13:1008–15.
9. Sörensson P, Heiberg E, Saleh N, Bouvier F, Caidahl K, Tornvall P, Rydén L, Pernow J, Arheden H. Assessment of myocardium at risk with contrast enhanced steady-state free precession cine cardiovascular magnetic resonance compared to single-photon emission computed tomography. J Cardiovasc Magn Reson. 2010;12:25.
10. Goldfarb JW, Arnold S, Han J. Recent myocardial infarction: assessment with unenhanced T1-weighted MR imaging. Radiology. 2007;245:245–50.
11. Nordlund D, Klug G, Heiberg E, Koul S, Larsen TH, Metzler B, Erlinge D, Atar D, Carlsson M, Engblom H, Arheden H. Performance of contrast enhanced SSFP and T2-weighted imaging for determining myocardium at risk in a multi-vendor, multi-center setting- data from the MITOCARE and CHILL-MI trials. J Cardiovasc Magn Reson. 2015;17 Suppl 1:194.
12. Alderman EL, Stadius M. The angiographic definitions of the Bypass Angioplasty Revascularization Investigation. Coron Artery Dis. 1992;3:1189–207.
13. Ortiz-Perez JT, Meyers SN, Lee DC, Kansal P, Klocke FJ, Holly TA, Davidson CJ, Bonow RO, Wu E. Angiographic estimates of myocardium at risk during acute myocardial infarction: validation study using cardiac magnetic resonance imaging. Eur Heart J. 2007;28:1750–8.

14. Sörensson P, Saleh N, Bouvier F, Böhm F, Settergren M, Caidahl K, Tornvall P, Arheden H, Rydén L, Pernow J. Effect of post-conditioning on infarct size in patients with ST elevation myocardial infarction. Heart. 2010;96:1710–5.

15. Kim RJ, Fieno DS, Parrish TB, Harris K, Chen EL, Simonetti O, Bundy J, Finn JP, Klocke FJ, Judd RM. Relationship of MRI delayed contrast enhancement to irreversible injury, infarct age, and contractile function. Circulation. 1999; 100:1992–2002.

16. Simonetti OP, Kim RJ, Fieno DS, Hillenbrand HB, Wu E, Bundy JM, Finn JP, Judd RM. An improved MR imaging technique for the visualization of myocardial infarction. Radiology. 2001;218:215–23.

17. Heiberg E, Sjögren J, Ugander M, Carlsson M, Engblom H, Arheden H. Design and validation of segment - a freely available software for cardiovascular image analysis. BMC Med Imaging. 2010;10:1.

18. Heiberg E, Ugander M, Engblom H, Götberg M, Olivecrona GK, Erlinge D, Arheden H. Automated quantification of myocardial infarction from MR images by accounting for partial volume effects: animal, phantom, and human study. Radiology. 2008;246:581–8.

19. Tufvesson J, Carlsson M, Aletras AH, Engblom H, Deux JF, Koul S, Sörensson P, Pernow J, Atar D, Erlinge D, Arheden H, Heiberg E. Automatic segmentation of myocardium at risk from contrast enhanced SSFP CMR: validation against expert readers and SPECT. BMC Med Imaging. 2016;16:19.

20. Brandt PW, Partridge JB, Wattie WJ. Coronary arteriography; method of presentation of the arteriogram report and a scoring system. Clin Radiol. 1977;28:361–5.

21. Kalbfleisch H, Hort W. Quantitative study on the size of coronary artery supplying areas postmortem. Am Heart J. 1977;94:183–8.

22. Graham MM, Faris PD, Ghali WA, Galbraith PD, Norris CM, Badry JT, Mitchell LB, Curtis MJ, Knudtson ML. (Alberta Provincial Project for Outcome Assessment in Coronary Heart Disease) Validation of three myocardial jeopardy scores in a population-based cardiac catheterization cohort. Am Heart J. 2001;142:254–61.

23. Engblom H, Heiberg E, Jensen SE, Nordrehaug JE, Dubois-Randé J-L, Halvorsen S, Koul S, Erlinge D, Atar D, Carlsson M, Arhedren H. Design of clinical cardioprotection trials using CMR: impact of myocardial salvage index and a narrow inclusion window on sample size. J Cardiovasc Magn Reson. 2015;17 Suppl 1:90.

24. Shayne AJ, Brown KA, Gupta SN, Chan CW, Luu TM, Di Carli MF, Reynolds HG, Stevenson WG, Kwong RY. Characterization of the peri-infarct zone by contrast-enhanced cardiac magnetic resonance imaging is a powerful predictor of post-myocardial infarction mortality. Circulation. 2006;114:32–9.

25. Erlinge D, Götberg M, Lang I, Holzer M, Noc M, Clemmensen P, Jensen U, Metzler B, James S, Bötker HE, Omerovic E, Engblom H, Carlsson M, Arheden H, Ostlund O, Wallentin L, Harnek J, Olivecrona GK. Rapid endovascular catheter core cooling combined with cold saline as an adjunct to percutaneous coronary intervention for the treatment of acute myocardial infarction. The CHILL-MI trial: a randomized controlled study of the use of central venous catheter core cooling combined with cold saline as an adjunct to percutaneous coronary intervention for the treatment of acute myocardial infarction. J Am Coll Cardiol. 2014;63:1857–65.

26. Atar D, Arheden H, Berdeaux A, Bonnet JL, Carlsson M, Clemmensen P, Cuvier V, Danchin N, Dubois-Randé JL, Engblom H, Erlinge D, Firat H, Halvorsen S, Hansen HS, Hauke W, Heiberg E, Koul S, Larsen AI, Le Corvoisier P, Nordrehaug JE, Paganelli F, Pruss RM, Rousseau H, Schaller S, Sonou G, Tuseth V, Veys J, Vicaut E, Jensen SE. Effect of intravenous TRO40303 as an adjunct to primary percutaneous coronary intervention for acute ST-elevation myocardial infarction: MITOCARE study results. Eur Heart J. 2015;36:112–9.

27. Moral S, Rodriguez-Palomares JF, Descalzo M, Marti G, Pineda V, Otaegui I, Garcia Del Blanco B, Evangelista A, Garcia-Dorado D. Quantification of myocardial area at risk: validation of coronary angiographic scores with cardiovascular magnetic resonance methods. Rev Esp Cardiol (Engl Ed). 2012;65:1010–7.

28. Aletras AH, Kellman P, Derbyshire JA, Arai AE. ACUT2E TSE-SSFP: a hybrid method for T2-weighted imaging of edema in the heart. Magn Reson Med. 2008;59:229–35.

29. Kellman P, Aletras AH, Mancini C, McVeigh ER, Arai AE. T2-prepared SSFP improves diagnostic confidence in edema imaging in acute myocardial infarction compared to turbo spin echo. Magn Reson Med. 2007;57:891–7.

30. Payne AR, Casey M, McClure J, McGeoch R, Murphy A, Woodward R, et al. Bright-blood T2-weighted MRI has higher diagnostic accuracy than dark-blood short tau inversion recovery MRI for detection of acute myocardial infarction and for assessment of the ischemic area at risk and myocardial salvage. Circ Cardiovasc Imaging. 2011;4:210–9.

31. Friedrich MG, Abdel-Aty H, Taylor A, Schulz-Menger J, Messroghli D, Dietz R. The salvaged area at risk in reperfused acute myocardial infarction as visualized by cardiovascular magnetic resonance. J Am Coll Cardiol. 2008;51:1581–7.

32. Wright J, Adriaenssens T, Dymarkowski S, Desmet W, Bogaert J. Quantification of myocardial area at risk with T2-weighted CMR: comparison with contrast-enhanced CMR and coronary angiography. JACC Cardiovasc Imaging. 2009;2:825–31.

33. Giri S, Chung YC, Merchant A, Mihai G, Rajagopalan S, Raman SV, Simonetti OP. T2 quantification for improved detection of myocardial edema. J Cardiovasc Magn Reson. 2009;11:56.

34. Ugander M, Bagi PS, Oki AJ, Chen B, Hsu LY, Aletras AH, Shah S, Greiser A, Kellman P, Arai AE. Myocardial edema as detected by pre-contrast T1 and T2 CMR delineates area at risk associated with acute myocardial infarction. JACC Cardiovasc Imaging. 2012;5:596–603.

35. Nordlund D, Klug G, Heiberg E, Koul S, Larsen TH, Hoffmann P, Metzler B, Erlinge D, Atar D, Aletras AH, Carlsson M, Engblom H, Arheden H. Multi-vendor, multicentre comparison of contrast-enhanced SSFP and T2-STIR CMR for determining myocardium at risk in ST-elevation myocardial infarction. Eur Heart J Cardiovasc Imaging. 2016;17:744–53.

36. Higgins CB, Herfkens R, Lipton MJ, Sievers R, Sheldon P, Kaufman L, Crooks LE. Nuclear magnetic resonance imaging of acute myocardial infarction in dogs: alterations in magnetic relaxation times. Am J Cardiol. 1983;52:184–8.

37. García-Dorado D, Oliveras J, Gili J, Sanz E, Pérez-Villa F, Barrabés J, Carreras MJ, Solares J, Soler-Soler J. Analysis of myocardial oedema by magnetic resonance imaging early after coronary artery occlusion with or without reperfusion. Cardiovasc Res. 1993;27:1462–9.

38. Aletras AH, Tilak GS, Natanzon A, Hsu LY, Gonzalez FM, Hoyt Jr RF, Arai AE. Retrospective determination of the area at risk for reperfused acute myocardial infarction with T2-weighted cardiac magnetic resonance imaging: histopathological and displacement encoding with stimulated echoes (DENSE) functional validations. Circulation. 2006;113:1865–70.

39. Diesbourg LD, Prato FS, Wisenberg G, Drost DJ, Marshall TP, Carroll SE, O'Neill B. Quantification of myocardial blood flow and extracellular volumes using a bolus injection of Gd-DTPA: kinetic modeling in canine ischemic disease. Magn Reson Med. 1992;23:239–53.

40. Saeed M, Wendland MF, Masui T, Higgins CB. Reperfused myocardial infarctions on T1- and susceptibility-enhanced MRI: evidence for loss of compartmentalization of contrast media. Magn Reson Med. 1994;31:31–9.

41. Arheden H, Saeed M, Higgins CB, Gao DW, Bremerich J, Wyttenbach R, Dae MW, Wendland MF. Measurement of the distribution volume of gadopentetate dimeglumine at echoplanar MR imaging to quantify myocardial infarction: comparison with 99mTc-DTPA autoradiography in rats. Radiology. 1999;211:698–708.

42. Arheden H, Saeed M, Higgins CB, Gao DW, Ursell PC, Bremerich J, Wyttenbach R, Dae MW, Wendland MF. Reperfused rat myocardium subjected to various durations of ischemia: estimation of the distribution volume of contrast material with echo-planar MR imaging. Radiology. 2000;215:520–8.

43. Thuny F, Lairez O, Roubille F, Mewton N, Rioufol G, Sportouch C, Sanchez I, Bergerot C, Thibault H, Cung TT, Finet G, Argaud L, Revel D, Derumeaux G, Bonnefoy-Cudraz E, Elbaz M, Piot C, Ovize M, Croisille P. Postconditioning reduces infarct size and edema in patients with ST-segment elevation myocardial infarction. J Am Coll Cardiol. 2012;59:2175–81.

44. White SK, Frohlich GM, Sado DM, Maestrini V, Fontana M, Treibel TA, Meier P, Ariti C, Davies JR, Moon JC, Yellon DM, Hausenloy DJ. Remote ischemic conditioning reduces myocardial infarct size and edema in patients with ST-segment elevation myocardial infarction. JACC Cardiovasc Interv. 2015;8:178–88.

45. Josephson ME. Use of the electrocardiogram in acute myocardial infarction. N Engl J Med. 2003;348:933–40.

11

Improving visualization of 4D flow cardiovascular magnetic resonance with four-dimensional angiographic data: generation of a 4D phase-contrast magnetic resonance CardioAngiography (4D PC-MRCA)

Mariana Bustamante[1,2], Vikas Gupta[1,2], Carl-Johan Carlhäll[1,3] and Tino Ebbers[1,2]*

Abstract

Magnetic Resonance Angiography (MRA) and Phase-Contrast MRA (PC-MRA) approaches used for assessment of cardiovascular morphology typically result in data containing information from the entire cardiac cycle combined into one 2D or 3D image. Information specific to each timeframe of the cardiac cycle is, however, lost in this process. This study proposes a novel technique, called Phase-Contrast Magnetic Resonance CardioAngiography (4D PC-MRCA), that utilizes the full potential of 4D Flow CMR when generating temporally resolved PC-MRA data to improve visualization of the heart and major vessels throughout the cardiac cycle. Using non-rigid registration between the timeframes of the 4D Flow CMR acquisition, the technique concentrates information from the entire cardiac cycle into an angiographic dataset at one specific timeframe, taking movement over the cardiac cycle into account. Registration between the timeframes is used once more to generate a time-resolved angiography. The method was evaluated in ten healthy volunteers. Visual comparison of the 4D PC-MRCAs versus PC-MRAs generated from 4D Flow CMR using the traditional approach was performed by two observers using Maximum Intensity Projections (MIPs). The 4D PC-MRCAs resulted in better visibility of the main anatomical regions of the cardiovascular system, especially where cardiac or vessel motion was present. The proposed method represents an improvement over previous PC-MRA generation techniques that rely on 4D Flow CMR, as it effectively utilizes all the information available in the acquisition. The 4D PC-MRCA can be used to visualize the motion of the heart and major vessels throughout the entire cardiac cycle.

Keywords: Computer-Assisted Image Analysis, 4D flow cardiovascular magnetic resonance (4D flow CMR), Phase-Contrast Magnetic Resonance Angiography (PC-MRA)

Introduction

Magnetic Resonance Angiography (MRA) is a commonly used technique for vessel visualization, utilized routinely to detect or evaluate pathologies such as stenoses, aneurysms or vascular anomalies. Conventional MRA commonly relies on the use of external agents for contrast enhancement, as opposed to Phase-Contrast MRA (PC-MRA) where the contrast is generated using phase differences in the MR signal [1, 2]. PC-MRA data are typically acquired without cardiac gating in a breath-hold. Consequently, any motion present during the cardiac cycle will be averaged in the resulting image, likely becoming difficult to perceive.

Three-dimensional (3D) cine (time-resolved) phase-contrast cardiovascular magnetic resonance (CMR) with three-directional velocity-encoding (4D Flow CMR) is a technique that permits visualization and evaluation of

* Correspondence: tino.ebbers@liu.se
[1]Division of Cardiovascular Medicine, Department of Medical and Health Sciences, Linköping University, Linköping, Sweden
[2]Center for Medical Image Science and Visualization (CMIV), Linköping University, Linköping, Sweden
Full list of author information is available at the end of the article

the pulsatile blood flows in the chambers of the heart and great thoracic vessels over the cardiac cycle in a single acquisition [3]. In 4D Flow CMR, data is acquired using cardiac electrocardiography (ECG) gating. Therefore, the resulting images also include information about the motion of the heart and vessels over the cardiac cycle. Considerably similar images to those obtained when using PC-MRA are often generated from the 4D Flow CMR data for orientation and visualization purposes. During this process, motion over the cardiac cycle is typically averaged and consequently lost.

Different methods for 3D PC-MRA data generation from 4D Flow CMR have been proposed and evaluated [4–6]. These methods combine and average the velocity and magnitude information over the cardiac cycle. The velocities yield higher intensities in the resulting image in areas of high blood flow, while the magnitude signal adds morphological information and mitigates noise in areas of very low signal, such as the lungs. For N timeframes, [3, 5], and [7], proposed the following equation:

$$3DPC\text{--}MRA = \frac{1}{N}\sum_{t=1}^{N}M^2(t) * \sqrt{\left(V_x^2(t) + V_y^2(t) + V_z^2(t)\right)}$$

(1)

While [6] proposed the following:

$$3DPC\text{--}MRA = \sqrt{\frac{1}{N}\sum_{t=1}^{N}M^2(t) * \left(V_x^2(t) + V_y^2(t) + V_z^2(t)\right)}$$

(2)

In these equations, t is the corresponding timeframe, V_x, V_y and V_z are the blood flow velocity components in three spatial directions, and M is the magnitude of the signals acquired during the 4D Flow CMR acquisition. The 3D PC-MRAs generated from 4D Flow CMR data are often visualized using Maximum Intensity Projections (MIPs) or isosurface renderings, resulting in slightly different angiographic images, as shown in Fig. 1.

In addition to vessel visualization, the generated data can also be used to segment the blood lumen, which may be necessary for further analyses, such as flow assessments [8–10], or wall shear stress (WSS) estimation [11]. A 3D PC-MRA generated from 4D Flow CMR using the described approaches will have the same features and limitations as a standard PC-MRA, such as the smoothing of moving structures. This hampers visualization of the heart chambers and can affect the calculation of parameters that rely on segmentation. For example, when estimating WSS from a time-averaged PC-MRA, the movement of the aortic wall due to the natural distension and recoil motion of the aorta over the cardiac cycle is usually not accounted for [12].

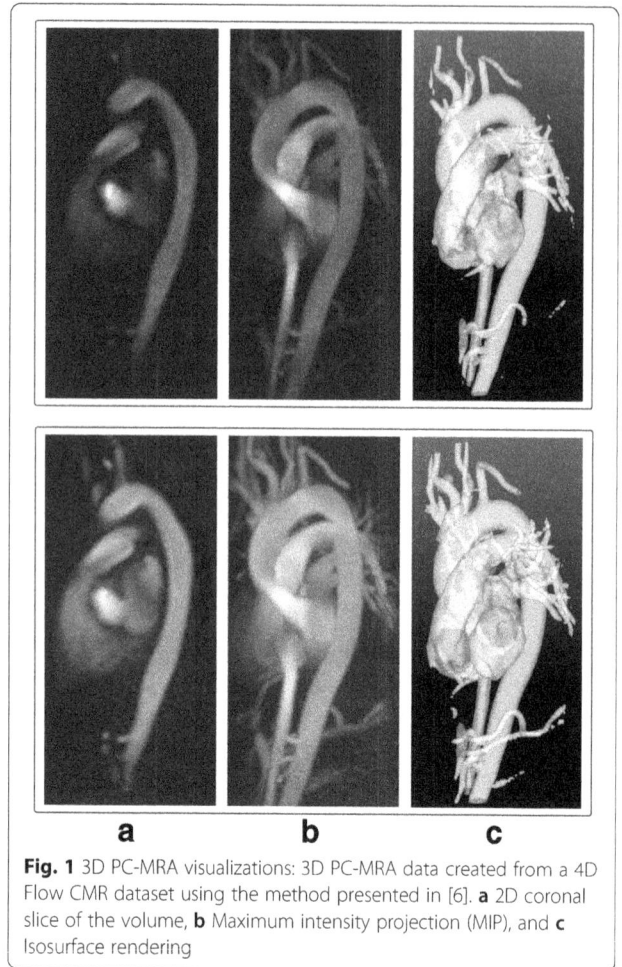

Fig. 1 3D PC-MRA visualizations: 3D PC-MRA data created from a 4D Flow CMR dataset using the method presented in [6]. **a** 2D coronal slice of the volume, **b** Maximum intensity projection (MIP), and **c** Isosurface rendering

The goal of this study is to present and evaluate a novel technique, called 4D Phase-Contrast Magnetic Resonance CardioAngiography (4D PC-MRCA), that utilizes the full potential of 4D Flow CMR for the visualization of heart chambers ("cardio") and vessels ("angio").

The purpose of creating a 4D PC-MRCA is two-fold: first, to allow the visualization of both the motion of the heart and major vessels throughout the cardiac cycle by generating an image that is time-resolved; and second, to enhance the intensities in the heart ventricles and atria to improve their discernibility. The 4D PC-MRCA is not intended to substitute the conventional contrast-enhanced MR angiography (CE-MRA); instead, it aims to improve the visualization of 4D Flow CMR.

Methods

Creation of a 4D Phase-Contrast Magnetic Resonance CardioAngiography (4D PC-MRCA)

A 4D Flow CMR dataset can be seen as a series of three-dimensional volumes over time (4D), where each volume contains magnitude information as well as three-directional velocity information.

In order to allow for visualization of temporal changes in the geometry of both the thoracic vessels and the heart over a cardiac cycle, the 4D PC-MRCAs were generated using the following steps:

1. PC-MRA data were generated for every available timeframe using equation 3 for each voxel in the magnitude and velocity data included in the 4D Flow CMR dataset.

$$PC-MRA(t) = M(t) * \left(V_x^2(t) + V_y^2(t) + V_z^2(t)\right)^\gamma \quad (3)$$

Gamma (γ) correction of 0.2 was used to enhance the velocity values and to make sure that the lower velocities, such as those present in the heart chambers, were also included in the image. The resulting 4D image retains the information specific to each timeframe of the cardiac cycle.

2. All the timeframes of the 4D Flow CMR magnitude image were aligned to one timeframe of the cardiac cycle using non-rigid registration. For the selected datasets belonging to healthy volunteers, this timeframe was chosen to be during mid-diastole (diastasis), when the heart was at an intermediate position between early and late ventricular diastole. For N timeframes in a cardiac cycle, this resulted in $N-1$ transformations, B_t, each corresponding to one timeframe, t. See Fig. 2 for further clarification of this step.

3. Each timeframe, t, of the PC-MRA data created in step 1 was transformed using the corresponding deformation field, B_t, to generate a set of images with intensities that depend on the blood flow patterns at each timeframe, but with the shape and morphology expected in the chosen diastasis timeframe.

4. A 3D PC-MRCA was calculated as an MIP of these images over time. These data contain high contrast in all sections of the cardiovascular system where high blood flow occurs at least once during the heartbeat, and morphologically corresponds to one specific timeframe of the cardiac cycle. The maximum of the

images over time was preferred over the average in order to preserve visibility in the heart chambers, where the contrast is usually lower.

5. A new set of registrations were executed. In this case, the magnitude image of the chosen diastasis timeframe was registered to the remaining timeframes of the cardiac cycle. This resulted in $N-1$ transformations, F_t, one for each timeframe, t, that were then applied to the 3D PC-MRCA in order to obtain a time-resolved (four-dimensional) PC-MRCA.

A non-rigid registration method based on the Morphon algorithm was used for this study [13]. The implementation uses diffeomorphic field accumulation, together with fluid and elastic regularization of the displacement fields in order to generate physically plausible deformations [14]. The regularization parameters were initially determined following the settings from a previous study where the same registration method was used on clinical computed tomography (CT) images [15]. Further tuning of these parameters for the current application resulted in the following settings:

- Number of scales: 2
- Number of iterations per scale: 3
- Gaussian kernel with σ of 1.5 pixels for both fluid and elastic regularization.

The 4D PC-MRCA generation tool created for this project was implemented using MATLAB (release 2015b, The MathWorks, Inc., Natick, Massachusetts, USA).

Study population

Evaluation of the proposed method was performed on ten 4D Flow CMR datasets acquired from healthy volunteers with no prior history of cardiovascular disease or cardiovascular medication. The group's mean age was 66±4, within the range 59–71, and included 9 females and 1 male.

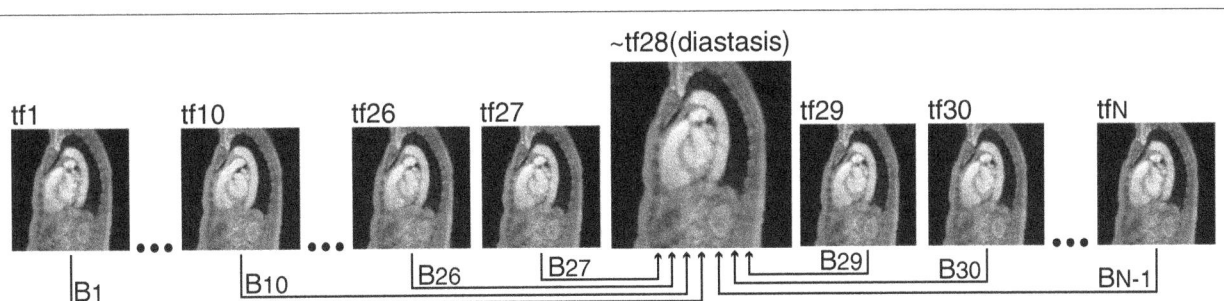

Fig. 2 4D PC-MRCA creation, step 2: Registration of every timeframe of the average magnitude image to a timeframe in mid-diastole (diastasis), resulting in $N-1$ transformations, B_t

4D Flow CMR examinations were performed on a clinical 3 T Philips Ingenia scanner (Philips Healthcare, Best, the Netherlands) and were acquired during free-breathing, using a navigator gated gradient-echo pulse sequence with interleaved three-directional flow-encoding and retrospective vector cardiogram controlled cardiac gating. All subjects were injected with a Gd contrast agent (Magnevist, Bayer Schering Pharma AG) prior to the acquisition for a late-enhancement study. Scan parameters included: Candy cane view adjusted to cover both ventricles, velocity encoding (VENC) 120 cm/s, flip angle 10°, echo time 2.6 ms, repetition time 4.4 ms, parallel imaging (SENSE) speed up factor 3 (AP direction), k-space segmentation factor 3, acquired temporal resolution of 52.8 ms, spatial resolution $2.7 \times 2.7 \times 2.7$ mm^3, and elliptical k-space acquisition. The typical scan time was 7–8 min excluding and 10–15 min including the navigator gating.

The 4D Flow CMR data were corrected for concomitant gradient fields on the CMR scanner. Offline processing corrected for phase wraps using a temporal phase unwrapping method [16], and background phase errors were corrected using a weighted 2nd order polynomial fit to the static tissue [17].

Noise caused by the presence of air in the velocity data was suppressed by thresholding the signal intensity in the magnitude data. Values lower than 10% of the maximum magnitude value were ignored, as proposed in [7]. Also, voxels with an absolute velocity value more than 50% higher than the velocity encoding (VENC) were ignored. This suppressed a few scattered voxels (on average 0.011% of all voxels) with very noisy velocity information but a magnitude value above the magnitude threshold.

Evaluation

4D PC-MRCA and 3D PC-MRA data were generated for each dataset, and MIPs of each method were used to assess the resulting images. Anatomical regions of the cardiovascular system were scored according to their visibility in the projections, emphasizing the diagnostic quality of the evaluated image. The scoring was performed independently by two observers: a clinician with 5 years of experience in cardiovascular imaging, and an image analyst with 3 years of experience in cardiovascular imaging. Each score was based on the following scale: 1 = poor, region not visible, of no diagnostic quality; 2 = fair, region faintly visible, but not of diagnostic quality; 3 = good, complete region visible, of diagnostic quality; 4 = excellent, region clearly defined, of excellent diagnostic quality. The scores for each method were compared using the Wilcoxon rank-sum test. A p-value < 0.05 was considered to represent a significant difference between techniques.

To serve as comparison to the proposed method, 3D PC-MRA data were generated for this study using the method presented by Hennemuth et al. (2) since, similar to the 4D PC-MRCA, this method also retains higher intensities inside the heart. In contrast, other previously proposed 3D PC-MRA techniques focus mostly on the vessels and apply strong background suppression, thereby leaving very low intensities in and around the heart.

Results

Figure 3 shows different visualization methods applied to a 4D PC-MRCA in parts (a), (b), and (c). Additionally, part (d) shows isosurface renderings for three different timeframes of the four-dimensional image in which the approximate contour of the left ventricle has been indicated in red for visualization purposes. The corresponding movies for the entire cardiac cycle, including all the available timeframes, have been included as supplementary material.

An MIP for each timeframe available in the dataset can be calculated from the 4D PC-MRCA. In contrast, the 3D PC-MRA results in a single volume not representing any particular timeframe. Videos corresponding to each MIP were created using 36 angle projections, and have been included as supplementary material.

Isosurface renderings generated from 3D PC-MRAs and 4D PC-MRCAs for two datasets are shown in Fig. 4, only three different timeframes of the 4D image are shown due to space constraints. The corresponding movies for the entire cardiac cycle have been included as supplementary material. Additionally, the boundaries of the isosurfaces of the PC-MRA and PC-MRCA at two timeframes are compared in Fig. 5. Videos including the entire cardiac cycle have been included as supplementary material. Note that the 3D PC-MRA data is not time-resolved; consequently, the same isosurface was used for the different timeframes pictured. In this image, discrepancies can be observed between the PC-MRA and the location of the vessels as a consequence of vessel motion, especially during end-diastole.

Figure 6 (top) shows the average scores from the MIPs of 3D PC-MRA and 4D PC-MRCA data at a mid-diastolic timeframe. Figure 6 (bottom) illustrates the differences between the angiographies according to the percentiles obtained by each score in the scale. Detailed scores can be seen in Table 1. The differences between the scores obtained by both techniques were highly significant (4.97), with p < 0.001.

The 4D PC-MRCAs received higher scores than the 3D PC-MRAs in most cases. Noteworthy results were the higher scores obtained when evaluating the left and right chambers of the heart.

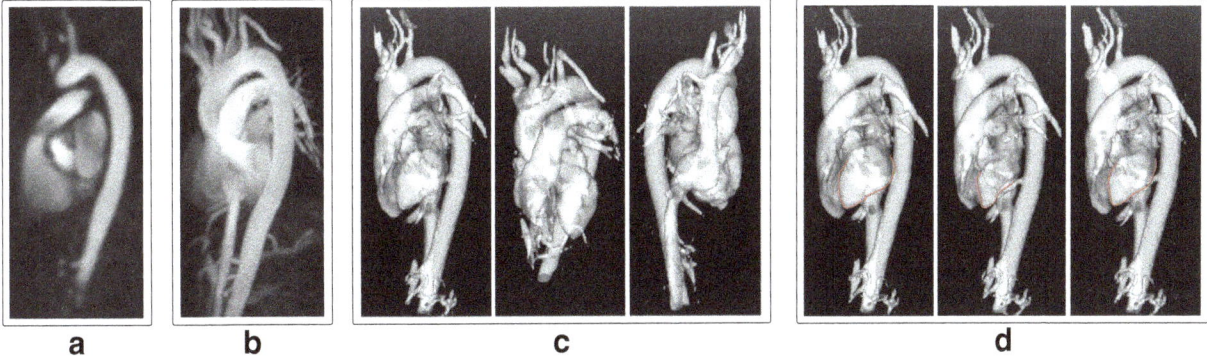

Fig. 3 Visualization of a 4D PC-MRCA: **a** Coronal slice at a mid-diastolic timeframe. **b** Maximum Intensity Projection (MIP) at a mid-diastolic timeframe. **c** Isosurface renderings from three different points of view at an end-diastolic timeframe. **d** Isosurface renderings for three timeframes of the cardiac cycle (end-diastole, systole, mid-diastole). For visualization purposes, the left ventricle has been delineated in red for each timeframe

Fig. 4 Method comparison using isosurfaces: 3D PC-MRA and 4D PC-MRCA isosurface renderings generated for two 4D Flow CMR datasets (*top and bottom*). The left ventricle has been highlighted in red in all the images for visualization purposes

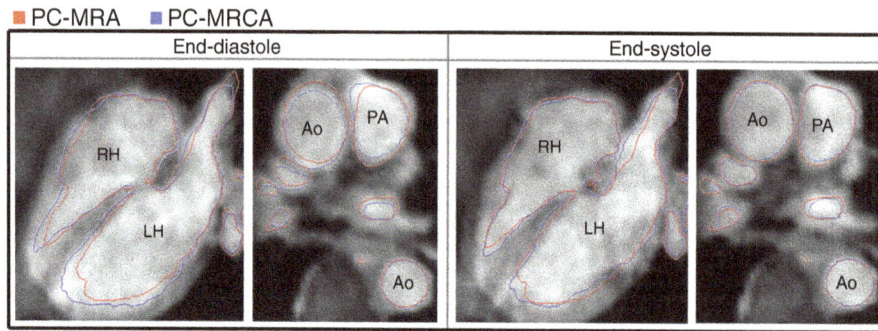

Fig. 5 Comparison of isosurface boundaries: PC-MRA (*red*) and PC-MRCA (*blue*) at two timeframes. The visible regions are: Left ventricle and atrium (*left heart*, LH), right ventricle and atrium (*right heart*, RH), aorta (Ao), and pulmonary artery (PA)

Discussion

The proposed method to calculate 4D PC-MRCA data from 4D Flow CMR permits visualization of the cardiovascular system from several viewpoints, together with the possibility of observing the motion of the heart and vessels during the entire cardiac cycle. This represents an improvement over the existing techniques for 3D PC-MRA generation from 4D Flow CMR and can be an advantage in clinical practice, particularly when the type of clinical question being assessed is influenced by cardiovascular wall motion.

During the visual evaluation, 4D PC-MRCA outperformed 3D PC-MRA obtaining higher averages and scores of mainly threes and fours on the defined scale, compared to mostly twos or threes for the PC-MRA (see Fig. 6). Furthermore, the movement of the myocardial and vascular walls over the cardiac cycle produced disparities in the 3D PC-MRA in several timeframes.

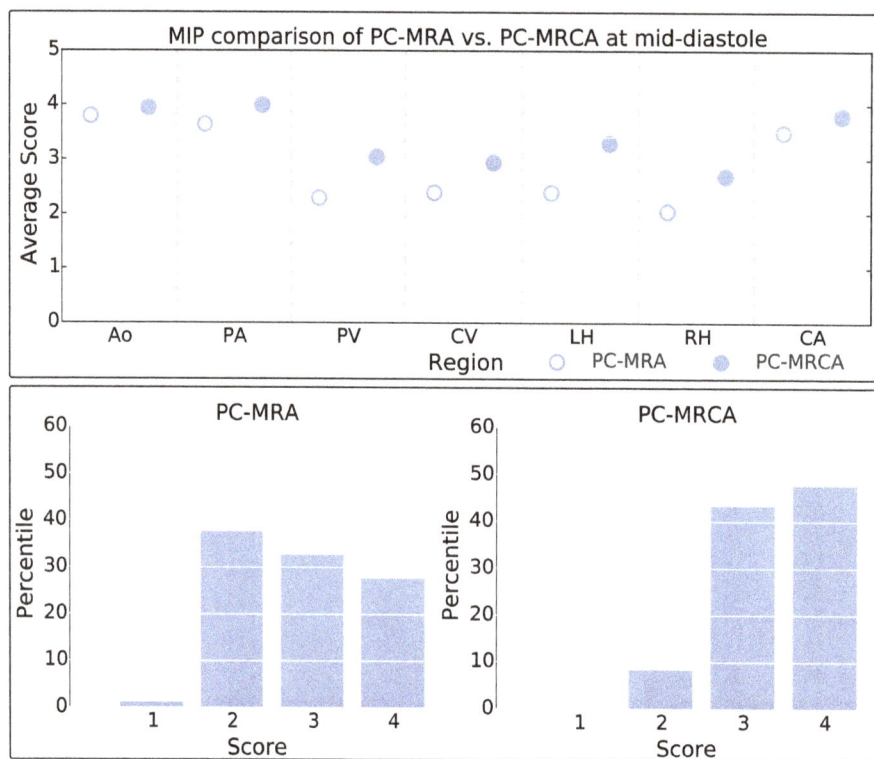

Fig. 6 Visual evaluation results: Top: Average scores obtained by the MIPs of the PC-MRA and PC-MRCA at mid-diastole. The regions evaluated were: Aorta (Ao), pulmonary arteries (PA), pulmonary veins (PV), caval veins (CV), left ventricle and atrium (LH), right ventricle and atrium (RH), and carotid arteries (CA). The differences for LH, RH, PV, and CV are statistically significant ($p < 0.05$). Bottom: Percentile of scores obtained for each value in the scale by the MIPs of the PC-MRA (*left*) and the PC-MRCA at mid-diastole (*right*). The difference between the scores obtained by the PC-MRA and those obtained by the PC-MRCA is statistically significant ($p < 0.001$)

Table 1 Detailed visual evaluation scores

Region	3D PC-MRA				4D PC-MRCA (mid-diastole)			
	Score:1	Score:2	Score:3	Score:4	Score:1	Score:2	Score:3	Score:4
Aorta	[0,0]	[0,0]	[2,2]	[8,8]	[0,0]	[0,0]	[1,0]	[9,10]
Pulmonary arteries	[0,0]	[0,0]	[2,5]	[8,5]	[0,0]	[0,0]	[0,0]	[10,10]
Pulmonary veins	[0,0]	[7,7]	[3,3]	[0,0]	[0,0]	[1,1]	[7,8]	[2,1]
Caval veins	[0,0]	[8,4]	[2,6]	[0,0]	[0,0]	[1,2]	[9,6]	[0,2]
Left ventricle and atrium	[0,0]	[5,7]	[5,3]	[0,0]	[0,0]	[0,1]	[5,7]	[5,2]
Right ventricle and atrium	[2,0]	[8,7]	[0,3]	[0,0]	[0,0]	[3,3]	[7,7]	[0,0]
Carotid arteries	[0,0]	[0,0]	[4,6]	[6,4]	[0,0]	[0,0]	[1,3]	[9,7]

Number of datasets that received the indicated score during visual evaluation of the MIP generated for the PC-MRA and PC-MRCA at mid-diastole. [Observer 1, Observer 2]. Scale: 1 = poor, region not visible, of no diagnostic quality; 2 = fair, region faintly visible, but not of diagnostic quality; 3 = good, complete region visible, of diagnostic quality; 4 = excellent, region clearly defined, of excellent diagnostic quality

These problems were especially visible in the ascending aorta and pulmonary artery, two regions frequently assessed with angiographic images. An example of such discrepancies can be seen in Fig. 5 at end-diastole.

Accurate depiction of the vessel wall over the cardiac cycle is important in obtaining accurate measurements of vessel size, as this can vary significantly throughout the cardiac cycle. It also enables an accurate computation of certain parameters, such as WSS, which has been studied intensively in the ascending aorta and carotid arteries. Furthermore, previous studies have emphasized the necessity for accurate vessel wall location for WSS calculation [12, 18]. Its analysis, however, has so far been focused on peak values. Accurate segmentation of the vessel wall over the complete cardiac cycle would allow for computation of additional interesting WSS parameters, such as oscillatory shear index (OSI) [19].

The presented method is completely automatic. Consequently, it can be easily added to the existing post-processing algorithms already required by 4D Flow CMR acquisitions, e.g., transformation from DICOM to other formats, background correction, phase unwrapping, etc.

Although the resulting images are not precise enough to be used directly in the segmentation of the cardiac ventricles and atria, the 4D PC-MRCAs enabled sufficient description of the location, motion, and size of the cardiac chambers to fulfill the goal of visualization of the cardiovascular system over the entire cardiac cycle. It was not the aim of this study to evaluate a potential segmentation method resulting from the PC-MRCA data. However, a combination of the PC-MRCA and advanced segmentation techniques is expected to result in better segmentation of the cardiac chambers on 4D Flow MR images.

We have evaluated the method on 10 healthy volunteers. The presented method is, however, also expected to be able to aid in the visualization of subjects with pathological features such as vascular disease, heart valve disease, and myocardial disease affecting the size or shape of the heart. The PC-MRCA generated from a dataset with a dilated left ventricle with at least moderately depressed systolic function has been included as supplementary material. In pathological cases involving severe jet flow, signal void may occur in the PC-MRI data, which is known to affect traditional PC-MRA. This signal void is also expected to affect the PC-MRCA, but possibly to a lesser extent. The concept used in computing the PC-MRCA allows for the utilization of information from the whole cardiac cycle. Jet flow typically only occurs in either systole or diastole. By utilizing information from the complete cardiac cycle, the cardiac phases without signal void can be used in the PC-MRCA. This could be a subject of future research.

The specific equation used to combine the magnitude and velocity images in step 1 of the described method should depend on the required aim of the PC-MRCA images. In this evaluation, we did not focus on background suppression in favor of increasing the intensities in areas of lower flow velocities. Changes to the proposed equation can be made in order to enhance different areas of the image or to achieve stronger background suppression. For instance, an optimal depiction of the aortic wall could be achieved by replacing equation (3) with an equation similar to equation (1). This might produce a slightly better delineation of the aorta, but at the cost of a lower quality depiction of other anatomical regions. Moreover, using average instead of maximum to create the diastasis-located image in step 4 of the PC-MRCA creation could be particularly useful if the input data is noisy.

The generation of one 4D PC-MRCA took on average twenty minutes on a system with 64GB of RAM and a 6-core 3.5GHz processor. The current implementation included parallel execution of multiple registrations. Further improvements to the running time can be achieved by employing GPU programming, or by taking advantage of the fact that the second set of registrations required (step 5 of the method) correspond to the inverse of the transformations obtained during the first set of registrations (step 2 of the method). Consequently, both sets of transformations, B_t and F_t for a timeframe t, could be calculated together in step 2.

As an additional measure of the accuracy of the non-rigid registration, the inverse consistency of the deformation fields B_t and F_t was assessed by comparing the image intensities of each timeframe of the magnitude image after applying both the backward and forward registrations. The magnitude images had intensities in the range [0-1], thus the maximum possible error is 1. The sum of squared errors (± standard deviation) obtained for all the datasets included in the study was $8.940 * 10^{-5} \pm 2.811 * 10^{-4}$. This inverse consistency error was considered to be sufficiently small to result in accurate registrations.

Limitations

Most of the structures fared well after registration was applied to them in order to represent the motion that occurs during a heartbeat. However, in the evaluated datasets, the caval veins and right atrium of the heart were located very close to the border of the 4D Flow CMR image, and were on a few occasions deformed incorrectly by the registration.

Currently, 4D Flow CMR images are often acquired after injection of a contrast agent for CE-MRA or delayed contrast-enhanced CMR studies. In some cases,

even blood pool agents are used [20, 21]. Also in this study, the 4D flow CMR acquisition was preceded by an injection of an extracellular contrast agent for delayed contrast-enhaced CMR. Traces of this contrast agent were still present during the 4D Flow CMR acquisitions, improving the contrast between the blood and the remaining tissues. The presented method was not evaluated in depth on images without any contrast agent. However, preliminary results on this type of datasets showed promising results, and example of such can be seen in Fig. 7. To generate angiographic data from 4D Flow CMR acquired without previous Gadolinium contrast injection, while still maintaining the same quality as the currently presented PC-MRCAs, would most likely require modifications on the technique in order to account for the lower contrast expected in these images.

Conclusions

The proposed technique to derive a time-resolved three-dimensional phase-contrast Magnetic Resonance CardioAngiography (4D PC-MRCA) outperformed previous techniques to obtain angiographic data from 4D Flow CMR during visual evaluation. The 4D PC-MRCA allows for visualization of the cardiovascular anatomy, including the heart chambers, over the cardiac cycle. This facilitates orientation and enhances visualization of 4D Flow CMR data. Moreover, it might also lead to time-resolved segmentation of this type of acquisitions, which may allow for improved analysis of useful hemodynamic parameters over the complete cardiac cycle.

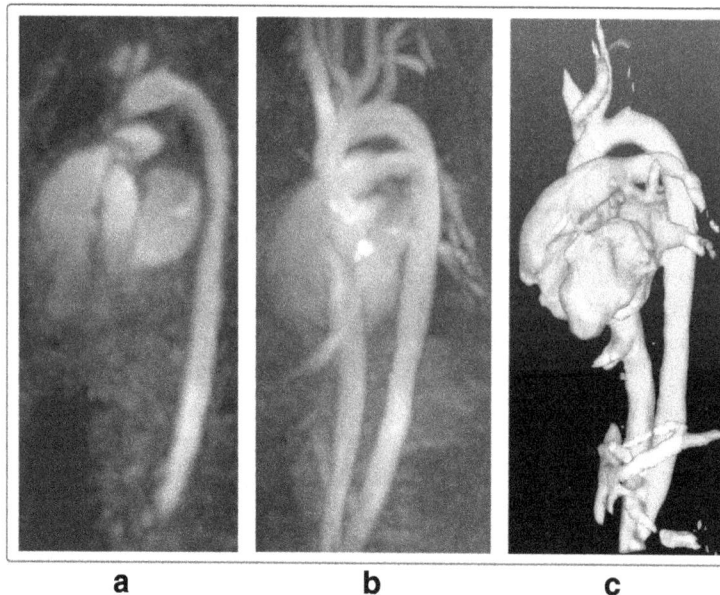

Fig. 7 4D PC-MRCA from a dataset acquired without contrast agent: Visualized at a mid-diastolic timeframe. **a** Coronal slice, **b** Maximum Intensity Projection (MIP), and **c** Isosurface rendering

Additional files

Additional file 1: 4D PC-MRCA, dataset 1. Isosurface rendering visualization of a 4D PC-MRCA throughout the cardiac cycle.

Additional file 2: 4D PC-MRCA, dataset 2. Isosurface rendering visualization of a 4D PC-MRCA throughout the cardiac cycle.

Additional file 3: 4D PC-MRCA MIP at end-diastole. Maximum Intensity Projection (MIP) of a 4D PC-MRCA at end-diastole created using 36 angle projections.

Additional file 4: 4D PC-MRCA MIP at mid-diastole. Maximum Intensity Projection (MIP) of a 4D PC-MRCA at mid-diastole created using 36 angle projections.

Additional file 5: 4D PC-MRCA MIP at end-systole. Maximum Intensity Projection (MIP) of a 4D PC-MRCA at end-systole created using 36 angle projections.

Additional file 6: Isosurface comparison of PC-MRA and PC-MRCA in the heart. Boundaries of the isosurfaces of the PC-MRA and PC-MRCA throughout the cardiac cycle superimposed in a four-chamber view of the 4D Flow CMR magnitude image.

Additional file 7: Isosurface comparison of PC-MRA and PC-MRCA in the major vessels. Boundaries of the isosurfaces of the PC-MRA and PC-MRCA throughout the cardiac cycle superimposed in a slice of the 4D Flow CMR magnitude image where the ascending aorta, descending aorta, and pulmonary artery are visible.

Additional file 8: 4D PC-MRCA, dataset 3. Isosurface rendering visualization of a 4D PC-MRCA throughout the cardiac cycle for a subject with an enlarged left ventricle and depressed systolic function (Ejection Fraction = 33%).

Abbreviations
CE-MRA: Contrast Enhanced Magnetic Resonance Angiography; CMR: Cardiovascular Magnetic Resonance; MIP: Maximum Intensity Projection; OSI: Oscillating Shear Index; PC-MRA: Phase-Contrast Magnetic Resonance Angiography; PC-MRCA: Phase-Contrast Magnetic Resonance CardioAngiography; WSS: Wall Shear Stress.

Acknowledgements
The authors would like to thank Alexandru Fredriksson for the valuable help provided during the evaluation of the results.

Funding
This work was supported by the European Research Council [grant number 310612], the Swedish Heart and Lung foundation [grant number 20140398], the Swedish Research Council [grant number 621-2014-6191].

Authors' contributions
All authors participated in the conception and design of the study. C.-J.C. preformed the recruitment of subjects and carried out the data acquisition. M.B. and V.G. participated in the implementation of the method. M.B. performed the evaluation of the results. M.B. drafted the manuscript. All authors edited and revised the manuscript. All authors read and approved the final manuscript.

Competing interests
The authors declare that they have no competing interests.

Author details
[1]Division of Cardiovascular Medicine, Department of Medical and Health Sciences, Linköping University, Linköping, Sweden. [2]Center for Medical Image Science and Visualization (CMIV), Linköping University, Linköping, Sweden. [3]Department of Clinical Physiology, Department of Medical and Health Sciences, Linköping University, Linköping, Sweden.

References
1. Dumoulin CL. Phase contrast MR angiography techniques. Magn Reson Imaging Clin N Am. 1995;3(3):399–411.
2. Gatehouse P, Keegan J, Crowe L, Masood S, Mohiaddin R, Kreitner K-F, Firmin D. Applications of phase-contrast flow and velocity imaging in cardiovascular MRI. Eur Radiol. 2005;15(10):2172–84. doi:10.1007/s00330-005-2829-3.
3. Markl M, Kilner PJ, Ebbers T. Comprehensive 4D velocity mapping of the heart and great vessels by cardiovascular magnetic resonance. J Cardiovasc Magn Reson. 2011;13(1):7. doi:10.1186/1532-429X-13-7.
4. Bock J, Wieben O, Johnson K, Hennig J, Markl M. Optimal processing to derive static PC-MRA from time-resolved 3D PC-MRI data. In: Proceedings 16th Scientific Meeting, International Society for Magnetic Resonance in Medicine. Toronto: The International Society for Magnetic Resonance in Medicine; 2008. p. 3053
5. Markl M, Harloff A, Bley TA, Zaitsev M, Jung B, Weigang E, Langer M, Hennig J, Frydrychowicz A. Time-resolved 3D MR velocity mapping at 3T: improved navigator-gated assessment of vascular anatomy and blood flow. J Magn Reson Imaging. 2007;25(4):824–31. doi:10.1002/jmri.20871.
6. Hennemuth A, Friman O, Schumann C, Bock J, Drexl J, Huellebrand M. Markl M. Peitgen H-O. Fast interactive exploration of 4D MRI flow data. In: Wong KH, Holmes III, DR. p. 79640. International Society for Optics and Photonics (2011). doi:10.1117/12.878202
7. Bock J, Frydrychowicz A, Stalder AF, Bley TA, Burkhardt H, Hennig J, Markl M. 4D phase contrast MRI at 3 T: Effect of standard and blood-pool contrast agents on SNR, PC-MRA, and blood flow visualization. Magn Reson Med. 2010;63(2):330–8. doi:10.1002/mrm.22199.
8. Frydrychowicz A, Berger A, MunozdelRio A, Russe MF, Bock J, Harloff A, Markl M. Interdependencies of aortic arch secondary flow patterns, geometry, and age analysed by 4-dimensional phase contrast magnetic resonance imaging at 3 Tesla. Eur Radiol. 2012;22(5):1122–30.
9. Schnell S, Entezari P, Mahadewia RJ, Malaisrie SC, McCarthy PM, Collins JD, Carr J, Markl M. Improved Semiautomated 4D Flow MRI Analysis in the Aorta in Patients With Congenital Aortic Valve Anomalies Versus Tricuspid Aortic Valves. J Comput Assist Tomogr. 2015;40(1):102–8. doi:10.1097/RCT.0000000000000312.
10. Bustamante M, Petersson S, Eriksson J, Alehagen U, Dyverfeldt P, Carlhäll C-J, Ebbers T. Atlas-based analysis of 4D flow CMR: Automated vessel segmentation and flow quantification. J Cardiovasc Magn Reson. 2015;17(1):87. doi:10.1186/s12968-015-0190-5.
11. Harloff A, Nussbaumer A, Bauer S, Stalder AF, Frydrychowicz A, Weiller C, Hennig J, Markl M. In vivo assessment of wall shear stress in the atherosclerotic aorta using flow-sensitive 4D MRI. Magn Reson Med. 2010; 63(6):1529–36. doi:10.1002/mrm.22383.
12. Petersson S, Dyverfeldt P, Ebbers T. Assessment of the accuracy of MRI wall shear stress estimation using numerical simulations. J Magn Reson Imaging. 2012;36(1):128–38. doi:10.1002/jmri.23610.
13. Knutsson H, Andersson M. Morphons: Segmentation using elastic canvas and paint on priors. In: Proceedings - International Conference on Image Processing. vol. 2. ICIP; 2005. pp. 1226–1229. doi:10.1109/ICIP.2005.1530283
14. Forsberg D, Andersson M, Knutsson H. Non-rigid Diffeomorphic Image Registration of Medical Images Using Polynomial Expansion. Berlin: Springer; 2012. pp. 304–12.
15. Forsberg D, Lundström C, Andersson M, Knutsson H. Model-based registration for assessment of spinal deformities in idiopathic scoliosis. Phys Med Biol. 2014;59(2):311–26. doi:10.1088/0031-9155/59/2/311.
16. Xiang QS. Temporal phase unwrapping for CINE velocity imaging. J Magn Reson Imaging. 1995;5(5):529–34. doi:10.1002/jmri.1880050509.
17. Ebbers T, Haraldsson H, Dyverfeldt P. Higher order weighted least-squares phase offset correction for improved accuracy in phase-contrast MRI. Proceedings of the International Society of Magnetic Resonance in Medicine 16 39(Cmiv), 1367 (2008)

18. Potters WV, van Ooij P, Marquering H, VanBavel E, Nederveen AJ. Volumetric arterial wall shear stress calculation based on cine phase contrast MRI. J Magn Reson Imaging. 2015;41(2):505–16. doi:10.1002/jmri.24560.

19. Stalder AF, Russe MF, Frydrychowicz A, Bock J, Hennig J, Markl M. Quantitative 2D and 3D phase contrast MRI: Optimized analysis of blood flow and vessel wall parameters. Magn Reson Med. 2008;60(5):1218–31. doi:10.1002/mrm.21778.

20. Vasanawala SS, Hanneman K, Alley MT, Hsiao A. Congenital heart disease assessment with 4D flow MRI. J Magn Reson Imaging. 2015;42(4):870–86. doi:10.1002/jmri.24856.

21. Dyverfeldt P, Bissell M, Barker AJ, Bolger AF, Carlh ̈all C-J, Ebbers T, Francios CJ, Frydrychowicz A, Geiger J, Giese D, Hope MD, Kilner PJ, Kozerke S, Myerson S, Neubauer S, Wieben O, Markl M. 4D flow cardiovascular magnetic resonance consensus statement. J Cardiovasc Magn Reson. 2015;17(1):72. doi:10.1186/s12968-015-0174-5.

12

Extra-cellular expansion in the normal, non-infarcted myocardium is associated with worsening of regional myocardial function after acute myocardial infarction

Pankaj Garg[1] (ID), David A. Broadbent[1,2], Peter P. Swoboda[1], James R.J. Foley[1], Graham J. Fent[1], Tarique A. Musa[1], David P. Ripley[1], Bara Erhayiem[1], Laura E. Dobson[1], Adam K. McDiarmid[1], Philip Haaf[1], Ananth Kidambi[1], Saul Crandon[1], Pei G. Chew[1], R. J. van der Geest[3], John P. Greenwood[1] and Sven Plein[1*]

Abstract

Background: Expansion of the myocardial extracellular volume (ECV) is a surrogate measure of focal/diffuse fibrosis and is an independent marker of prognosis in chronic heart disease. Changes in ECV may also occur after myocardial infarction, acutely because of oedema and in convalescence as part of ventricular remodelling. The objective of this study was to investigate changes in the pattern of distribution of regional (normal, infarcted and oedematous segments) and global left ventricular (LV) ECV using semi-automated methods early and late after reperfused ST-elevation myocardial infarction (STEMI).

Methods: Fifty patients underwent cardiovascular magnetic resonance (CMR) imaging acutely (24 h–72 h) and at convalescence (3 months). The CMR protocol included: cines, T2-weighted (T2 W) imaging, pre–/post-contrast T1-maps and LGE-imaging. Using T2 W and LGE imaging on acute scans, 16-segments of the LV were categorised as normal, oedema and infarct. 800 segments (16 per-patient) were analysed for changes in ECV and wall thickening (WT).

Results: From the acute studies, 325 (40.6%) segments were classified as normal, 246 (30.8%) segments as oedema and 229 (28.6%) segments as infarct. Segmental change in ECV between acute and follow-up studies (Δ ECV) was significantly different for normal, oedema and infarct segments ($0.8 \pm 6.5\%$, $-1.78 \pm 9\%$, $-2.9 \pm 10.9\%$, respectively; $P < 0.001$). Normal segments which demonstrated deterioration in wall thickening at follow-up showed significantly increased Δ ECV compared with normal segments with preserved wall thickening at follow up ($1.82 \pm 6.05\%$ versus $-0.10 \pm 6.88\%$, $P < 0.05$).

Conclusion: Following reperfused STEMI, normal myocardium demonstrates subtle expansion of the extracellular volume at 3-month follow up. Segmental ECV expansion of normal myocardium is associated with worsening of contractile function.

Keywords: Acute myocardial infarction, CT and MRI, Cardiovascular imaging agents/techniques, Extracellular matrix

* Correspondence: S.Plein@leeds.ac.uk
Dr. Stefan Neubaurer served as a Guest Editor for this manuscript.
[1]Division of Biomedical Imaging, Leeds Institute of Cardiovascular and Metabolic Medicine (LICAMM) & Multidisciplinary Cardiovascular Research Centre, University of Leeds, Leeds LS2 9JT, UK
Full list of author information is available at the end of the article

Background

Following ST-elevation myocardial infarction (STEMI), even with immediate mechanical reperfusion therapy, 24–30% patients develop adverse left ventricular (LV) remodelling [1, 2]. LV remodelling is a predictor of heart failure, and hence is associated with morbidity and mortality. Post infarct, the acute loss of myocardial function results in an abrupt increase in LV loading conditions that induces a unique pattern of remodelling involving the normal (non-infarcted non-oedematous myocardium), oedematous (injured with oedematous myocardium) and infarcted myocardium [3].

The chronic phase of LV remodelling involves compensatory myocyte hypertrophy and alterations in ventricular geometry to distribute the increased wall stresses more evenly [4]. Early pre-clinical studies have speculated that the 'normal' non-infarcted myocardium also undergoes changes due to increased wall stress [5, 6]. There is limited evidence to support these concepts in humans. Additionally, it remains unknown if these changes in tissue composition of normal myocardium have any impact on regional contractility.

Cardiovascular magnetic resonance (CMR) offers comprehensive multi-parametric structural and functional assessment in patients with STEMI [7]. Using early gadolinium enhancement (EGE) and late gadolinium enhancement (LGE) imaging, accurate assessment of infarct characteristics (infarct size, transmurality of scar, presence of microvascular obstruction and LV thrombus) can be made. T2-weighted (T2 W) imaging allows to diagnose and quantify the extent of myocardial oedema following acute ischaemic injury [8, 9]. Native T1-mapping can also detect acute ischaemia and combined with post contrast T1 mapping allows quantification of the extra-cellular volume (ECV) [10–13].

This study aimed to investigate whether ECV expansion of normal myocardium occurs after STEMI and whether it is associated with a reduction in contractile function between baseline and follow up assessment. We also sought to determine the baseline CMR parameters that are most strongly associated with segmental functional change at follow up.

Methods

Study population

Patients with acute STEMI were prospectively enrolled from a single UK tertiary centre. The study design is detailed in Fig. 1.

The inclusion criteria were as follows: patients with first time acute STEMI treated by primary percutaneous

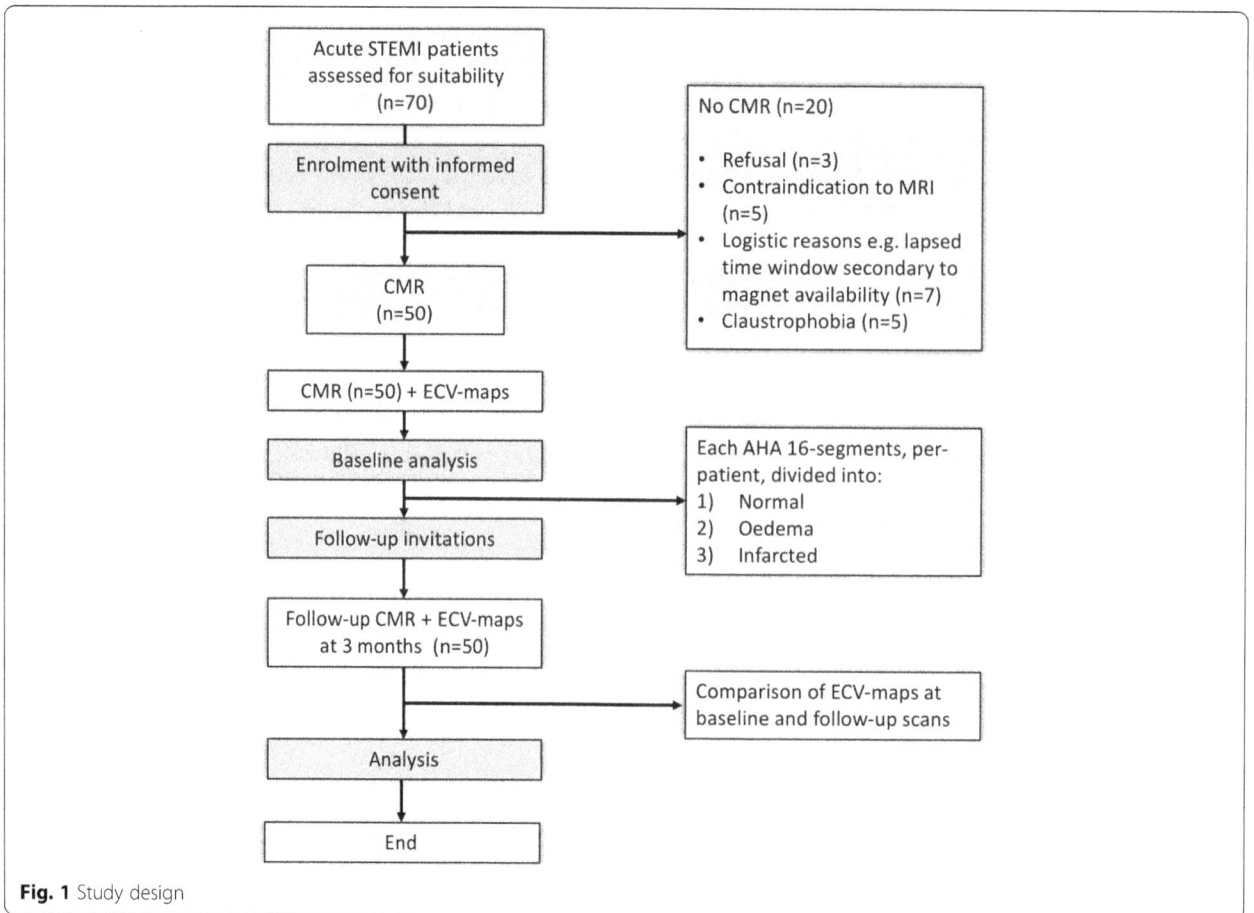

Fig. 1 Study design

coronary intervention (PPCI) within 12-h of onset of chest pain. Acute STEMI was defined as per current international guidelines [14]. Exclusion criteria included: previous myocardial infaction, coronary artery bypass grafting, known cardiomyopathy, estimated glomerular filtration rate < 30 ml/min/1.73 m2, haemodynamic instability (requiring on-going intravenous therapy or respiratory support) and contraindication to CMR imaging. After revascularization, all patients received standard post-myocardial infarction secondary prevention therapy at the discretion of the treating physician, and were enrolled in a cardiac rehabilitation programme if they were deemed suitable [15].

Cardiac catheterization
Coronary angiography and revascularisation were performed in a standard fashion as per current best practice guidelines [15, 16]. TIMI flow grades were assessed visually as described previously following coronary angioplasty [17].

Cardiovascular magnetic resonance
All patients underwent CMR imaging at either 1.5 Tesla (Ingenia CV, Philips Healthcare, Best, The Netherlands) or 3.0 Tesla (Achieva TX, Philips Healthcare, Best, The Netherlands). The choice of field strength was arbitrary and was predominantly dictated by availability of the scanners. A dedicated cardiac phased array receiver coil was used (1.5 T: 24-channel equipped with d-stream; 3 T: 32-channel). Acute CMR imaging was scheduled within 72-h of the index presentation and patients were invited to attend for a further CMR study at 3-months follow-up. The same field strength scanners were used for respective patients as for the acute scans.

Image acquisition
Cine, T2 W-imaging, EGE and LGE imaging were performed in contiguous stacks of short-axis slices covering the entire LV for each acquisition. The same slice geometry, position and 10 mm slice thickness were used for all pulse sequences.

T1-maps acquisition
Native and post-contrast T1-maps were planned using the '3-of-5' approach [18]. Post-contrast T1-maps were timed at 15 min after contrast administration and LGE-imaging was performed at 16–20 min.

Image analysis
For each pulse sequence, images with artefact were repeated until any artefact was removed or minimized. The highest quality images were used for analysis. Cine, T2 W-images, EGE-images and LGE-images were evaluated offline using MASS research software (Version

2016EXP, Leiden University Medical Centre, Leiden, The Netherlands).

Basic CMR image analysis, T1-maps quality assurance checks, pulse sequence parameters and imaging protocol are described in the online Additional file 1.

Categorising of left ventricular segments
Sixteen segments of the LV excluding the apex, adapted from the 17 segments of the American Heart Association (AHA) model [19], were visually assessed on acute CMR scans and labelled as 1) normal segment (no oedema on T2 W-imaging and no infarct on LGE-imaging), 2) oedema segment (predominantly oedema on T2 W-imaging with no infarct on LGE-imaging 3) infarct segment (presence of any infarction on LGE-imaging with/without oedema on T2 W-imaging).

Myocardial wall thickening analysis
Segmental myocardial systolic wall thickening (WT) analysis was performed for each slice based on endo- and epicardial contours. For each segment, end-diastolic and end-systolic wall thickness (EDWT and ESWT, respectively [mm]) were recorded as per previously published literature [20]. This method has demonstrated high intra-inter-observer agreement [21]. Myocardial systolic segmental WT ([mm]) was calculated as absolute change in EDWT and ESWT. For each LV segment, delta change of WT was derived. Functional improvement of segments was defined as positive delta change of WT from baseline to follow-up and vice versa. Additionally, radial strain was computed using endo–/epi- cardial contours through-out the complete cardiac cycle as per previously described methods [22].

Extracellular volume map analysis
ECV maps were generated for the 3 slices (base, mid and apex) from pre–/post-contrast T1-maps and haematocrit as per the standard techniques [10]. The endocardial and epicardial contours were outlined to define myocardium in the 3 slices. Microvascular obstruction (MVO) contours were imported from EGE imaging. Mean ECV values were generated for each segment of the 16 segments excluding the MVO in the infarct zone. Left ventricular global ECV was calculated by multiplication of the averaged per-patient ECV values (for all the 16 segments) and indexed LV end-diastolic volume (LVEDV). Similarly, left ventricular myocyte cell volume was calculated by using the previously published formula: (1-*global ECV*)*(*indexed* LVEDV) [23]. For each patient, mean ECV values for different types of segments (normal, oedema and infarct) were generated on both acute and follow-up studies. For each patient, increase or decrease of ECV of all non-infarcted, healthy myocardium was defined as the change in the mean ECV of all

segments and this was investigated for its association with patient characteristics (Table 1).

Adverse LV remodelling was defined as an absolute increase of LV end-systolic volumes >15% at 3 months follow-up [24, 25].

Intra–/inter-observer segmental ECV assessment

For intra–/inter-observer assessments, 48 segments were selected from three randomly chosen scans. To test the inter-observer reliability of segmental ECV values, two blinded observers carried out independent segmentation of ECV-maps (PG and SC) in these segments. To test intra-observer reliability, one observer (PG) undertook a second blinded analysis after three months.

Statistical analysis

Statistical analysis was performed using SPSS® Statistics 21.0 (International Business Machines, Inc., Chicago, Illinois, USA). Normality of quantitative data was established using the Shapiro-Wilk test. Normally distributed continuous variables are expressed as mean ± SD and non-normally distributed are expressed as median (25th–75th quartile ranges). Demographic comparisons between patients with rise and fall of ECV at follow-up, in the normal myocardial segments, were performed with an independent samples t-test for normally distributed variables and by Mann-Whitney independent t-test for not normally distributed. For paired comparison in Table 2, Wilcoxon test was used. A repeated-measures analysis of variance (ANOVA) was performed on demographic and global ECV (rise/fall) at follow-up. Linear regression was used to investigate which baseline study parameter was most strongly associated with number of segments with functional recovery at follow-up. Univariate analysis was performed for each variable separately. Step-wise multivariate linear regression was used for parameters with statistical significance from one-way analysis ($p < 0.1$). Intra–/inter-observer agreement was assessed by investigating the coefficient of variability (CV), concordance correlation coefficient (CCC), precision and accuracy. All statistical tests were 2-tailed; p values <0.05 were considered significant.

Sample size calculations

We used data of remote zone ECV from published literature using to inform the sample size calculations for this study. In a previous study, delta remote zone ECV in patients with/without adverse LV remodelling were: 0.9 ± 2.2% (with adverse LV remodelling, $n = 8$) versus 0.9 ± 0.9% (without adverse LV remodelling, $n = 32$) [26]. Using these data, as per the mean comparison method described by Machin et al., 295 normal segments were needed to investigate functional changes. [27]. Presuming 40% of myocardium is normal post STEMI, the study thus needed to recruit at least 46 patients to give a power of 80% at an alpha of 0.05.

Results

Patient characteristics

Seventy patients were considered for inclusion, of which 50 had baseline and follow-up CMR (Fig. 1). Acute scans were performed at a median of 48 h after the index presentation. 32 patients had CMR at 1.5 Tesla and 18 patients had CMR at 3 Tesla. All 50 patients were included in the statistical analysis. Clinical and patient demographics are detailed in Table 1.

Per-patient analysis

Patients were categorised into two groups depending on the rise/fall of normal myocardial ECV between baseline and follow-up studies (Table 1). Twenty-eight patients (56%) demonstrated an increase in average normal myocardial ECV at follow-up when compared to acute ECV. No significant differences were seen in baseline demographics between the two groups of patients with a rise or fall of delta-ECV. Patients with triple vessel disease were more prevalent in the group that showed a rise in ECV in normal segments (1 patient versus 7 patients, $P = 0.05$). There were no differences relating to the field strength of the scanner that was use and the 3 T patients, 10 patients (55.6%) demonstrated ECV expansion in normal myocardial versus 18 (56.2%) on the 1.5 T ($P = 0.96$ for comparison of 3 T and 1.5 T). LV mass reduced significantly from baseline to follow-up, but global ECV and myocyte cell volume showed no significant change (Table 2).

Per-segment analysis

800 segments were analysed acutely and at follow-up. From the acute studies, 325 (40.6%) segments were classified as normal, 246 (30.8%) segments were classified as oedema and 229 (28.6%) segments were classified as infarct segments. Myocardial oedema was only seen in the peri-infarct zone of the culprit vessel.

Intra–/inter-observer checks for segmental ECV

For the 48 segments which were analysed, intra-observer CV was 6%, with excellent CCC (0.94, 95% CI 0.90–97), high precision (0.95) and accuracy (0.99). For the inter-observer analysis, CV was 7%, with good CCC (0.92, 95% CI 0.87–95) and high precision (0.93) and accuracy (0.99).

Pattern of ECV change

Oedema and infarct segments demonstrated significant reductions in ECV at follow-up (Table 2). Conversely, there was a smaller but statistically significant rise in the ECV of normal myocardium at follow-up ($P = 0.03$).

Segmental change in ECV between acute and follow-up studies was significantly different for normal, oedema

Table 1 Clinical and angiographic characteristics in patients with change of normal segment ECV per-patient between acute and follow-up scan

	Normal segment ECV ↓ (n = 22)		Normal segment ECV ↑ (n = 28)		
	Mean/Median/Count	SD/ 25%–75%/%	Mean/Median/Count	SD/25%–75%/%	p-value
Patient Demographics					
Age, yrs	60	11	58	11	0.39
Sex (Male)[c]	20	40	22	44	0.24
Smoker[c]	14	28	16	32	0.65
Hypertension[c]	5	10	3	6	0.25
Hyperlipidaemia[c]	9	18	8	16	0.37
Diabetes Mellitus[c]	4	8	2	4	0.24
Stroke[c]	1	2	0	0	0.26
Presenting Characteristics					
Systolic Blood Pressure, mmHg	137	24	134	36	0.88
Heart rate, beats/min	73	14	74	16	0.95
Time from onset of CP to reperfusion, min[c]	261	158–454	222	149–344	0.43
Heart Failure Killip Class[a]					
I[c]	20	40	26	52	0.80
II[c]	1	2	2	4	0.70
III-IV[c]	1	2	0	0	0.26
Ventricular fibrillation at presentation[c]	0	0	3	6	0.11
Angiographic Characteristics					
Number of diseased arteries[b]					
Single vessel disease[c]	16	30	16	32	0.26
Two vessel disease[c]	5	10	5	10	0.67
Three vessel disease[c]	1	2	7	14	**0.05**
Culprit Vessel					
Left main stem[c]	0	0	1	2	0.37
Left anterior descending[c]	14	28	15	30	0.48
Left circumflex[c]	2	4	2	4	0.80
Right coronary[c]	6	12	11	22	0.38
QRS duration, msec[c]	90	86–110	94	82–100	0.86
TIMI coronary flow pre-PCI (<2)[c]	18	36	26	52	0.15
TIMI coronary flow post-PCI (<3)[c]	2	4	2	4	0.77
Laboratory results					
White blood cells[c], ×10^9/l	11	10–15	11	10–13	0.86
Estimated Glomerular Filtration Rate[c], ml/min/1.73m^2	88	77–90	90	78–90	0.47
Creatine kinase[c], U/l	1493	786–2400	1584	867–2570	0.75
Troponin[c],	50,000	16,441–50,000	50,000	48,335–50,000	0.34
HBA1c[c], mmol/mol	41	36–44	40	36–44	0.77

Table 1 Clinical and angiographic characteristics in patients with change of normal segment ECV per-patient between acute and follow-up scan *(Continued)*

Infarct characteristics					
Infarct size, volume in %	30	17	26	12	0.42
Area at risk, volume in %	49	19	46	17	0.46
Presence of Microvascular Obstruction (MVO)	13	59	16	57	0.89

[a]Killip classification of heart failure after acute myocardial infarction: class I = no heart failure; class II = pulmonary rales or crepitations, a third heart sound, and elevated jugular venous pressure; class III = acute pulmonary edema; and class IV = cardiogenic shock
[b]Multi-vessel coronary artery disease was defined according to the number of stenoses of at least 50% of the reference vessel diameter by visual assessment and whether or not there was left main stem involvement
Abbreviations: BMI = body mass index; CMR = cardiac magnetic resonance; CP = chest pain; ECV = extracellular volume; HBA1c = glycated haemoglobin; PCI = percutaneous coronary intervention; STEMI = ST-segment elevation myocardial infarction; TIMI = Thrombolysis In Myocardial Infarction
[c]Non-normally distributed

and infarct segments ($0.8 \pm 6.5\%$ versus $-1.78 \pm 9\%$ or $-2.9 \pm 10.9\%$; $P < 0.001$) (Fig. 2).

Temporal changes in normal segmental ECV did not demonstrate any significant association with number of >50% transmural scar segments (Fig. 3).

Segmental ECV and WT

Acute segmental ECV demonstrated significant correlation to both acute segmental WT ($P < 0.0001$) and to follow-up segmental WT ($P < 0.0001$) (Table 3). There was a significant increase in ΔECV in normal segments which

Table 2 Baseline and follow-up CMR parameters

	Acute CMR		Follow-up CMR		P-value[a]
	Median	25%–75% quartiles	Median	25%–75% quartiles	
Baseline CMR characteristics					
LVEDVi, ml/m2	79.1	71–87	80.45	70–89	0.41
LVESVi, ml/m2	42	36–50	38.7	31–47	0.02
LV MASSi, grams/m2	55.45	48–64	48.55	43–55	<0.0001
EF, %	45.65	36–51	52.35	43–59	<0.0001
IS, volume in %	23.9	17–38	13.75	9–27	<0.0001
Segmental myocardial tissue composition and function					
	Median	25% - 75% Quartiles	Median	25% - 75% Quartiles	
Normal ECV, % (n = 325)	27.5	24.8–3 0.5	27.7	25.2–32	0.03
Oedema ECV, % (n = 246)	34	29–39.3	32	28–37	0.0002
Infarct ECV, % (n = 229)	44	37.4–49	41	33.6–46	<0.0001
Normal WT (mm) (n = 325)	3.7	2.7–4.8	3.8	2.0–4.7	0.81
Oedema WT (mm) (n = 246)	2.9	1.8–4.3	3.3	2.4–4.3	0.02
Infarct WT (mm) (n = 229)	1.6	0.47–2.8	2.4	1.1–3.6	<0.0001
Normal EDT (mm)	7.3	6–8	6.7	6–7.5	<0.0001
Oedema EDT (mm)	7.4	6–8.5	6.5	5–7.6	<0.0001
Infarct EDT (mm)	7.9	7–9	6.4	56–7.6	<0.0001
Global myocardial tissue composition					
Total LV myocyte volume, mL/m2	51.2	45.7–57.4	53.6	46.3–61	0.14
Total LV extracellular matrix, ml/m2	25.8	22.7–32.8	26.1	21.8–32.8	0.68

LV measurements are indexed to body surface area (BSA), infarct volumes are unindexed. LVEDVi = Left ventricular end-diastolic volume (indexed), LVESVi = Left ventricular end-systolic volume (indexed), LVMi = Left ventricular mass (indexed), RS = peak systolic radial strain (%)
[a]Wilcoxon test (paired samples)

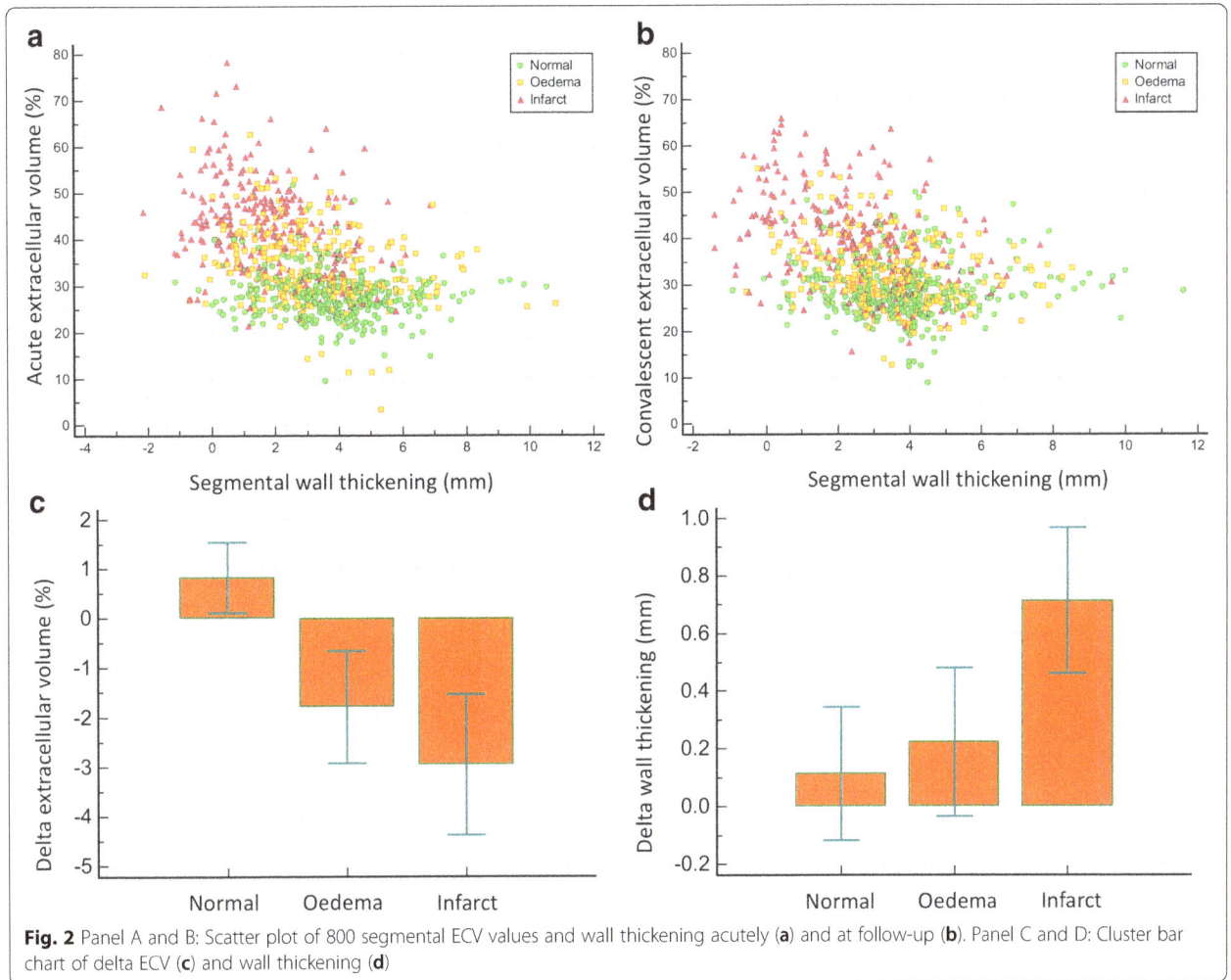

Fig. 2 Panel A and B: Scatter plot of 800 segmental ECV values and wall thickening acutely (**a**) and at follow-up (**b**). Panel C and D: Cluster bar chart of delta ECV (**c**) and wall thickening (**d**)

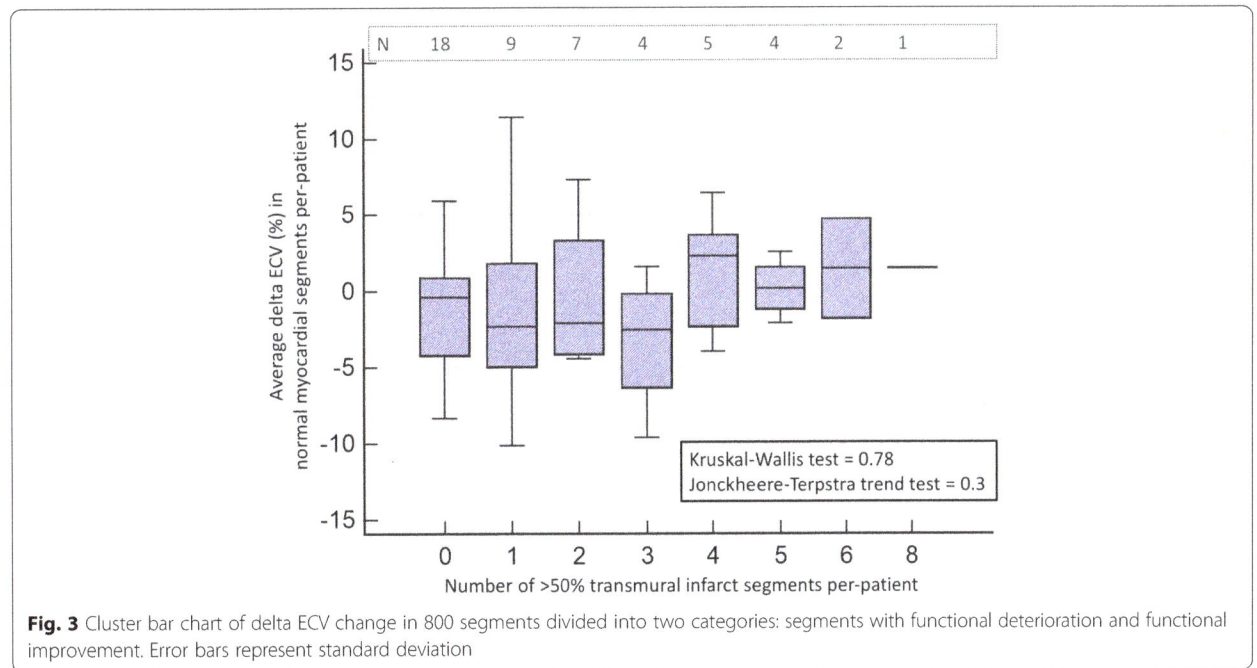

Fig. 3 Cluster bar chart of delta ECV change in 800 segments divided into two categories: segments with functional deterioration and functional improvement. Error bars represent standard deviation

Table 3 Segmental function and extracellular volume (ECV) results

Left Ventricular Segmental Function (800 segments)

		Acute WT			Follow-up WT		
		Spearman rank correlation coefficient		*P*-value	Spearman rank correlation coefficient		*P*-value
Acute ECV		−0.46		<0.0001	−0.32		<0.0001
Follow-up ECV		−0.34		<0.0001	−0.35		<0.0001
		Function Deteriorated			Function Improved		
		Mean	SD	n (%)	Mean	SD	n (%)
Delta ECV[a] (%)	Normal	1.82	6.05	158 (19.8)	−0.10	6.88	167 (20.9)	*P* < 0.05
	Oedematous	0.12	8.72	107 (13.4)	−3.25	9.05	139 (17.4)	*P* < 0.05
	Infarct	−0.34	9.35	80 (10.0)	−4.36	11.42	149 (18.6)	*P* < 0.05

[a]Tests are adjusted for all pairwise comparisons within a row of each innermost sub-table using the Bonferroni correction

demonstrated deterioration in wall thickening (Table 3, Fig. 4). For the oedema and infarct segments, ΔECV was significantly different (less or no improvement) in segments with a decrease in wall thickening versus segments that demonstrated improvement in wall thickening (*P* < 0.05, Table 3, Fig. 5). All segments with functional improvement showed a reduction in follow-up ECV. The percentage of "normal" myocardial segments that demonstrated functional improvement and greater than normal acute baseline ECV (>28%) was not significantly different to "normal" segments with no functional recovery (54% versus 53%, *P* = 0.33).

Peak systolic radial strain results are detailed in the online '**Supplementary material**'. Acute ECV of the normal, oedema and infarct segments demonstrated

an inverse relation to final follow-up radial strain (Fig. 6).

By univariable analysis of all demographic and CMR parameters, acute oedema and infarct segment ECVs demonstrated association to number of segments (per-patient) that had improvement in function (Table 4). On multivariable linear regression analysis, infarct ECV was most strongly associated with number of segments with functional improvement (beta = 0.4, *P* = 0.037).

Adverse LV remodelling

Acute myocardial ECV of normal segments was significantly higher in patients who demonstrated adverse LV remodelling (*P* = 0.04) (Table 5). Infarct and oedema

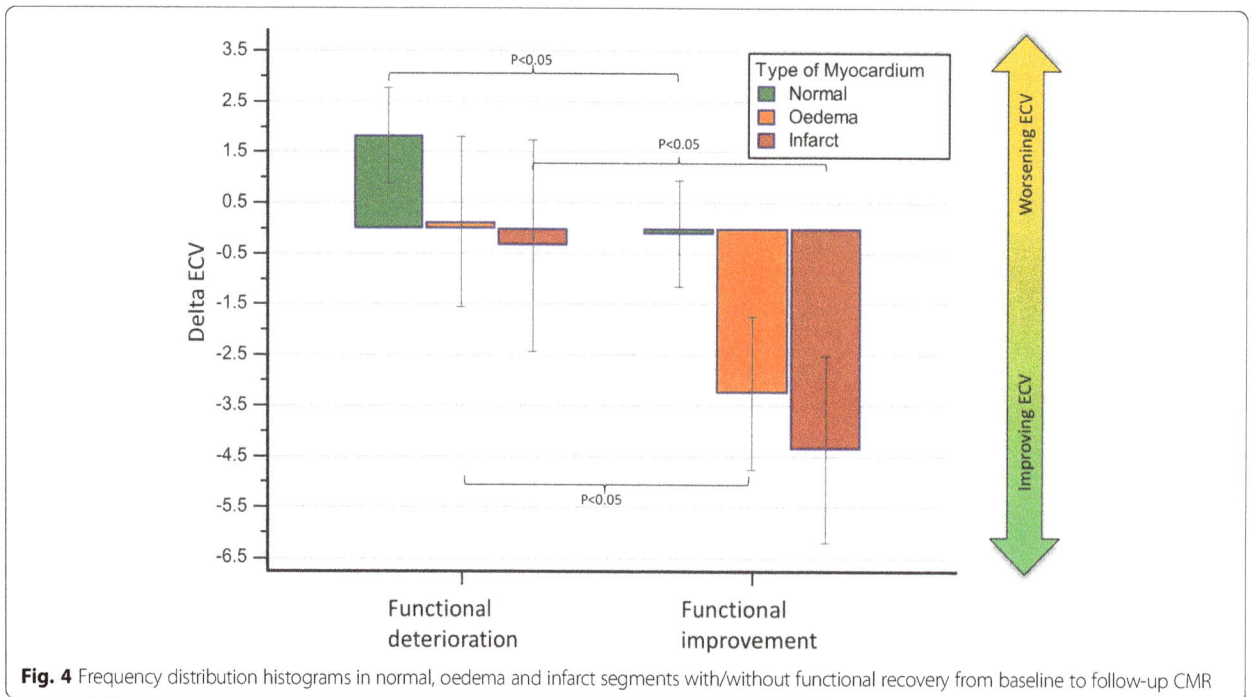

Fig. 4 Frequency distribution histograms in normal, oedema and infarct segments with/without functional recovery from baseline to follow-up CMR

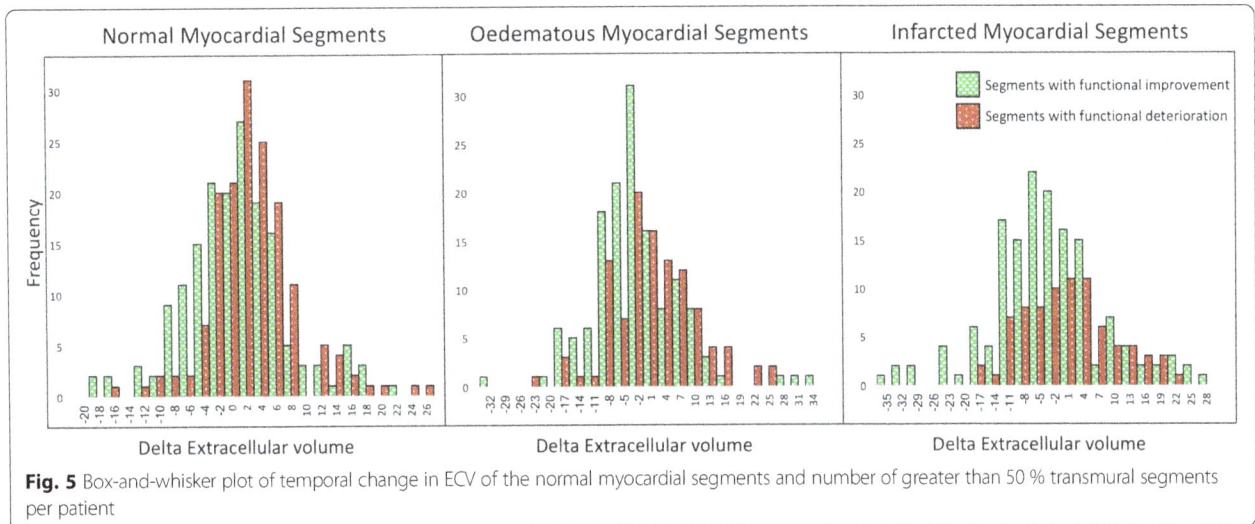

Fig. 5 Box-and-whisker plot of temporal change in ECV of the normal myocardial segments and number of greater than 50 % transmural segments per patient

acute ECV did not demonstrate a difference depending on the presence of adverse LV remodelling at follow-up.

Discussion

The present study demonstrates that 1) in reperfused STEMI, normal myocardial segments show a subtle expansion of the ECV between baseline and 3 month follow-up; 2) conversely, oedematous and infarcted segments show a significant reduction in ECV at follow up; 3) normal segments that demonstrate deterioration in

segmental function at follow-up show a substantial increase in delta-ECV from baseline to follow up; 4) acute infarct ECV demonstrates the best association with the number of segments with functional recovery (Fig. 3) and 5) high acute normal myocardial segmental ECV is associated with adverse LV remodelling at follow-up.

Previous studies have already shown that ECV is raised in 'remote' myocardium in acute STEMI [26, 28]. Remote myocardium is defined as the AHA segment 180-degrees from the infarct territory with normal motion

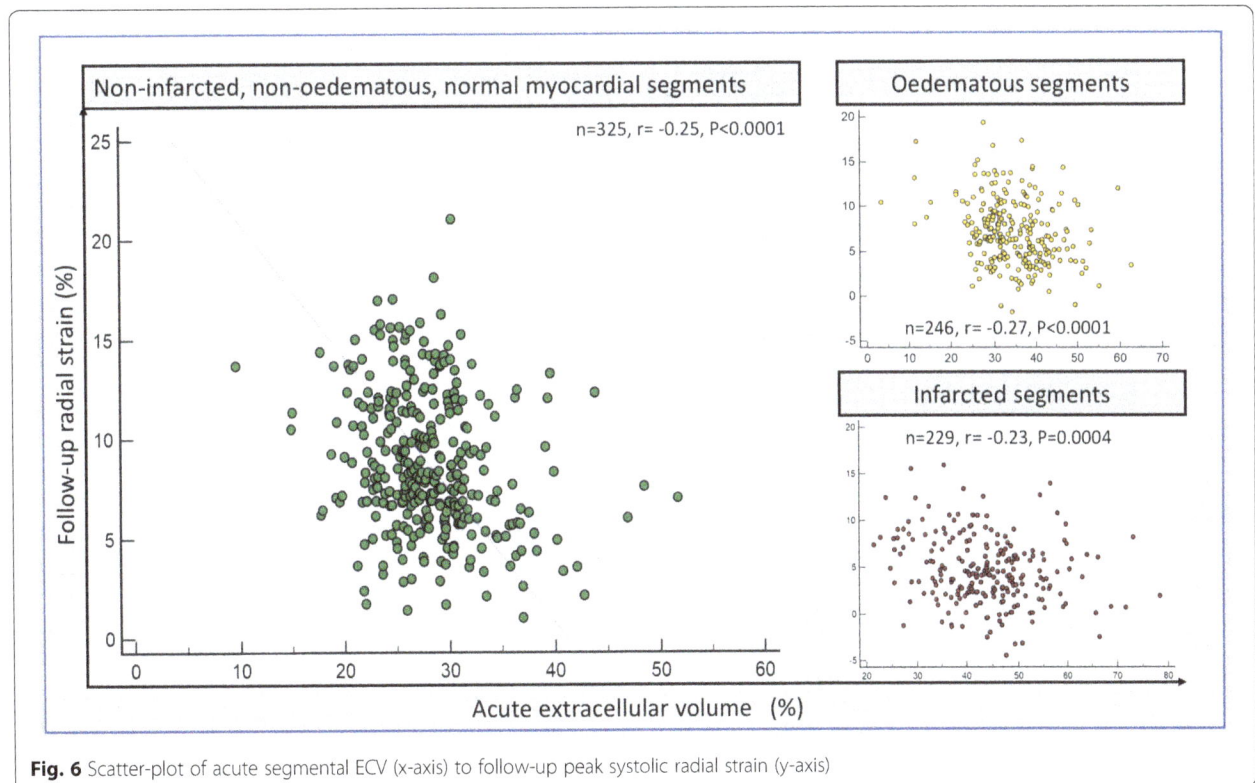

Fig. 6 Scatter-plot of acute segmental ECV (x-axis) to follow-up peak systolic radial strain (y-axis)

Table 4 Linear regression of baseline patient parameters to number of myocardial segments with improved function at follow-up study

Number of myocardial segments (per-patient) with improved function			
	Univariate P-Value	Multivariate P-Value	Beta
Age	0.11		
Sex	0.99		
Diabetes Mellitus	0.57		
Hypertension	0.69		
Smoker	0.53		
Time from onset of CP to reperfusion	0.93		
Killip Class I	0.76		
Killip Class II	0.85		
Killip Class III-IV	0.79		
Left main stem disease	0.14		
1-vessel disease	0.48		
2-vessel disease	0.67		
3-vessel disease	0.87		
TIMI flow pre-intervention	0.47		
TIMI flow post intervention	0.47		
LVEDV	0.74		
LVESV	0.76		
LV Mass	0.39		
LV ejection fraction	0.51		
Stroke volume	0.43		
Infarct size	0.57		
Area at risk (AAR)	0.18		
Acute non-infarcted normal myocardial ECV	0.89		
Acute AAR ECV	0.05	0.32	
Acute Infarct ECV	0.04	0.037	0.29

and no LGE [26, 28]. In the present study, we chose to assess all segments that did not have evidence of oedema or infarction and in order to avoid misinterpretation with the standard definition of 'remote' myocardium, defined these as 'normal' segments. Carberry et al.

Table 5 Association of acute myocardial ECV to adverse LV remodelling

	LV AVR -ve	LV AVR + ve	P-value
Number of patients (n)	40	10	
Acute non-oedematous, non-infarcted healthy myocardial ECV (%)	27.9 ± 3	30.4 ± 3.6	0.04
Acute infarct ECV (%)	43 ± 8	42 ± 6	0.61
Acute oedema ECV (%)	35.1 ± 6	33.3 ± 4	0.41

demonstrated that acute remote zone ECV post STEMI is associated with certain baseline patient characteristics (male gender, body mass index and history of diabetes) [28]. They also showed that the remote zone ECV was associated with the level of baseline N-terminal pro b-type natriuretic peptide (NT-proBNP). In our study the number of patients with angiographic triple vessel disease was marginally higher in patients with increased normal myocardial ECV when compared to patients with 0–/1–/2-vessel disease (Table 1, $P = 0.05$). We speculate that in triple vessel disease, coronary steal may reduce flow in non-culprit vessels due to better flow down the revascularised culprit vessel, which may cause adverse tissue level remodelling [29–31]. Other possible mechanisms which influence non-infarcted myocardium include increased loading conditions secondary to infarct characteristics. For example, Litwin et al.'s pre-clinical work demonstrated that the extra-cellular matrix of the non-infarcted normal myocardium undergoes expansion mainly due to increased wall stresses [6].

Associations of segmental ECV and segmental and global function have been studied previously [26, 32, 33]. Collins et al. demonstrated that the segmental extent of fibrosis is associated with segmental function in non-ischaemic cardiomyopathy [33]. Additionally, they demonstrated that this linear association was still relevant in patients with preserved global function and in patients with no late gadolinium enhancement. Our study has now shown that mean ECV is also associated with segmental function in patients with acute STEMI. Bulluck et al. demonstrated that mean segmental ECV in the remote myocardium is raised acutely post STEMI (18). Their mean segmental remote myocardial ECV values are comparable to the present study's 'normal' myocardial segment ECV (27.9 ± 2.1%).

Remote (defined as normal myocardium in this study) myocardial dysfunction after STEMI is considered the main reason why some patients demonstrate function loss that is disproportionate to infarct size [30, 34]. Bogaert et al. demonstrated that remote myocardial dysfunction contributes significantly to the loss in global ventricular function. The present study confirms that normal myocardium with no obvious oedema or infarction can also be affected by functional loss measured by either LV wall thickening or radial strain. Additionally, this study further shows that normal myocardial segments after acute MI which demonstrate dysfunction also have significant extracellular matrix expansion. This could be explained by increased reactive fibrosis during the proliferative and maturation phase of remodelling, in the extracellular matrix of the normal myocardial segments, mainly due to higher wall shear stresses [35].

A recent study from our group demonstrated that acute 'infarct zone' ECV is predictive of regional and global LV functional recovery, and adds prognostic value over LGE

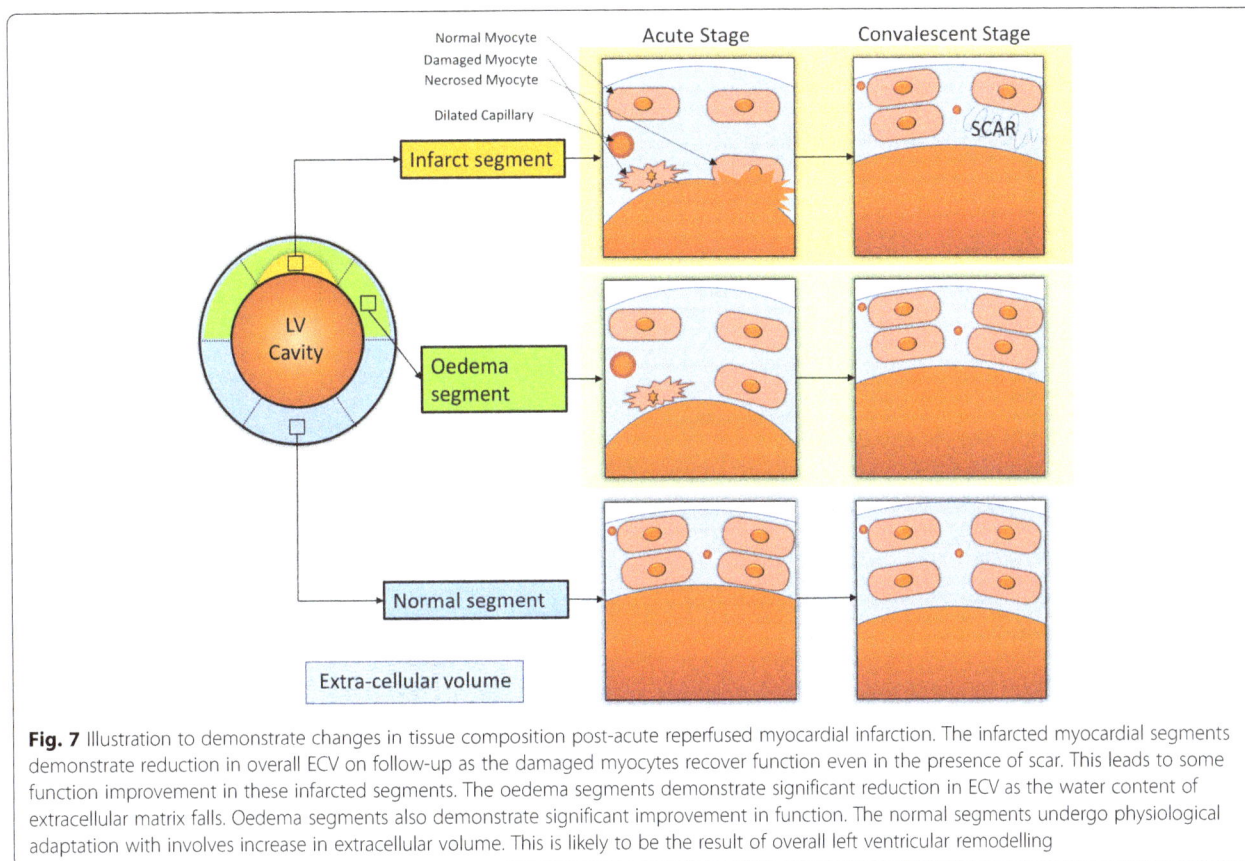

Fig. 7 Illustration to demonstrate changes in tissue composition post-acute reperfused myocardial infarction. The infarcted myocardial segments demonstrate reduction in overall ECV on follow-up as the damaged myocytes recover function even in the presence of scar. This leads to some function improvement in these infarcted segments. The oedema segments demonstrate significant reduction in ECV as the water content of extracellular matrix falls. Oedema segments also demonstrate significant improvement in function. The normal segments undergo physiological adaptation with involves increase in extracellular volume. This is likely to be the result of overall left ventricular remodelling

[36]. Particularly for infarcts with higher transmural extent, acute infarct ECV was an additional predictor of functional recovery that can complement transmural infarct extent by LGE. In addition to these previously reported findings, we have now shown that acute infarct mean segmental ECV correlates with segmental functional recovery at follow-up and that a reduction in ECV in infarct segments is associated with improvement in regional function at follow-up.

This is the first in-vivo study that reports longitudinal changes in segmental ECV in non-infarcted normal, oedema and infarcted LV segments. Our data suggest that non-oedematous, non-infarcted normal LV myocardium undergoes remodelling with a subtle expansion of the extracellular matrix (Fig. 7). In particular, normal myocardial segments which demonstrate myocardial functional loss at follow-up have an increase in ECV.

Limitations

Of 70 patients that underwent initial screening for recruitment only 50 patients underwent the entire protocol possibly introducing an element of selection bias. However, in a clinical study of acutely ill patients, exclusion or drop out of patients is common and our exclusion rate is within that reported in similar previous reports [9, 37]. There were other caveats to the present

study: firstly, segments specifically classified as infarct also conceivably had oedema, which may have altered the results for respective segments. An important limitation of T1-mapping for clinical application is possible partial volume contamination from blood. Nevertheless, MOLLI sequences used in the present study, have been shown to be precise and reproducible [38]. The results of this study may be influenced by the tethering and local interaction of "adjacent" (to peri-infarct zone) normal myocardium. Changes in the adjacent normal myocardium may demonstrate a different pattern of temporal changes when compared to remote myocardium.

Conclusion

This study suggests that following reperfused STEMI, the 'normal' LV myocardium undergoes remodelling with a subtle expansion of the extracellular matrix. In particular, normal segments which have functional loss demonstrate significant expansion of the extracellular space. Additionally, acute myocardial ECV of normal segments was significantly higher in patients who experienced adverse LV remodelling. Myocardial segments with oedema and infarction demonstrate significant reduction in ECV.

Abbreviations

AHA: American Heart Association; ANOVA: a repeated-measures analysis of variance; CCC: concordance correlation coefficient; CMR: cardiovascular magnetic resonance; CV: coefficient of variability; ECV: extracellular volume; EDWT: end-diastolic wall thickness; EGE: early gadolinium enhancement; ESWT: end-systolic wall thickness; LGE: late gadolinum enhancement; LV: left ventricle/left ventricular; LVEDV: left ventricular end-distolic volume; MVO: microvascular obstruction; NT-proBNP: N-terminal pro b-type natriuretic peptide; PPCI: primary percutaneous coronary intervention; STEMI: ST-elevation myocardial infarction; T2 W: T2-weighted; TIMI: Thrombolysis In Myocardial Infarction; WT: wall thickening

Acknowledgements

S.P. was funded by a British Heart Foundation fellowship (FS/10/62/28409) and by a British Heart Foundation chair (CH/16/2/32089). We thank Gavin Bainbridge, Caroline Richmond, Margaret Saysell and Petra Bijsterveld for their assistance in recruiting and collecting data for this study.

Funding

This work was supported by the British Heart Foundation [FS/10/62/28409 and CH/16/2/32089to S.P.].

Authors' contributions

PG was involved in recruitment, CMR analysis, statistics and drafted the study manuscript. DAB developed CMR protocol for the study. PPS, JRJF, GJF, TAM, DPR, BE, LED, AKM, PH, PGC and AK were major contributors in writing the manuscript. SC did CMR and basic statistical analysis. RJvG contributed substantially in smooth running of the core lab at Leiden (LUMC) and automated analysis. JPG and SP provided senior review of the final drafted manuscript. All authors read and approved the final manuscript and agreed to be accountable for all aspects of the work.

Competing interests

The authors declare that they have no competing interests.

Author details

[1]Division of Biomedical Imaging, Leeds Institute of Cardiovascular and Metabolic Medicine (LICAMM) & Multidisciplinary Cardiovascular Research Centre, University of Leeds, Leeds LS2 9JT, UK. [2]Medical Physics and Engineering, Leeds Teaching Hospitals NHS Trust, Leeds, UK. [3]Division of Image Processing, Leiden University Medical Centre, Leiden, The Netherlands.

References

1. Galli A, Lombardi F. Postinfarct Left Ventricular Remodelling: A Prevailing Cause of Heart Failure. Cardiol. Res. Pract. [Internet]. Hindawi Publishing Corporation; 2016 [cited 2016 Nov 20];2016:1–12 Available from: http://www.hindawi.com/journals/crp/2016/2579832/
2. Velagaleti RS, Pencina MJ, Murabito JM, Wang TJ, Parikh NI, D'Agostino RB, et al. Long-term trends in the incidence of heart failure after myocardial infarction. Circulation [Internet]. 2008 [cited 2016 Nov 20];118:2057–2062. Available from: http://www.ncbi.nlm.nih.gov/pubmed/18955667.
3. Sutton MGSJ, Sharpe N. Left ventricular remodeling after myocardial infarction. Circulation. 2000;101
4. Konstam MA, Kramer DG, Patel AR, Maron MS, Udelson JE. Left ventricular remodeling in heart failure: current concepts in clinical significance and assessment. JACC. Cardiovasc Imaging. [Internet]. 2011 [cited 2016 Nov 20]; 4:98–108. Available from: http://www.ncbi.nlm.nih.gov/pubmed/21232712.
5. Pfeffer MA, Braunwald E. Ventricular remodeling after myocardial infarction. Experimental observations and clinical implications. Circulation [Internet]. 1990 [cited 2016 Sep 23];81:1161–1172. Available from: http://www.ncbi.nlm.nih.gov/pubmed/2138525.
6. Litwin SE, Litwin CM, Raya TE, Warner AL, Goldman S. Contractility and stiffness of noninfarcted myocardium after coronary ligation in rats. Effects of chronic angiotensin converting enzyme inhibition. Circulation. 1991 [cited 2016 Nov 20];83:1028–1037. Available from: http://www.ncbi.nlm.nih.gov/pubmed/1999008.
7. Garg P, Underwood SR, Senior R, Greenwood JP, Plein S. Noninvasive cardiac imaging in suspected acute coronary syndrome. Nat. Rev. Cardiol. [Internet]. 2016 [cited 2017 Feb 11];13:266–275. Available from: http://www.ncbi.nlm.nih.gov/pubmed/26911331.
8. Garg P, Kidambi A, Swoboda PP, Foley JRJ, Musa TA, Ripley DP, et al. The role of left ventricular deformation in the assessment of microvascular obstruction and intramyocardial haemorrhage. Int. J. Cardiovasc Imaging. Springer Netherlands; 2016 [cited 2016 Nov 6];1–10 Available from: http://link.springer.com/10.1007/s10554-016-1006-x
9. Garg P, Kidambi A, Foley JRJ, Musa T AI, Ripley DP, Swoboda PP, et al. Ventricular longitudinal function is associated with microvascular obstruction and intramyocardial haemorrhage. Open Hear. British Cardiovascular Society; 2016 [cited 2016 may 18];3:e000337. Available from: http://www.ncbi.nlm.nih.gov/pubmed/27175286.
10. Moon JC, Messroghli DR, Kellman P, Piechnik SK, Robson MD, Ugander M, et al. Myocardial T1 mapping and extracellular volume quantification: a Society for Cardiovascular Magnetic Resonance (SCMR) and CMR Working Group of the European Society of Cardiology consensus statement. J. Cardiovasc. Magn. Reson. [Internet]. BioMed Central; 2013 [cited 2016 Feb 27];15:92 Available from: http://www.pubmedcentral.nih.gov/articlerender.fcgi?artid=3854458&tool=pmcentrez&rendertype=abstract
11. Kellman P, Wilson JR, Xue H, Ugander M, Arai AE. Extracellular volume fraction mapping in the myocardium, part 1: evaluation of an automated method. J. Cardiovasc. Magn. Reson. [Internet]. 2012 [cited 2016 Nov 20];14:63 Available from: http://jcmr-online.biomedcentral.com/articles/10.1186/1532-429X-14-63
12. Kellman P, Wilson JR, Xue H, Bandettini WP, Shanbhag SM, Druey KM, et al. Extracellular volume fraction mapping in the myocardium, part 2: initial clinical experience. J. Cardiovasc. Magn. Reson. [Internet]. 2012 [cited 2014 Sep 27];14:64 Available from: http://www.jcmr-online.com/content/14/1/63
13. Garg P, Broadbent DA, Swoboda PP, Foley JRJ, Fent GJ, Musa TA, et al. Acute Infarct Extracellular Volume Mapping to Quantify Myocardial Area at Risk and Chronic Infarct Size on Cardiovascular Magnetic Resonance ImagingCLINICAL PERSPECTIVE. Circ. Cardiovasc. Imaging [Internet]. 2017 [cited 2017 Jul 22];10:e006182. Available from: http://www.ncbi.nlm.nih.gov/pubmed/28674085.
14. Thygesen K, Alpert JS, Jaffe AS, Simoons ML, Chaitman BR, White HD, et al. Third universal definition of myocardial infarction. J. Am. Coll. Cardiol. [Internet]. 2012 [cited 2014 Nov 10];60:1581–1598. Available from: http://www.ncbi.nlm.nih.gov/pubmed/22958960.
15. Steg PG, James SK, Atar D, Badano LP, Blömstrom-Lundqvist C, Borger MA, et al. ESC Guidelines for the management of acute myocardial infarction in patients presenting with ST-segment elevation. Eur. Heart J. [Internet]. 2012 [cited 2014 Jul 9];33:2569–2619. Available from: http://www.ncbi.nlm.nih.gov/pubmed/22922416.
16. Levine GN, Bates ER, Bittl JA, Brindis RG, Fihn SD, Fleisher LA, et al. 2016 ACC/AHA Guideline Focused Update on Duration of Dual Antiplatelet Therapy in Patients With Coronary Artery Disease: A Report of the American College of Cardiology/American Heart Association Task Force on Clinical Practice Guidelines: An Update of the. Circulation [Internet]. 2016 [cited 2016 Apr 8];134:e123–e155 Available from: http://circ.ahajournals.org/lookup/doi/10.1161/CIR.0000000000000404
17. The Thrombolysis in Myocardial Infarction (TIMI) trial. Phase I findings. TIMI Study Group. N. Engl. J. Med. [Internet]. 1985 [cited 2015 Dec 25];312:932–936. Available from: http://www.ncbi.nlm.nih.gov/pubmed/4038784.
18. Messroghli DR, Bainbridge GJ, Alfakih K, Jones TR, Plein S, Ridgway JP, et al. Assessment of regional left ventricular function: accuracy and reproducibility of positioning standard short-axis sections in cardiac MR imaging. Radiology. 2005 [cited 2015 Aug 12];235:229–236. Available from: http://www.ncbi.nlm.nih.gov/pubmed/15731374.
19. Cerqueira MD, Weissman NJ, Dilsizian V, Jacobs AK, Kaul S, Laskey WK, et al. Standardized myocardial segmentation and nomenclature for tomographic imaging of the heart. A statement for healthcare professionals from the Cardiac Imaging Committee of the Council on Clinical Cardiology of the American Heart Association. Circulation. 2002 [cited 2014 Nov 15];105:539–542. Available from: http://www.ncbi.nlm.nih.gov/pubmed/11815441.
20. Nowosielski M, Schocke M, Mayr A, Pedarnig K, Klug G, Köhler A, et al. Comparison of wall thickening and ejection fraction by cardiovascular

magnetic resonance and echocardiography in acute myocardial infarction. J. Cardiovasc. Magn. Reson. [Internet]. 2009 [cited 2016 Apr 10];11:22 Available from: http://www.pubmedcentral.nih.gov/articlerender.fcgi?artid=2717065&tool=pmcentrez&rendertype=abstract

21. Rodrigues JCL, Rohan S, Dastidar AG, Trickey A, Szantho G, Ratcliffe LEK, et al. The Relationship Between Left Ventricular Wall Thickness, Myocardial Shortening, and Ejection Fraction in Hypertensive Heart Disease: Insights From Cardiac Magnetic Resonance Imaging. J. Clin. Hypertens. [Internet]. 2016 [cited 2017 mar 4];18:1119–1127. Available from: http://www.ncbi.nlm.nih.gov/pubmed/27316563.

22. Russo C, Jin Z, Homma S, Rundek T, Elkind MS V, Sacco RL, et al. Relationship of multidirectional myocardial strain with radial thickening and ejection fraction and impact of left ventricular hypertrophy: a study in a community-based cohort. Echocardiography [Internet]. NIH Public Access; 2013 [cited 2017 Jul 7];30:794–802. Available from: http://www.ncbi.nlm.nih.gov/pubmed/23360509.

23. Fontana M, Banypersad SM, Treibel TA, Abdel-Gadir A, Maestrini V, Lane T, et al. Differential Myocyte Responses in Patients with Cardiac Transthyretin Amyloidosis and Light-Chain Amyloidosis: A Cardiac MR Imaging Study. Radiology Radiological Society of North America. 2015 [cited 2016 Dec 20];277:388–397 Available from: http://pubs.rsna.org/doi/10.1148/radiol.2015141744

24. Gerbaud E, Montaudon M, Chasseriaud W, Gilbert S, Cochet H, Pucheu Y, et al. Effect of ivabradine on left ventricular remodelling after reperfused myocardial infarction: A pilot study. Arch. Cardiovasc Dis.2014 [cited 2017 Jul 7];107:33–41. Available from: http://www.ncbi.nlm.nih.gov/pubmed/24440004.

25. Huttin O, Coiro S, Selton-Suty C, Juillière Y, Donal E, Magne J, et al. Prediction of Left Ventricular Remodeling after a Myocardial Infarction: Role of Myocardial Deformation: A Systematic Review and Meta-Analysis. PLoS One [Internet]. Public Library of Science; 2016 [cited 2017 Jul 7];11:e0168349. Available from: http://www.ncbi.nlm.nih.gov/pubmed/28036335.

26. Bulluck H, Rosmini S, Abdel-Gadir A, White SK, Bhuva AN, Treibel TA, et al. Automated Extracellular Volume Fraction Mapping Provides Insights Into the Pathophysiology of Left Ventricular Remodeling Post-Reperfused ST-Elevation Myocardial Infarction. J. Am. Heart Assoc. [Internet]. Lippincott Williams & Wilkins; 2016 [cited 2016 Oct 13];5:e003555. Available from: http://www.ncbi.nlm.nih.gov/pubmed/27402229.

27. Machin D, Campbell M, Fayers P PA. Sample Size Tables for Clinical Studies. Second Ed. Blackwell Sci. IBSN. 1997;18–20.

28. Carberry J, Carrick D, Haig C, Rauhalammi SM, Ahmed N, Mordi I, et al. Remote Zone Extracellular Volume and Left Ventricular Remodeling in Survivors of ST-Elevation Myocardial Infarction. Hypertens. (Dallas, Tex. 1979) [Internet]. 2016 [cited 2016 Oct 13];68:385–391. Available from: http://www.ncbi.nlm.nih.gov/pubmed/27354423.

29. Epstein FH, Wijns W, Vatner SF, Camici PG. Hibernating Myocardium. N. Engl. J. Med. 1998 [cited 2017 Jul 7];339:173–181. Available from: http://www.ncbi.nlm.nih.gov/pubmed/9664095.

30. Hassell MECJ, Vlastra W, Robbers L, Hirsch A, Nijveldt R, Tijssen JGP, et al. Long-term left ventricular remodelling after revascularisation for ST-segment elevation myocardial infarction as assessed by cardiac magnetic resonance imaging. Open Hear. [Internet]. 2017;4. Available from: http://openheart.bmj.com/content/4/1/e000569.abstract

31. Carluccio E, Biagioli P, Alunni G, Murrone A, Giombolini C, Ragni T, et al. Patients With Hibernating Myocardium Show Altered Left Ventricular Volumes and Shape, Which Revert After Revascularization. J. Am. Coll. Cardiol. [Internet]. 2006 [cited 2017 Jul 7];47 Available from: http://www.onlinejacc.org/content/47/5/969?ijkey=13b01788051362944e2c90202bc381cfe1c3504e&keytype2=tf_ipsecsha

32. Levine JM, Collins JD, Murtagh G, Markl M, Carr JC, Choudhury L. Segmental late gadolinium enhancement and gadolinium extracellular volume in hypertrophic cardiomyopathy. J. Cardiovasc. Magn. Reson. [Internet]. BioMed Central; 2016 [cited 2016 Oct 12];18:P155 Available from: http://jcmr-online.biomedcentral.com/articles/10.1186/1532-429X-18-S1-P155

33. Collins J, Sommerville C, Magrath P, Spottiswoode B, Freed BH, Benzuly KH, et al. Extracellular volume fraction is more closely associated with altered regional left ventricular velocities than left ventricular ejection fraction in nonischemic cardiomyopathy. Circ. Cardiovasc. Imaging [Internet]. 2015 [cited 2016 Oct 12];8.

Available from: http://www.ncbi.nlm.nih.gov/pubmed/25552491.

34. Bogaert J, Bosmans H, Maes A, Suetens P, Marchal G, Rademakers FE. Remote myocardial dysfunction after acute anterior myocardial infarction: impact of left ventricular shape on regional function: a magnetic resonance myocardial tagging study. J. Am. Coll. Cardiol. [Internet]. 2000 [cited 2017 Jul 7];35:1525–1534. Available from: http://www.ncbi.nlm.nih.gov/pubmed/10807456.

35. Talman V, Ruskoaho H. Cardiac fibrosis in myocardial infarction-from repair and remodeling to regeneration. Cell Tissue Res. [Internet]. Springer; 2016 [cited 2017 Jul 7];365:563–581. Available from: http://www.ncbi.nlm.nih.gov/pubmed/27324127.

36. Kidambi A, Motwani M, Uddin A, Ripley DP, McDiarmid AK, Swoboda PP, et al. Myocardial extracellular volume estimation by CMR predicts functional recovery following acute MI. JACC Cardiovasc Imaging. 2016;2071

37. Garg P, Kidambi A, Swoboda PP, Foley JRJ, Musa TA, Ripley DP, et al. The role of left ventricular deformation in the assessment of microvascular obstruction and intramyocardial haemorrhage. Int. J. Cardiovasc. Imaging. 2017 [cited 2016 Nov 22];33:361–370 Available from: http://link.springer.com/10.1007/s10554-016-1006-x

38. Kellman P, Hansen MS, Moon J, Messroghli D, Kellman P, Piechnik S, et al. T1-mapping in the heart: accuracy and precision. J. Cardiovasc. Magn. Reson. [Internet]. BioMed Central; 2014 [cited 2016 Dec 8];16:2 Available from: http://jcmr-online.biomedcentral.com/articles/10.1186/1532-429X-16-2

13

Non-contrast MR angiography at 1.5 Tesla for aortic monitoring in Marfan patients after aortic root surgery

Simon Veldhoen[1,2]* (iD), Cyrus Behzadi[1], Alexander Lenz[1], Frank Oliver Henes[1], Meike Rybczynski[3], Yskert von Kodolitsch[3], Thorsten Alexander Bley[2], Gerhard Adam[1] and Peter Bannas[1]

Abstract

Background: Contrast-enhanced cardiovascular magnetic resonance angiography (CE-CMRA) is the established imaging modality for patients with Marfan syndrome requiring life-long annual aortic imaging before and after aortic root replacement. Contrast-free CMRA techniques avoiding side-effects of contrast media are highly desirable for serial imaging but have not been evaluated in the postoperative setup of Marfan patients. The purpose of this study was to assess the feasibility of non-contrast balanced steady-state free precession (bSSFP) magnetic resonance imaging for aortic monitoring of postoperative patients with Marfan syndrome.

Methods: Sixty-four adult Marfan patients after aortic root replacement were prospectively included. Fourteen patients (22%) had a residual aortic dissection after surgical treatment of type A dissection. bSSFP imaging and CE-CMRA were performed at 1.5 Tesla. Two radiologists evaluated the images regarding image quality (1 = poor, 4 = excellent), artifacts (1 = severe, 4 = none) and aortic pathologies. Readers measured the aortic diameters at defined levels in both techniques. Statistics included observer agreement for image scoring and diameter measurements and ROC analyses for comparison of the diagnostic performance of bSSFP and CE-CMRA.

Results: Both readers observed no significant differences in image quality between bSSFP and CE-CMRA and found a median image quality score of 4 for both techniques (all $p > .05$). No significant differences were found regarding the frequency of image artifacts in both sequences (all $p > .05$). Sensitivity and specificity for detection of aortic dissections was 100% for both readers and techniques. Compared to bSSFP imaging, CE-CMRA resulted in higher diameters (mean bias, 0.9 mm; $p < .05$). The inter-observer biases of diameter measurements were not significantly different (all $p > .05$), except for the distal graft anastomosis ($p = .001$). Using both techniques, the readers correctly identified a graft suture dehiscence with aneurysm formation requiring surgery.

Conclusion: Unenhanced bSSFP CMR imaging allows for riskless aortic monitoring with high diagnostic accuracy in Marfan patients after aortic root surgery.

Background

Marfan syndrome is a genetic disorder of the connective tissue with autosomal dominant inheritance. Its prevalence has been indicated by one in 5.000–10.000 individuals [1, 2]. Mutations in the FBN1 gene encoding the protein Fibrillin cause general connective tissue insufficiency [3, 4]. Progressive dilation of the aortic root at the sinuses of Valsalva is the most common cardiovascular complication of Marfan syndrome [5, 6]. Aortic root aneurysms may cause aortic dissection and represent the main cause of death in undetected Marfan syndrome [5–7]. Nowadays, pharmacotherapies reduce the progression rate of aortic dilation, and elective repair of the aortic root has significantly improved the survival of Marfan patients [8, 9]. However, life-long annual aortic imaging is mandatory for Marfan patients to determine if and when aortic root replacement is indicated [8, 10].

* Correspondence: veldhoen_s@ukw.de
[1]Department of Diagnostic and Interventional Radiology and Nuclear Medicine, University Medical Center Hamburg-Eppendorf, Hamburg, Germany
[2]Department of Diagnostic and Interventional Radiology, University Hospital Würzburg, Bavaria, Germany
Full list of author information is available at the end of the article

Cardiovascular magnetic resonance angiography (CMRA) has been established for serial monitoring of aortic pathologies [11, 12]. Contrast-enhanced CMRA (CE-CMRA) is considered the reference technique in CMRA imaging [11, 12]. However, gadolinium based contrast agents bear the risk of side effects such as hypersensitivity, nephrogenic systemic fibrosis or cerebral gadolinium deposition [13, 14]. This highlights the need for non-contrast CMRA techniques for lifelong annual imaging of Marfan patients. Several non-contrast CMRA techniques have been evaluated for imaging the aorta [15, 16]. Among these, balanced steady-state with free precession (bSSFP) sequences offer inherent high contrast between blood and background tissues, thereby allowing for optimal delineation of the aortic wall [15, 17, 18]. Recent studies confirmed that bSSFP sequences allow for accurate pre-operative monitoring of aortic root diameters in Marfan patients [19–21].

Prolonged survival after aortic surgery has led to an increase of Marfan patients with aortic complications beyond the root [22]. Elective replacement of the aortic root removes the most important predilection site for aneurysms, but the distal aorta remains at risk for dilation [9, 23]. Complications such as aneurysms and dissections in the distal aorta are doubled in Marfan patients with previous elective aortic surgery [9]. However, even after aortic root replacement the ascending aorta remains in focus of interest as life-threatening complications such as suture dehiscence with development of aneurysm in the graft region may occur [24, 25]. Thus, life-long annual aortic imaging is mandatory before and after aortic root replacement for early detection of proximal as well as distal aortic complications [6, 8, 9, 26–28].

Thorough evaluation of non-contrast bSSFP sequences for imaging in the post-operative set up of Marfan has not yet been performed. However, minimizing the risks of contrast media associated side-effects is highly desirable in Marfan patients undergoing lifelong annual aortic imaging also after aortic surgery. Therefore, we aimed to assess the feasibility of non-contrast bSSFP imaging for monitoring of aortic diameters and dissections in Marfan patients after aortic root replacement.

Methods
Study population
The prospective cohort study was approved by the institutional review board. All patients provided written informed consent. We included 64 adult patients (42 men; 22 women; age range 19–73 years; mean age 44 ± 13 years) with confirmed Marfan after aortic root surgery. Forty-six patients (72%; 30 men; 16 women; age range 19–73 years; mean age 44 ± 13 years) underwent prophylactic aortic root surgery due to increased aortic root diameters. Eighteen patients (28%; 12 men; 6 women; age range 34–72 years; mean age 47 ± 9 years) underwent aortic root replacement

due to acute type A dissection. At the time of CMR imaging, 50 patients (78%) had no dissection, while 14 patients (22%) had a known residual aortic dissection after surgical treatment of type A dissection. These dissections were confirmed by previous cross sectional imaging examinations and/or known from surgical reports. Eleven patients (17%) underwent additional aortic surgery distally to the aortic root: Five patients had aortic arch replacement, two had prosthesis of the descending aorta, and four had thoracic endovascular aortic repair of the descending aorta.

All included Marfan patients underwent CMR imaging as part of their routine postoperative follow-up. The mean interval between aortic root surgery and CMR study was 6.9 ± 5.9 years. Minors and patients with contraindications for CMR were not included. The local Universitary Marfan Center associated with the University Heart Center established the Marfan diagnosis in each subject based on evaluation according to the latest Ghent nosology as well as genetic analyses with sequencing of the FBN1 gene [2, 11, 29].

CMR imaging
CMR imaging was performed using a 1.5 Tesla scanner equipped with a five-channel coil for cardiac imaging (Achieva, Philips Medical Systems, The Netherlands). Electrocardiography (ECG)-leads were placed in typical manner for cardiac triggering.

ECG-gated non-contrast 2D bSSFP imaging with sensitivity encoding (SENSE) was triggered to the end-diastolic phase of the cardiac cycle for minimization of motion artefacts and acquired during end-expiratory breath-hold as recommended by current guidelines [11]. Images were acquired in the transversal and coronal plane as well as in para-sagittal orientation aligned with the curvature of the aortic arch during a single breath-hold for each orientation. [19, 21]. Image parameters were as follows: TR/TE, 3.2/1.6 ms; flip angle, 90°; field of view, 430 mm × 302 mm; matrix, 256 × 180; number of slices, 20; in-plane resolution, 1.7 mm × 1.7 mm; slice thickness, 10 mm; SENSE-factor, 2; acquisition time for each stack, 12–16 s (depending on the individual heart rate).

Contrast-enhanced 3D CMRA of the entire aorta was performed after automatic injection (2 ml/s) of gadopentetate dimeglumine (Gd-DTPA, Magnevist, Bayer-Schering Pharma AG, Germany) at a dose of 0.1 mmol/kg bodyweight into an antecubital vein. Scanning parameters of the gradient-echo T1-weighted sequence were as follows: TR/TE, 4.8/1.4 ms; flip angle, 40°; field of view, 450x360x90–130 mm; matrix, 368x189x25–36. True spatial resolution was 1.2 × 1.9 × 3.6 mm³, interpolated to 0.9 × 0.7 × 3.6 mm (512 × 512 matrix). To determine the scan delay after contrast injection a 2 ml test bolus was used. Imaging was started at the time of contrast arrival in the descending aorta during end-expiratory breath hold. Two separate post-contrast datasets were acquired with a 10-s respiration interval. The series with superior illustration of the contrast bolus was picked for image analyses. Total acquisition time, including the test bolus, ranged from 90s to 120 s depending on the patient anatomy and the field of view.

Qualitative image analyses

Two radiologists ((S.V and C.B.) with five and four years of experience in cardiovascular imaging, respectively) performed individual reading of anonymized and randomized images acquired with bSSFP and CE-CMRA sequences. Readers evaluated entire series of all imaging planes.

First, the overall subjective image quality of the aorta was rated based on a four-point scale: Score of 1 = poor image quality, poorly defined anatomic details, poor diagnostic confidence; score of 2 = reduced image quality, limitations in anatomic detail, impairment of diagnostic confidence; score of 3 = good image quality, clear anatomic details, no impairment of diagnostic confidence; score of 4 = excellent image quality, distinct anatomic details, full diagnostic confidence [30].

Second, the presence of image artifacts at the site of the aortic root graft was scored on a four-point scale: Score of 1 = severe artifacts; score of 2 = moderate artifacts; score of 3 = minor artifacts; score of 4 = no artifacts [31].

Third, the presence of aortic dissection was scored on a five-point scale (score of 1 = certainly dissection, full diagnostic confidence; score of 2 = probably dissection, impairment of diagnostic confidence; score of 3 = unsure; score of 4 = probably no dissection, impairment of diagnostic confidence; score of 5 = certainly no dissection, full diagnostic confidence) [31, 32].

Fourth, the readers were asked to note the presence of any other relevant aortic pathology such as aneurysms.

Quantitative image analyses

Both readers performed aortic diameter measurements on identically orientated para-sagittal source images of non-contrast bSSFP and CE-CMRA sequences. Aortic diameters were measured perpendicular to the blood-filled lumen [21]. Readers were free to choose appropriate slices displaying the maximal profile of the aorta from the stacks of para-sagittal images [21]. The following measuring points were determined: i) middle of the aortic root graft, ii) distal anastomosis of the graft, iii) ascending aorta at the level of the pulmonary trunk, iv) mid aortic arch between the branching of the left carotid and the left subclavian artery, v) descending aorta at the level of the pulmonary trunk, vi) aorta at the level of the diaphragm, and vii) aorta proximal to the coeliac trunk

(Fig. 1) [6, 11]. Defined aortic measuring levels that were replaced by implanted grafts were skipped and excluded from further analyses. Diameters were measured three times in each image series: Reader 1 performed two measurements with an interval of 6 weeks for assessment of the intra-observer agreement. Reader 2 performed a third measurement for assessment of the inter-observer agreement.

Statistical analysis

Wilcoxon signed-rank test was used to assess differences in the subjective scoring of the image quality and the degree of artifacts in bSSFP imaging and CE-CMRA. Intraclass correlation coefficient (ICC) was calculated to assess inter-observer agreement regarding these subjective scorings. Sensitivity and specificity regarding detection of aortic dissection in bSSFP imaging and CE-CMRA was assessed using receiver operating characteristic (ROC) analyses. Scorings were clustered in identified dissections with high levels of confidence (scores of 4 and 5) vs. no dissection (scores 1–3). The resulting areas under the curve (AUC) with corresponding 95% confidence intervals (CI) were used to compare the performance of the techniques regarding detection of aortic dissections.

Bland–Altman and ICC analyses were used to assess intra- and inter-observer agreement regarding diameter measurements obtained from bSSFP imaging and CE-CMRA. A paired t-test was performed for comparison of mean differences and F-test for comparison of variances. Pearson's correlation was calculated to determine the correlation between diameters assessed by bSSFP and CE-CMRA. P-values <.05 were considered as statistically significant. Statistical analyses were performed using SPSS v. 20.0 (International Business Machines, Inc., Chicago, Illinois, USA) and Excel v. 15.26 (Microsoft, Redmond, Washington, USA).

Results

All CMR studies were performed without periprocedural complications and all examinations were included into the evaluation.

Overall aortic image quality

All examinations were diagnostic. None of the CMR examinations resulted in poor diagnostic confidence (score 1) regarding the overall image quality. Reader 1 and reader 2 found good to excellent image quality in 97 and 95% of the bSSFP examinations and in 98% of CE-CMRA scans, respectively. There was no significant difference in image quality scores between SSFP imaging and CE-CMRA (reader 1, p = .37; reader 2, p = .16). The median image quality score was 4 for both readers and techniques. The inter-rater agreement was comparable

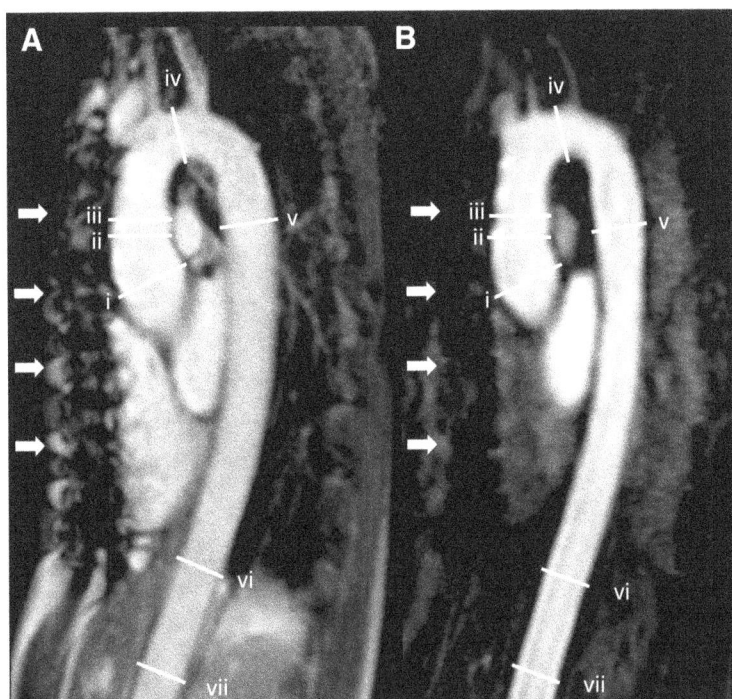

Fig. 1 Aortic diameter measurements: Parasagittal (**a**) non-contrast 2D bSSFP and (**b**) 3D CE-CMRA of a 37-year-old woman with Marfan syndrome 5 years after valve-sparing aortic root replacement (David procedure). White lines indicate the seven measurement levels along the aorta. From proximal to distal: i) middle of the aortic root graft, ii) distal anastomosis of the graft, iii) ascending aorta at the level of the pulmonary trunk, iv) mid aortic arch, v) descending aorta at the level of the pulmonary trunk, vi) aorta at the level of the diaphragm, and vii) aorta proximal to the celiac trunk. Both readers rated the image quality and artifact level as 4 points (best quality and no diagnosis interfering artifacts, respectively) for both bSSFP and CE-CMRA. However, note the presence of artifacts caused by sternal cerclages in both examinations (white arrows)

(ICC = 0.63 for bSSFP vs. 0.56 for CE-CMRA). Detailed results of image quality ratings are provided in Table 1.

Artifact scoring at the level of the aortic root graft

Reader 1 found severe or moderate artifacts in 9% of bSSFP scans (0% in CE-CMRA) and scored 91% with minor or no artifacts (100% in CE-CMRA). Reader 2 found severe or moderate artifacts in 13% of bSSFP scans (11% in CE-CMRA) and scored 88% with minor or no artifacts (89% in CE-CMRA). The higher frequency of artifacts observed in bSSFP imaging did not reach the level of significance for both readers (reader 1, $p = .18$; reader 2, $p = .12$). ICC analyses showed superior inter-rater agreement in bSSFP imaging (bSSFP, 0.81; CE-CMRA, 0.65). Detailed results of image artifact ratings are given in Table 1.

Scoring of aortic dissection

Reader 1 and reader 2 detected all of the 14 dissections with both bSSFP and CE-CMRA, resulting in a sensitivity of 100% for both readers and techniques. There were no false-positive ratings regarding both readers and techniques resulting in a specificity of 100%. Corresponding AUCs of reader 1 and reader 2 were 1.00 (CI: 1.00–1.00) for both techniques. The inter-rater agreement was

excellent in both bSSFP (ICC 0.98, CI: 0.97–0.99) and CE-CMRA (ICC 0.99, CI: 0.99–1.00). Figure 2 shows the comparison of bSSFP and CE-CMRA in a patient with known residual type A aortic dissection.

Aortic diameter measurements and observer agreement

CE-CMRA resulted in statistically significant larger diameters at all aortic levels (bias: 0.5–1.3 mm) when compared to non-contrast bSSFP imaging (all $p < .05$). Pearson's correlation analyses revealed moderate to strong correlation of diameters obtained by bSSFP imaging and CE-CMRA at all aortic levels ($r = 0.66$–0.96). Detailed results of diameter measurements are provided in Table 2.

The mean intra-observer biases of the diameter measurements ranged between -0.1 mm and 0.6 mm in bSSFP imaging vs. -0.2 mm and 0.7 mm in CE-CMRA without a statistically significant difference (all $p > .05$). Also, there was no statistically significant difference between the variances of both bSSFP imaging and CE-CMRA (all $p > .05$). Detailed results of the intra-observer analyses are given in Table 3.

The mean inter-observer bias of the diameter measurements ranged between –3.9 mm and 2.1 mm in bSSFP imaging vs. -3.3 mm and 2.7 mm in CE-CMRA. There was

Table 1 Results of the qualitative measurements

Qualitative Reading and Technique	Reader 1		Reader 2		ICC
Overall aortic image quality					
2D bSSFP	n	%	n	%	0.63 [0.45–0.76]
Score 1 – Poor	0	0.0	0	0.0	
Score 2 – Reduced	2	3.1	3	4.7	
Score 3 – Good	11	17.2	20	31.3	
Score 4 – Excellent	51	79.7	41	64.1	
Median score	4		4		
3D CE-CMRA	N	%	n	%	0.56 [0.37–0.71]
Score 1 – Poor	0	0.0	0	0.0	
Score 2 – Reduced	1	1.6	1	1.6	
Score 3 – Good	10	15.6	16	25.0	
Score 4 – Excellent	53	82.8	47	73.4	
Median score	4		4		
P (Wilcoxon)	0.37		0.16		
Artifact scoring at the aortic root					
2D bSSFP	n	%	n	%	0.81 [0.62–0.90]
Score 1 - Severe	2	3.1	2	3.1	
Score 2 - Moderate	4	6.3	6	9.4	
Score 3 - Minor	9	14.1	20	31.3	
Score 4 - Absent	49	76.6	36	56.3	
Median score	4		4		
3D CE-CMRA	n	%	n	%	
Score 1 - Severe	0	0.0	0	0.0	0.65 [0.46–0.78]
Score 2 - Moderate	0	0.0	7	10.9	
Score 3 - Minor	14	21.9	11	17.2	
Score 4 - Absent	50	78.1	46	71.9	
Median score	4		4		
P (Wilcoxon)	0.18		0.12		

Categorial rating of non-contrast 2D–balanced steady state free precession (bSSFP) imaging and 3D contrast-enhanced cardiovascular magnetic resonance angiography (CE-CMRA) regarding diagnostic image quality and image artifacts was performed using Likert scales. The scoring data of the two readers are given as absolute frequencies and percentages. Wilcoxon signed rank test was used to intraindividually compare the two sequence techniques. $P < .05$ indicated significant differences. The Intraclass Correlation Coefficient (ICC) was used to assess the interrater agreement. Its 95% confidence interval is given in square brackets

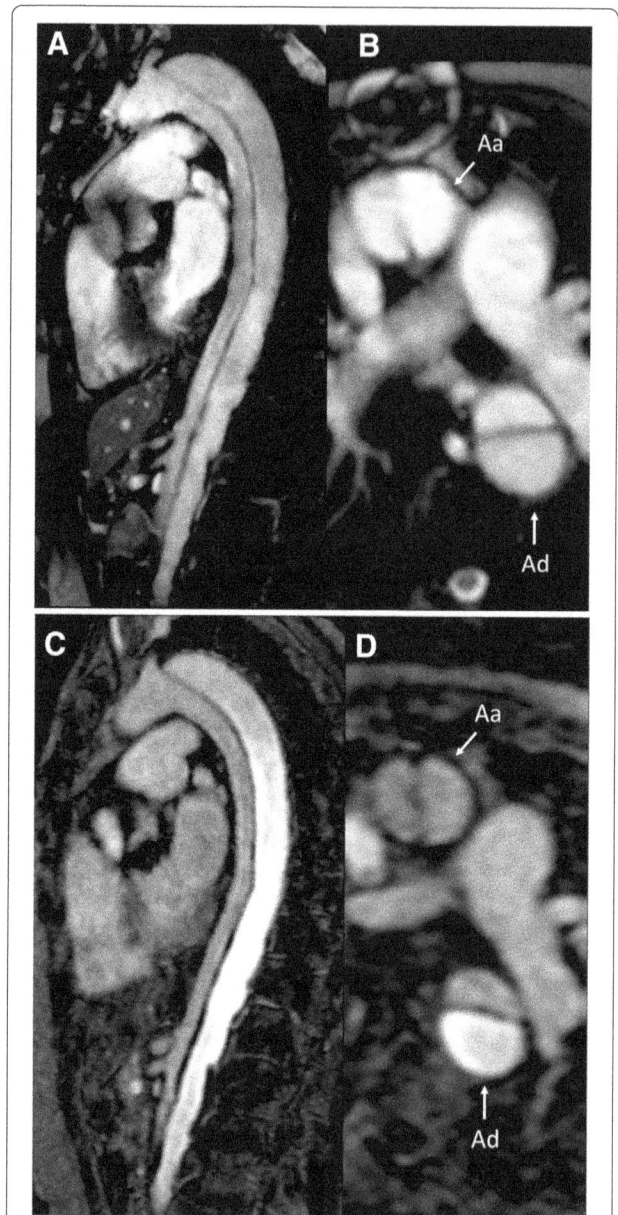

Fig. 2 Aortic dissection in bSSFP and CE-CMRA: Residual aortic dissection 18-years after aortic root replacement due to acute type A dissection in a 72 year-old woman with Marfan syndrome. Both non-contrast 2D SSFP in (**a**) parasagittal and (**b**) transversal plane as well as 3D CE-CMRA in (**c**) parasagittal and (**d**) transversal orientation clearly display the dissection membrane visible in the ascending (Aa) and descending aorta (Ad) with high image quality (4 points by both readers). The CE-CMRA provides additional information regarding the perfusion of lumens and shows hyperperfusion of the larger false lumen in the descending aorta in this case

no statistically significant difference between the biases of bSSFP imaging and CE-CMRA (all p > .05), except for the level of the distal anastomosis of the aortic root graft (mean difference, bSSFP 0.1 mm vs. 1.4 mm in CE-CMRA; $p = .02$). There was no statistically significant difference between the variances of both bSSFP imaging and CMRA (all p > .05), except for the level of the distal anastomosis of the aortic root graft (bSSFP, 95% limits of agreement, ±4.5 mm vs. CE-CMRA, ±7.9 mm; $p = .001$), the descending aorta (bSSFP, 95% limits of agreement ±6.1 mm vs. CE-CMRA, ±12.0 mm; p = <.001), and the celiac trunk (bSSFP, 95% limits of agreement ±14.3 mm vs. CE-CMRA, ±5.3 mm; p = <.001). Detailed results of the inter-observer analyses are given in Table 4.

Table 2 Comparison of aortic diameters as determined by 2D bSSFP and 3D CE-CMRA imaging

2D bSSFP vs. 3D CE-CMRA	Mid Graft	Distal anastomosis	Ascending aorta	Aortic arch	Descending aorta	Diaphragm	Coelic trunk
Mean diameter 2D bSSFP (mm)	32.9	29.1	31.7	27.9	28.0	26.4	25.8
Mean diameter 3D CE-CMRA (mm)	33.5	30.2	32.9	28.9	28.8	26.9	26.7
Mean difference (mm)	−0.5	−1.1	−1.3	−1.0	−0.8	−0.6	−0.9
Limits of agreement (mm)	−5.7 to 4.6	−7.1 to 4.9	−4.9 to 2.4	−7.1 to 5.0	−10.5 to 8.9	−5.2 to 4.0	−5.1 to 3.2
Standard deviation (mm)	2.6	3.0	1.9	3.1	4.9	2.3	2.1
Variance (mm^2)	7.0	9.3	3.5	9.46	24.4	5.4	4.5
Pearson's correlation (r)	0.75	0.66	0.89	0.74	0.79	0.96	0.96
P value (t-test)	**0.005**	**0.009**	**0.011**	**0.011**	**0.042**	**<0.001**	**<0.001**

Comparison of aortic diameters as determined by 2D bSSFP and 3D CE-CMRA imaging as described by Bland and Altman. Provided measurements are the average of reader 1 and reader 2. Pearson's correlation coefficient (r) for the different imaging modalities is indicated. Paired t-test was performed for comparison of mean diameters. Significant differences are in bold

Other findings

Both readers correctly identified a postoperative aneurysm at the distal aortic suture line of the aortic root graft in both non-contrast bSSFP and CE-CMRA in one of the 64 included patients (1.6%) (Fig. 3). Following computed tomography angiography for validation of this finding, the patient underwent surgical revision with re-replacement of the aortic root. No other pathology of the aortic graft region was found in any of the remaining 63 patients (98.4%).

Discussion

We successfully demonstrated non-contrast bSSFP imaging to provide high image quality, precise and reproducible aortic diameter measurements, and high diagnostic performance in detection of relevant aortic pathologies in Marfan patients after aortic root replacement.

All patients were correctly scored regarding presence of aortic dissections by both readers using both non-contrast bSSFP imaging and CE-CMRA, resulting in 100% sensitivity and specificity for both imaging techniques. Moreover, both readers correctly detected a postoperative aneurysm at the distal aortic suture line with both imaging techniques in a patient after David procedure (Fig. 3). Thus, both bSSFP and CE-CMRA provided comparable diagnostic performance regarding monitoring of aortic dissection and detection of other potentially life-threating complications in postoperative Marfarn patients.

Both observers found no significant differences in overall image quality regarding the two imaging techniques. Former studies in pre-operative patients found superior image quality of bSSFP sequences when compared to CE-CMRA [19, 21]. However, this superior image quality was

Table 3 Intra-observer variance

	Mid-Graft	Distal anastomosis	Ascending aorta	Aortic arch	Descending aorta	Diaphragm	Celiac trunk
Intra-observer variance							
2D SSFP							
Mean difference (mm)	0.22	0.38	0.56	0.14	−0.05	0.29	−0.07
Limits of agreement (mm)	−3.18 to 3.62	−4.39 to 5.14	−3.59 to 4.70	−5.22 to 5.49	−4.21 to 4.10	−6.55 to 7.13	−7.64 to 7.51
Standard deviation (mm)	1.74	2.43	2.11	2.73	2.12	3.49	3.87
Variance (mm^2)	3.01	5.92	4.47	7.47	4.50	12.17	14.95
ICC	0.95	0.88	0.94	0.89	0.98	0.96	0.94
3D CE-CMRA							
Mean difference (mm)	0.03	−0.23	0.17	0.58	0.19	0.33	0.73
Limits of agreement (mm)	−3.60 to 3.66	−5.54 to 5.07	−2.55 to 2.88	−3.82 to 4.97	−4.32 to 4.72	−5.31 to 5.98	−6.69 to 8.16
Standard deviation (mm)	1.85	2.71	1.38	2.24	2.31	2.88	3.79
Variance (mm^2)	3.44	7.34	1.92	5.02	5.31	8.29	14.35
ICC	0.92	0.84	0.97	0.93	0.95	0.96	0.92
p-value (t test)	0.491	0.140	0.480	0.367	0.589	0.922	0.869
p-value (F test)	0.605	0.398	0.089	0.133	0.530	0.144	0.870

Intra-observer variance of measured aortic diameters as determined by non-contrast 2D bSSFP imaging and 3D CE-CMRA as described by Bland and Altman. Intraclass correlation coefficients (ICC) are given for both sequence types. Paired t-test was performed for comparison of mean differences and F test for comparison of variances

Table 4 Inter-observer variance

	Inter-observer variance						
	Mid-Graft	Distal anastomosis	Ascending aorta	Aortic arch	Descending aorta	Diaphragm	Celiac trunk
	2D SSFP						
Mean difference (mm)	2.08	0.08	1.17	0.10	1.97	1.10	0.79
Limits of agreement (mm)	−4.45 to 8.61	−4.43 to 4.59	−4.87 to 7.20	−5.04 to 5.24	−4.10 to 8.03	−6.34 to 8.55	−8.64 to 10.21
Standard deviation (mm)	3.33	2.30	3.1	2.62	3.10	3.80	4.81
Variance (mm^2)	11.1	5.29	9.47	6.87	9.59	14.43	23.13
ICC	0.69	0.83	0.86	0.90	0.95	0.89	0.85
	3D CE-CMRA						
Mean difference (mm)	2.34	1.38	1.44	0.41	2.69	1.62	0.95
Limits of agreement (mm)	−4.8 to 9.56	−5.72 to 8.47	−3.54 to 6.43	−5.68 to 6.49	−9.31 to 14.70	−5.39 to 8.62	−4.34 to 6.25
Standard deviation (mm)	3.68	3.62	2.54	3.10	6.13	3.57	2.70
Variance (mm^2)	13.57	13.11	6.47	9.63	37.53	12.77	7.29
ICC	0.48	0.68	0.84	0.78	0.75	0.87	0.88
p-value (t test)	0.543	**0.023**	0.385	0.549	0.350	0.064	0.069
p-value (F test)	0.443	**0.001**	0.440	0.220	**<0.001**	0.641	**<0.001**

Inter-observer variance of measured aortic diameters as determined by non-contrast 2D bSSFP imaging and 3D CE-CMRA as described by Bland and Altman. Intraclass correlation coefficients (ICC) are given for both sequence types. Paired t-test was performed for comparison of mean differences and F test for comparison of variances. Significant differences are in bold (significant at $p < .05$)

limited to the aortic root and the ascending aorta. These aortic levels are permanently in motion due to the cardiac cycle and therefore benefit most from ECG-gating, resulting in less blurring of the aortic wall structures in bSSFP images. In contrast, rather motionless distal aortic parts showed comparable image quality in the mentioned pre-operative studies, matching the observations in this report of postoperative Marfarn patients. Moreover, it is likely that the advantage of ECG-gating in bSSFP imaging regarding image quality at the aortic root is mitigated by artifacts caused by the implanted graft. Indeed, results of the subjective scoring of both readers revealed more artifacts at the aortic root graft when using the non-contrast bSSFP sequence at 1.5 Tesla, however, without reaching a statistical significant difference. As bSSFP techniques are prone to off-resonance effects typically manifesting as banding artifacts, more and stronger artifacts caused by surgical material at the stent graft implantation site and the surgical entryway are to be expected [17, 33]. Therefore, unfortunate localization of banding artifacts in bSSFP sequences may require alternative sequences for correct evaluation of the proximal and distal aortic anastomosis in particular cases. As off-resonance artifacts are pronounced at higher field strengths [33, 34], future studies need to address the image quality and artifacts of bSSFP imaging in postoperative Marfarn patients at 3 Tesla.

The diameter measurements revealed a good correlation between bSSFP and CE-CMRA. However, CE-CMRA revealed significantly larger diameters (0.5–1.3 mm) at all measurement points compared to the non-contrast bSSFP sequence. This may be explained by acquisition of the CE-CMRA throughout the cardiac cycle, comprising information from systole and diastole, during which the aortic diameter changes. The resulting blurred aortic wall structures may lead to overestimation of the diameters compared to bSSFP imaging, which was triggered to the diastole as recommended by current guidelines [11]. Previous studies have shown that ECG-gating also improves the image quality of CE-CMRA [35]. However, we do not pursue these ECG-gated contrast-enhanced techniques at our institution, as we strive to avoid the use of contrast material for repeated life-long imaging of Marfan patients.

Both, bSFFP imaging and CE-CMRA revealed excellent intra-rater agreement of diameter measurements at all aortic levels, serving as marker for high reproducibility. Regarding inter-rater agreement, a significant higher variability was found for CE-CMRA than for bSSFP imaging at the distal graft anastomosis. This difference is likely explained by blurring of aortic wall structures due to cardiac motion in CE-CMRA, making reliable and exact measurements challenging.

The results acknowledge bSSFP imaging as an equivalent imaging technique when compared to CE-CMRA regarding aortic monitoring in postoperative Marfan patients. The reported observations have important clinical implications: At our institution, we stopped application of intravenous contrast for routine MR imaging of the thoracic aorta at 1.5 Tesla in asymptomatic postoperative Marfarn patients without known aortic dissection and perform bSSFP imaging only. Only if aortic dissection is known to be present or newly found on non-contrast SSFP, we continue to acquire a CE-CMRA to assess contrast dynamics within the

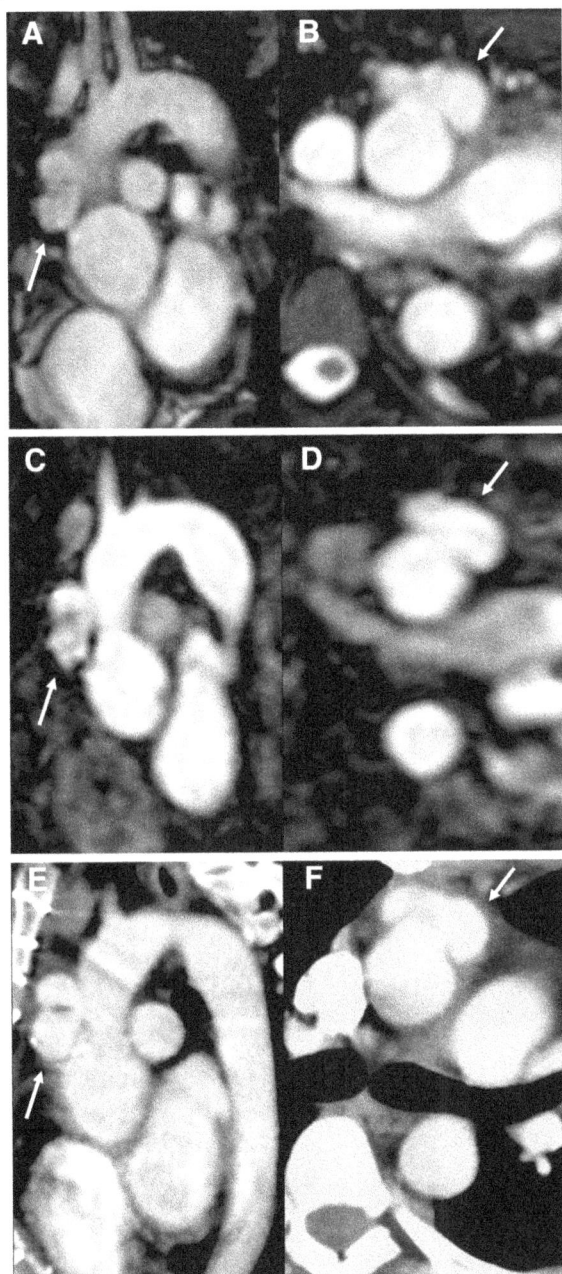

Fig. 3 Postoperative suture dehiscence: Postoperative suture dehiscence with consecutive aneurysm at the distal aortic suture line 1-year after David procedure in a 20-year-old man with Marfan syndrome. Both (**a**, **b**) non-contrast 2D bSSFP and (**c**, **d**) 3D CE-CMRA demonstrate the aneurysm (arrows) with high image quality (4 points by both readers). The CMR-based diagnosis was confirmed with (**e**, **f**) computed tomography angiography. The patient underwent immediate surgical revision with re-replacement of the aortic root for treatment of his potentially life-threating complication.

Beside the patients with aortic dissection, only one other aortic complication after root surgery was observed in the study population (patient with aneurysm at the distal aortic suture line). This limits the validity of the sequence comparison regarding diagnostics of aortic pathologies other than aortic dissection. However, both readers correctly identified this severe complication with both imaging techniques. The reoperation rate over 10 years after aortic root replacement due to postoperative complications has been indicated with 6% in Marfan patients, matching the observed single complication in this study population [36].

Some technical parameters of the used 2D bSFFP and the 3D CE-CMRA sequences did not fully match. This is the case, because a product sequence was used for bSSFP imaging without further adjusting resolution and volumetric coverage to the preset of the CE-CMRA sequence used in our institution, which was also a product sequence. It may be regarded as another study limitation that measurements were performed in para-sagittal planes (along the flow axis of the aorta) without using secondary multiplanar reformations. However, as the orientation of both 2D bSSFP and 3D CE-CMRA were identical, we believe that secondary reformations would not have provided significantly different results. In clinical practice, particularly when the aortic diameters reach threshold values, secondary reformations can be performed to assess the maximal diameter of the aorta in different orientations.

Last, it should be recognized that although the readers performed individual reading of anonymized and randomized images acquired with bSSFP and CE-CMRA sequences, a true blinding was not possible since it is obvious to a reader whether a contrast agent was administered.

Conclusion

In summary, 2D bSSFP imaging and 3D CE-CMRA resulted in equivalent image quality, thereby providing comparable performance regarding detection of aortic dissection and aneurysm as well as reliable aortic diameter assessment in Marfan patients after aortic root replacement. The results acknowledge non-contrast bSSFP imaging of the thoracic aorta as an appropriate alternative for serial monitoring of patients with Marfan syndrome after aortic root surgery. Renouncement of intravenous gadolinium contrast avoids adverse effects and facilitates patient management. Only when aortic dissection is known to be present or newly detected on unenhanced bSSFP images, additional acquisition of a CE-CMRA is recommended.

Abbreviations
AUC: Area under the curve; bSSFP: balanced steady state with free precision; CE-CMRA: Contrast-enhanced CMRA; CI: Confidence interval;

true and false lumens of the dissected aorta (Fig. 3) and for improved three-dimensional visualization of the exact extent of the dissection e.g. within the supraaortic branches.

CMRA: Cardiovascular magnetic resonance angiography;
ECG: Electrocardiogram; ROC: Receiver operating characteristic; TE: Echo time;
TR: Repetition time

Acknowledgements
Not applicable

Funding
Nothing to declare

Authors' contributions
SV and PB were responsible for the conception of the work, for data acquisition, analysis, interpretation and for the manuscript draft. CB, FH and AL substantially contributed to the acquisition and analysis of data for the work. MR and YK were responsible for establishing the Marfan diagnosis and patient selection. TB and GA critically revised the manuscript. All authors read and approved the final manuscript.

Competing interests
All authors declare that they have no competing interests.

Author details
[1]Department of Diagnostic and Interventional Radiology and Nuclear Medicine, University Medical Center Hamburg-Eppendorf, Hamburg, Germany. [2]Department of Diagnostic and Interventional Radiology, University Hospital Würzburg, Bavaria, Germany. [3]Department of General and Interventional Cardiology, University Medical Center Hamburg-Eppendorf, Hamburg, Germany.

References
1. Rimoin DL, Pyeritz RE, Korf B. Emery and Rimoin's Principles and Practice of Medical Genetics. 6th Edition. Academic Press: Oxford; 2013.
2. Loeys BL, Dietz HC, Braverman AC, Callewaert BL, De Backer J, Devereux RB, et al. The revised Ghent nosology for the Marfan syndrome. J Med Genet. 2010;47:476–85.
3. Kodolitsch von Y, Robinson PN. Marfan syndrome: an update of genetics, medical and surgical management. Heart. BMJ Pub Group Ltd and Br Cardiovasc Soc. 2007;93:755–60.
4. Sheikhzadeh S, Brockstaedt L, Habermann CR, Sondermann C, Bannas P, Mir TS, et al. Dural ectasia in Loeys-Dietz syndrome: comprehensive study of 30 patients with a TGFBR1 or TGFBR2 mutation. Clin Genet. 2014;86:545–51. Blackwell Pub Ltd
5. Murdoch JL, Walker BA, Halpern BL, Kuzma JW, McKusick VA. Life expectancy and causes of death in the Marfan syndrome. N Engl J Med. 1972;286:804–8.
6. Judge DP, Dietz HC. Marfan's syndrome. Lancet. 2005;366:1965–76.
7. Holloway BJ, Rosewarne D, Jones RG. Imaging of thoracic aortic disease. Br J Radiol. 2011;84 Spec No 3:S338–S354.
8. Kodolitsch von Y, Rybczynski M, Detter C, Robinson PN. Diagnosis and management of Marfan syndrome. Futur Cardiol. 2008;4:85–96.
9. Engelfriet PM, Boersma E, Tijssen JGP, Bouma BJ, Mulder BJM. Beyond the root: dilatation of the distal aorta in Marfan's syndrome. Heart BMJ Pub Group Ltd and Br Cardiovasc Soc. 2006;92:1238–43.
10. von Kodolitsch Y, Robinson PN, Berger J. When should surgery be performed in Marfan syndrome and other connective tissue disorders to protect against type a dissection? In: Bonser RS, Pagano D, Haverich A, Mascaro J, editors. Controversies in aortic dissection and aneurysmal disease. New York: Springer; 2014. p. 17.
11. Hiratzka LF, Bakris GL, Beckman JA, Bersin RM, Carr VF, Casey DE, et al. 2010 ACCF/AHA/AATS/ACR/ASA/SCA/SCAI/SIR/STS/SVM guidelines for the diagnosis and management of patients with thoracic aortic disease. A report of the American College of Cardiology Foundation/American Heart Association task force on practice guidelines, American Association for Thoracic Surgery, American College of Radiology, American Stroke Association, Society of Cardiovascular Anesthesiologists, Society for Cardiovascular Angiography and Interventions, Society of Interventional Radiology, Society of Thoracic Surgeons, and Society for Vascular Medicine. J Am Coll Cardiol. 2010;55:e27–e129.

12. François CJ, Hartung MP, Reeder SB, Nagle SK, Schiebler ML. MRI for acute chest pain: current state of the art. J Magn Reson Imaging. 2013;37:1290–300.
13. Vitti RA. Gadolinium-based contrast agents and nephrogenic systemic fibrosis. Radiology. Radiol Soc North Am. 2009;250:959–60. 959–authorreply
14. McDonald RJ, McDonald JS, Kallmes DF, Jentoft ME, Murray DL, Thielen KR, et al. Intracranial gadolinium deposition after contrast-enhanced MR imaging. Radiology. 2015;275:772–82.
15. Gebker R, Gomaa O, Schnackenburg B, Rebakowski J, Fleck E, Nagel E. Comparison of different MRI techniques for the assessment of thoracic aortic pathology: 3D contrast enhanced MR angiography, turbo spin echo and balanced steady state free precession. Int J Cardiovasc Imaging. 2007;23:747–56.
16. Krishnam MS, Tomasian A, Deshpande V, Tran L, Laub G, Finn JP, et al. Noncontrast 3D steady-state free-precession magnetic resonance angiography of the whole chest using nonselective radiofrequency excitation over a large field of view: comparison with single-phase 3D contrast-enhancing magnetic resonance angiography. Investig Radiol. 2008;43:411–20.
17. Krishnam MS, Tomasian A, Malik S, Desphande V, Laub G, Ruehm SG. Image quality and diagnostic accuracy of unenhanced SSFP MR angiography compared with conventional contrast-enhanced MR angiography for the assessment of thoracic aortic diseases. Eur Radiol. 2010;20:1311–20.
18. Groth M, Henes FO, Müllerleile K, Bannas P, Adam G, Regier M. Accuracy of thoracic aortic measurements assessed by contrast enhanced and unenhanced magnetic resonance imaging. Eur J Radiol. 2012;81:762–6.
19. Veldhoen S, Behzadi C, Derlin T, Rybczinsky M, Kodolitsch von Y, Sheikhzadeh S, et al. Exact monitoring of aortic diameters in Marfan patients without gadolinium contrast: intraindividual comparison of 2D SSFP imaging with 3D CE-MRA and echocardiography. Eur Radiol. 2015;25:872–82. Springer Berlin Heidelberg
20. Bannas P, Rybczynski M, Sheikhzadeh S, von Kodolitsch Y, Derlin T, Yamamura J, et al. Comparison of cine-MRI and transthoracic echocardiography for the assessment of aortic root diameters in patients with suspected Marfan syndrome. Rofo © Georg Thieme Verlag KG. 2015;187:1022–8.
21. Bannas P, Groth M, Rybczynski M, Sheikhzadeh S, von Kodolitsch Y, Graessner J, et al. Assessment of aortic root dimensions in patients with suspected Marfan syndrome: intraindividual comparison of contrast-enhanced and non-contrast magnetic resonance angiography with echocardiography. Int J Cardiol. 2013;167:190–6. Elsevier B.V
22. Carrel T, Beyeler L, Schnyder A, Zurmühle P, Berdat P, Schmidli J, et al. Reoperations and late adverse outcome in Marfan patients following cardiovascular surgery. Eur J Cardiothorac Surg. 2004;25:671–5. Oxford Univ Press
23. Mimoun L, Detaint D, Hamroun D, Arnoult F, Delorme G, Gautier M, et al. Dissection in Marfan syndrome: the importance of the descending aorta. European heart journal. The Oxford Univ Press. 2011;32:443–9.
24. Jacobs NM, Godwin JD, Wolfe WG, Moore AV, Breiman RS, Korobkin M. Evaluation of the grafted ascending aorta with computed tomography. Complications caused by suture dehiscence. Radiology. 1982;145:749–53.
25. Treasure T, Pepper JR. Aortic root surgery in Marfan syndrome. Heart Ltd. 2011;97:951–2. BMJ Pub Group
26. Russo V, Renzulli M, La Palombara C, Fattori R. Congenital diseases of the thoracic aorta. Role of MRI and MRA. Eur Radiol. 2006;16:676–84.
27. Girdauskas E, Kuntze T, Borger MA, Falk V, Mohr FW. Distal aortic Reinterventions after root surgery in Marfan patients. Ann Thorac Sur. 2008;86:1815–9.
28. de Oliveira NC, David TE, Ivanov J, Armstrong S, Eriksson MJ, Rakowski H, et al. Results of surgery for aortic root aneurysm in patients with Marfan syndrome. J Thorac Cardiovasc Surg. 2003;125:789–96.
29. Kodolitsch von Y, De Backer J, Schüler H, Bannas P, Behzadi C, Bernhardt AM, et al. Perspectives on the revised Ghent criteria for the diagnosis of Marfan syndrome. Appl Clin Genet. 2015;8:137–55. Dove Press
30. Veldhoen S, Laqmani A, Derlin T, Karul M, Hammerle D, Buhk J-H, et al. 256-MDCT for evaluation of urolithiasis: iterative reconstruction allows for a significant reduction of the applied radiation dose while maintaining high subjective and objective image quality. J Med Imaging Radiat Oncol. 2014;58:283–90.
31. Bannas P, Bell LC, Johnson KM, Schiebler ML, François CJ, Motosugi U, et al. Pulmonary embolism detection with three-dimensional Ultrashort Echo time MR imaging: experimental study in canines. Radiol Radiol Soc North Am. 2016;278:413–21.

32. Bannas P, Bookwalter CA, Ziemlewicz T, Motosugi U, Munoz Del Rio A, Potretzke TA, et al. Combined gadoxetic acid and gadofosveset enhanced liver MRI for detection and characterization of liver metastases. Eur Radiol; 2017;27:32–40.. Springer Berlin Heidelberg.

33. Bangerter NK, Hargreaves BA, Vasanawala SS, Pauly JM, Gold GE, Nishimura DG. Analysis of multiple-acquisition SSFP. Magn Reson Med. 2004;51:1038–47. Wiley Subscription Services, Inc., A Wiley Company

34. Tyler DJ, Hudsmith LE, Petersen SE, Francis JM, Weale P, Neubauer S, et al. Cardiac cine MR-imaging at 3T: FLASH vs SSFP. J Cardiovasc Magn Reson. 2006;8:709–15. Taylor & Francis

35. Groves EM, Bireley W, Dill K, Carroll TJ, Carr JC. Quantitative analysis of ECG-gated high-resolution contrast-enhanced MR angiography of the thoracic aorta. American journal of Roentgenology. Am Roentgen Ray Soc. 2007;188:522–8.

36. Price J, Magruder JT, Young A, Grimm JC, Patel ND, Alejo D, et al. Long-term outcomes of aortic root operations for Marfan syndrome: a comparison of Bentall versus aortic valve-sparing procedures. J Thorac Cardiovasc Surg Elsevier. 2016;151:330–6.

14

Additive value of 3T cardiovascular magnetic resonance coronary angiography for detecting coronary artery disease

Lijun Zhang[1], Xiantao Song[2], Li Dong[1], Jianan Li[2], Ruiyu Dou[1], Zhanming Fan[1*], Jing An[3] and Debiao Li[4]

Abstract

Background: The purpose of the work was to evaluate the incremental diagnostic value of free-breathing, contrast-enhanced, whole-heart, 3 T cardiovascular magnetic resonance coronary angiography (CE-MRCA) to stress/rest myocardial perfusion imaging (MPI) and late gadolinium enhancement (LGE) imaging for detecting coronary artery disease (CAD).

Methods: Fifty-one patients with suspected CAD underwent a comprehensive cardiovascular magnetic resonance (CMR) examination (CE-MRCA, MPI, and LGE). The additive diagnostic value of MRCA to MPI and LGE was evaluated using invasive x-ray coronary angiography (XA) as the standard for defining functionally significant CAD ($\geq$ 50% stenosis in vessels > 2 mm in diameter).

Results: 90.2% (46/51) patients (54.0 $\pm$ 11.5 years; 71.7% men) completed CE-MRCA successfully. On per-patient basis, compared to MPI/LGE alone or MPI alone, the addition of MRCA resulted in higher sensitivity (100% vs. 76.5%, $p < 0.01$), no change in specificity (58.3% vs. 66.7%, $p = 0.6$), and higher accuracy (89.1% vs 73.9%, $p < 0.01$) for CAD detection (prevalence = 73.9%). Compared to LGE alone, the addition of CE-MRCA resulted in higher sensitivity (97.1% vs. 41.2%, $p < 0.01$), inferior specificity (83.3% vs. 91.7%, $p = 0.02$), and higher diagnostic accuracy (93.5% vs. 54.3%, $p < 0.01$).

Conclusion: The inclusion of successful free-breathing, whole-heart, 3 T CE-MRCA significantly improved the sensitivity and diagnostic accuracy as compared to MPI and LGE alone for CAD detection.

Keywords: 3 Tesla, Contrast enhanced, Coronary magnetic resonance angiography, Stress-rest perfusion imaging, Late gadolinium enhancement, Coronary artery disease

Background

Coronary artery disease (CAD) is a leading cause of mortality and morbidity around the world [1, 2]. Accurate diagnosis of CAD is important in risk stratification and in guiding clinical management [3–5]. Cardiovascular magnetic resonance (CMR) has emerged as an effective tool for the detection of CAD. CMR at both 1.5 T and 3 T has increasingly been used in clinical routine to assess myocardial ischemia and infarction caused by coronary artery stenosis using stress-rest myocardial perfusion imaging (MPI) and late gadolinium enhancement (LGE) imaging [6]. However, it is highly desirable to directly visualize coronary artery stenoses. CMR coronary angiography (MRCA) is technically challenging but has seen steady improvement in the last decade with highly promising clinical results [7–11]. At 1.5 T, several studies have shown the incremental value of MRCA when added to CMR MPI and LGE [12, 13]. The combined use of MRCA and CMR stress perfusion improved specificity for the detection of significant CAD [12]. Contrast-enhanced MRCA (CE-MRCA) at 3 T has shown excellent results in preliminary patient studies [10]. The purpose of this study was to evaluate the incremental value of CE-MRCA for the detection of CAD when added to routine CMR on 3 T.

Methods

Patient population

From October 2015 to February 2017, consecutive patients with suspected CAD were prospectively recruited. Inclusion criteria were: (1) age 30 years or older, (2)

* Correspondence: fanzm120@126.com
[1]Department of Radiology, Beijing Anzhen Hospital, Capital Medical University, Anzhenli Avenue, Chao Yang District, Beijing 100029, China
Full list of author information is available at the end of the article

presence of at least one major cardiovascular risk factor (smoking, diabetes, hypertension, or dyslipidemia), (3) documented stable angina. Figure 1 summarizes the study flow chart and the reasons for the exclusion of patients.

The study protocol was approved by the Ethics Committee of Beijing Anzhen Hospital. Written informed consent was obtained from the participants for publication of their individual details and images in this manuscript. The consent forms are held at the authors' institution and are available for review by the Editor-in-Chief.

CMR protocol

All examinations were performed on a 3 T whole-body scanner (MAGNETOM Verio, A Tim System; Siemens Healthineers, Erlangen, Germany) with a 32-element matrix coil. Detailed protocols with CE-MRCA and CMR are given in Fig. 2.

For CE-MRCA, a navigator-gated, electrocardiogram (ECG)-triggered, fat-saturated, inversion-recovery prepared segmented 3D gradient-echo sequence was employed [10]. Before examination, patients were trained to perform regular, shallow breathing and to avoid changes in depth of breathing during data acquisition [10]. Sixty seconds after the initiation of contrast agent administration (Magnevist, Bayer Healthcare,Berlin, Germany; 0.1 mmol/kg, 0.2 ml/sec), whole-heart CE-MRCA data acquisition was started. The imaging volume was prescribed in the axial plane to cover the entire heart. Prospective real-time adaptive motion correction was applied in the superior-inferior direction to compensate the respiratory motion based on the navigator signal with a correction factor of 0.6 [10]. Imaging parameters included: TR/TE = 3.0/1.4 ms, flip angle = 20°,

readout bandwidth = 610 Hz/pixel, acquired voxel size = $1.3 \times 1.3 \times 1.3$ mm^3 and interpolated to $0.65 \times 0.65 \times 0.65$ mm^3. Data acquisition was accelerated by employing generalized autocalibrating partially parallel acquisitions (GRAPPA) in the phase-encoding direction with a factor of 2. A non-selective inversion pulse was applied prior to the navigator gating and data acquisition to suppress background tissues. The inversion recovery time (TI) was 200 msec.

For CMR MPI, a T1-weighted saturation-recovery fast gradient echo sequence was used with TR/TE = 165.0/1.1 ms, flip angle =12°, TI = 100 ms, FOV = 350 × 450 mm^2, slice thickness = 8 mm. Three left ventricular (LV) short-axis slices (basal, midventricular, and apical) were acquired under maximal hyperemia achieved with 140 μg/kg/min IV adenosine infusion for 5 min, during the first pass of a bolus of 0.05 mmol/kg of contrast media (Magnevist, Bayer Healthcare) injected at 5 ml/s. During the examination, blood pressure and ECG were continuously recorded. Ten minutes after the stress perfusion, the same scan was repeated at rest.

For LGE imaging, a 2D phase-sensitive inversion recovery breath-hold sequence was used at least 10 min after the last administration of gadolinium (TR/TE = 4.1/1.56 ms, flip angle = 20°, FOV = 350 × 284 mm^2, slice thickness = 8 mm). LGE images were acquired in two LV long-axis (two-chamber and four-chamber) views and in multiple short-axis views with a slice distance of 8 mm, covering the whole LV from base to apex.

Imaging analysis

CE-MRCA was assessed by 2 experienced readers who were blinded to the patient information. Axial source

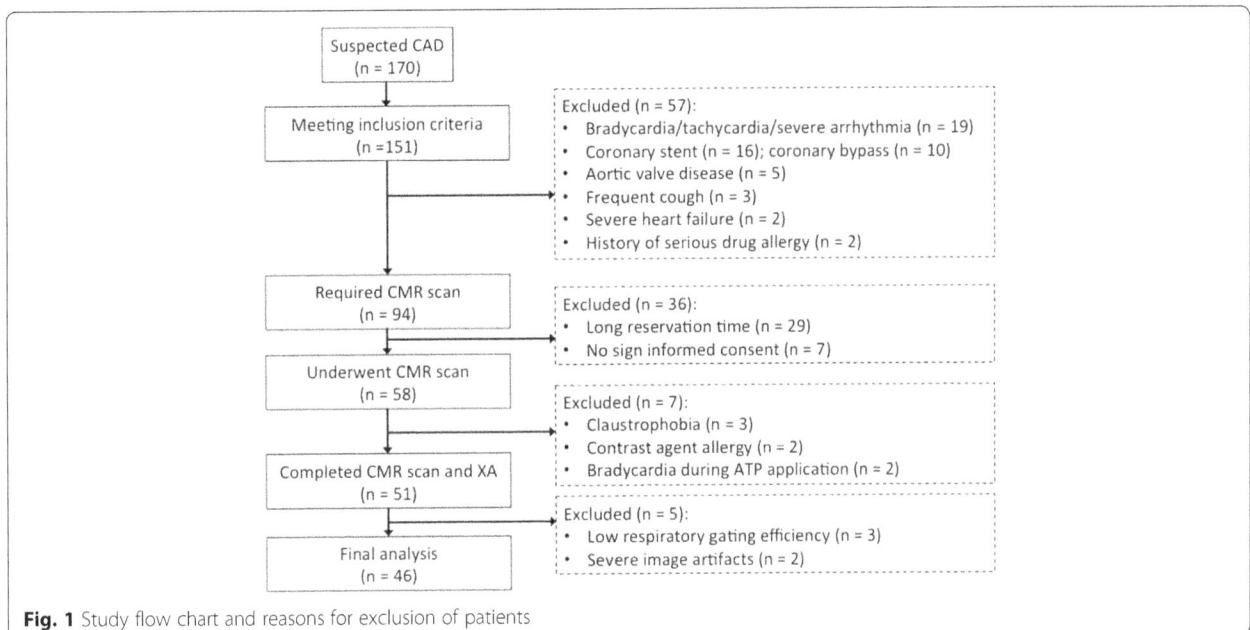

Fig. 1 Study flow chart and reasons for exclusion of patients

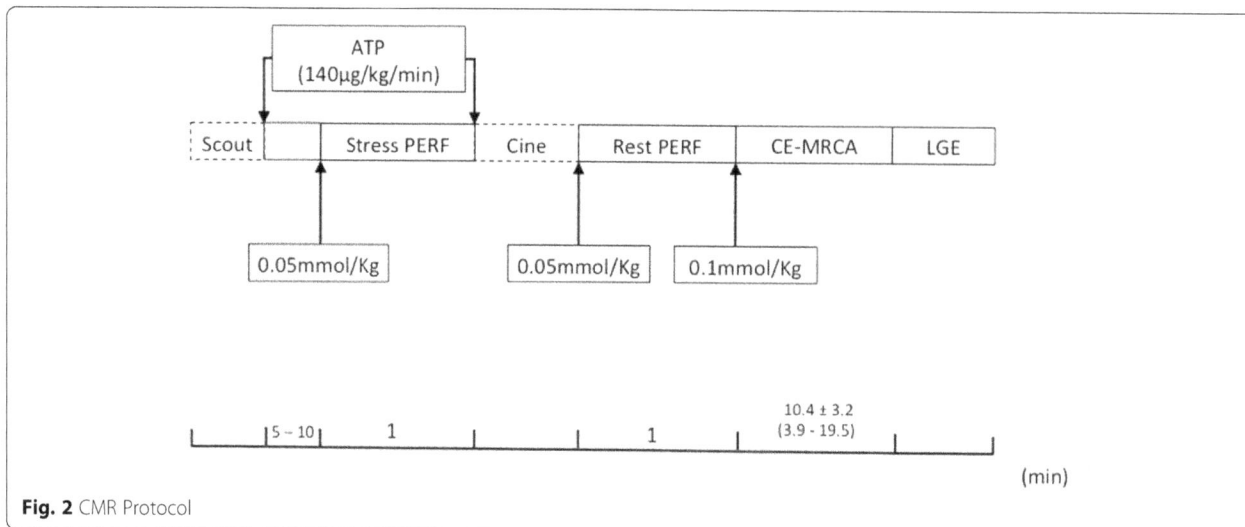

Fig. 2 CMR Protocol

images were assessed on a per-segment basis. The 15-segment American Heart Association (AHA) classification system was used for CAD diagnosis. Examples of various CE-MRCA image qualities (ImQ) are shown in Fig. 3. Images with ImQ 2 to 4 were evaluated for stenosis, and ImQ 1 was deemed non-assessable. CE-MRCA at each segment was graded on 5-point scale: 0 = normal; 1 = mild stenosis (< 50%); 2 = significant stenosis ≥50%; 3 = uninterpretable (cannot exclude significant stenosis); 4 = not visible. Segments with grades 0 and 1 were classified as negative and those with grade 2 were classified as positive. Segments with grades 3 and 4 were classified as negatives or positive depending on the results of MPI or LGE. When combining CE-MRCA and MPI or LGE, if any of the tests was positive, the overall result was deemed positive; if all were negative, the overall result was negative.

CMR perfusion images were assessed by visual comparison of stress and rest scans (17 segment American Heart Association (AHA) model, excluding the apex [14]). A perfusion deficit was determined if there were ten or more consecutive frames of apparent signal reduction. LGE images were analyzed visually using AHA segmentation, and bright segments were classified as positive.

Patients underwent x-ray coronary angiography (XA) within 1 week after CMR. The 15-segment AHA classification system was used for CAD diagnosis. Stenoses were quantitatively evaluated for segments with a diameter of > 2 mm (QuantCor software, QCA, Siemens Healthineers). Functionally significant CAD was defined as the presence of luminal stenosis ≥50%. Correspondence between LV myocardial segments and coronary arteries was determined based on the AHA model [14].

Statistical analysis
Continuous data are reported as mean ± standard deviation. Data analysis was performed on both patient- and vessel-bases. Sensitivity and specificity were calculated using true positive (TP), true negative (TN), false positive (FP), and false negative (FN) rates using XA as reference. The McNemar test was used to calculate differences between proportions (sensitivity, specificity, and accuracy) obtained from paired observations. Receiver operating characteristic (ROC) curves were calculated to assess the diagnostic efficacy and the area under the ROC curves (AUC) were compared between different imaging methods. Cohen's kappa statistic was used to assess inter-observer agreements. SPSS

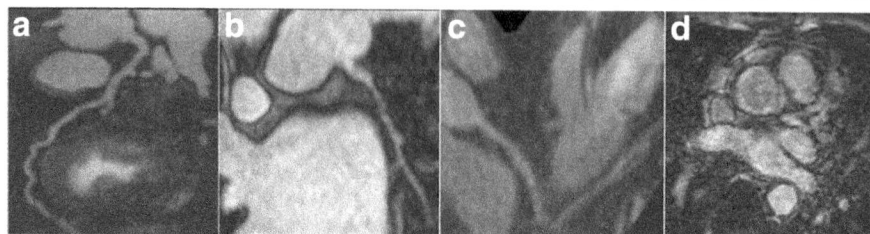

Fig. 3 Examples of contrast enhanced magnetic resonance coronary angiography (CE-MRCA) imaging quality grades, Grade 4 = minimal artifacts, excellent signal and contrast on left anterior descending coronary artery (LAD) (**a**); Grade 3 = slight artifacts and good signal and contrast on the left circumflex coronary artery (LCX) (**b**); Grade 2 = moderate artifacts and fair signal and contrast on the right coronary artery (RCA) (**c**); Grade 1 = severe image artifacts and poor signal and contrast on LAD (**d**)

statistics (version 21, International Business Machines, Armonk, New York, USA) was used for data analysis. $P < 0.05$ was considered a significant difference.

Results

One hundred and fifty one patients met the inclusion criteria of which 51 underwent CMR scanning. Detailed exclusion reasons were summarized in Fig. 1. The mean exam duration was 58.0 ± 7.9 min. The final analysis included 46 individuals (54.0 ± 11.5 years, 71.7% males) after excluding incomplete CE-MRCA ($n = 5$). Patient characteristics are shown in Table 1.

Image quality and assessability of MRCA

A total of 90.2% (46/51) of CE-MRCA studies were included in data analysis. Five patients were excluded: CE-MRCA was aborted in three patients due to extremely low respiratory gating efficiency (navigator efficiency< 20% by the time half of the imaging data were collected); severe motion artifacts were present in two patients as evaluated by an experienced radiologist. The mean scan time was 10.4 ± 3.2 min, ranging from 3.9 to 19.5 min. Patients did not receive medicine to reduce their heart rate (HR), thus 22 patients had a HR > 65 bpm and 24 patients had HR ≤ 65 bpm, with a mean HR of 67.3 ± 9.6 bpm. The average navigator respiratory gating efficiency was $35.0 \pm 9.1\%$. CE-MRCA was acquired during diastole in 21 patients (77% with HR ≤ 65 bpm) and during systole in 25 (67% with HR > 65 bpm). The average scan time of patients with diastolic acquisition was similar to that of systolic acquisition (10.3 ± 2.6 min vs. 10.4 ± 3.8 min, $p = 0.28$).

Significant stenosis was found in 73.9% patients (34/46) based on MRCA. The kappa value for inter-observer agreement on per-patient basis for the identification of

significant stenosis was 0.78 (95% CI, 0.55–1.0). Of the 34 patients, 16 (47.1%) had 1-vessel CAD, 11 (32.4%) had 2-vessel CAD, and 7 (20.6%) had 3-vessel CAD. On per-vessel basis, 42.8% (59/138) vessels had significant stenosis detected by MRCA, including 30.5% right coronary artery (RCA) (18/59), 40.7% left anterior descending artery (LAD) (24/59), and 28.8% left circumflex artery (LCX) (17/59).

Of the total 690 segments, 529 segments had diameter > 2 mm and 96.4% (510/529) were judged to have adequate image quality (ImQ 4 = 391, ImQ 3 = 101, ImQ 2 = 18) with an average ImQ of 3.7 ± 0.5. For stenosis grade, of 510 segments, 410 (80.4%) had grade 0 or 1, 89 (17.5%) had grade 2. Eleven segments had grades 3 (uninterpretable) or 4 (invisible).

On per-patient basis, CE-MRCA had a sensitivity of 97.1%, specificity of 91.7%, accuracy of 95.7%, and AUC of 0.94 (95% CI, 0.83–0.99). On per-vessel basis, CE-MRCA had a sensitivity of 89.3%, specificity of 89.0%, accuracy of 89.1%, and AUC of 0.89 (95% CI, 0.83–0.94).

Combination of CE-MRCA with MPI

The mean heart rates were 91 ± 11.4 bpm (ranging from 70 to 120 bpm) during stress perfusion and 67 ± 9.5 bpm (ranging from 50 to 86 bpm) during rest perfusion. The average increased HR was 23 ± 8.5 bpm (ranging from 9 to 42 bpm). On per-patient basis, the kappa value for inter-observer agreement for the identification of perfusion defect was 0.73 (95% CI, 0.52–0.93).

Of the total 736 segments in the 46 patients, 23.2% (171/736) was positive on MPI alone, corresponding to 52 main branches (RCA 21, LAD 16, and LCX 15). After adding CE-MRCA, the positive results increased to 75 main branches (RCA 25, LAD 29, and LCX 21).

The diagnostic performance of combined CE-MRCA and MPI compared to MPI alone was assessed in 46 patients and 138 vessels respectively. Results are given in Table 2. Compared to MPI alone, adding CE-MRCA to MPI showed higher sensitivity (100% vs. 76.5%, $p < 0.01$), similar specificity (58.3% vs. 66.7%, $p = 0.6$), and higher accuracy (89.1% vs. 73.9%, $p < 0.01$) on per-patient basis (Fig. 4). ROC analysis showed that there was no significant difference between the combination of CE-MRCA and MPI (AUC =0.79; 95% CI, 0.65–0.90), compared with MPI alone (AUC = 0.72; 95% CI, 0.56–0.84) ($p = 0.17$). AUC was improved in vessel-based analysis (0.84 [95% CI, 0.77–0.90] vs. 0.75 [95% CI, 0.67–0.82], $p = 0.01$) (Fig. 5).

In MPI alone, 4 patients were FPs and 8 patients were FNs. By adding CE-MRCA, the number of FPs was increased by 1 and number of FNs was decreased from 8 to 0 (Fig. 6).

Combination of MRCA with LGE

Based on LGE alone, 15 patients were founded positive and 31 patients were negative. Adding CE-MRCA to LGE,

Table 1 Characteristics of the study population

	Sensitivity (%)	Specificity (%)	Accuracy (%)
Patient Basis (N = 46, CAD 73.9%)			
MPI	76.5 (26/34)	66.7 (8/12)	73.9 (34/46)
MPI/LGE	76.5 (26/34)	66.7 (8/12)	73.9 (34/46)
MRCA	97.1 (33/34)	91.7 (11/12)	95.7 (44/46)
CE-MRCA+MPI/LGE	100 (34/34)	58.3 (7/12)	89.1 (41/46)
LGE	41.2 (14/34)	91.7 (11/12)	54.3 (25/46)
CE-MRCA+LGE	97.1 (33/34)	83.3 (10/12)	93.5 (43/46)
Vessel Basis (N = 138, CAD 30.4%)			
MPI	67.9 (38/56)	82.9 (68/82)	76.8 (106/138)
MPI/LGE	67.9 (38/56)	82.9 (68/82)	76.8 (106/138)
CE-MRCA	89.3 (50/56)	89.0 (73/82)	89.1 (123/138)
CE-MRCA+MPI/LGE	94.6 (53/56)	73.2 (60/82)	81.9 113/138)
LGE	28.6 (16/56)	95.1(78/82)	68.1 (94/138)
CE-MRCA+LGE	89.3 (50/56)	84.1(69/82)	86.2 (119/138)

Table 2 Diagnostic accuracy of the different imaging methods and their combination on per-patient and per-vessel bases

Number of patients (n)	46
Male sex	33 (71.7%)
Age (yrs)	54 ± 11.5
Body-mass index (kg/m²)	26 ± 3.2
Hypercholesterolemia	13 (28.2%)
Hypertension	29 (63.0%)
Diabetes mellitus	8 (17.4%)
Positive smoking history	17 (37.0%)
Current smoker	16 (34.8%)
Family history of CAD	6 (13.0%)

CAD coronary artery disease, *MPI* stress-rest myocardial perfusion imaging, *LGE* late gadolinium enhancement, *CE-MRCA* contrast enhanced magnetic resonance coronary angiography

35 patients were founded positive and 11 patients were negative. Although the number of FPs was slightly increased (from 1 to 2), the number of FNs was dramatically decreased from 20 to 1, compared to LGE alone (Fig. 6).

Adding CE-MRCA to LGE showed significantly higher sensitivity (97.1% vs. 41.2%, $p < 0.01$) translating into better diagnostic performance (AUC = 0.90 [95% CI, 0.78–0.97] vs. 0.66 [95% CI, 0.51–0.80], $p < 0.01$) (Fig. 7). Although specificity was inferior (83.3% vs. 91.7%, $p = 0.02$), diagnostic accuracy was significantly increased from 54.3% to 93.5%, compared to LGE alone (Fig. 4). The same trends were also found in vessel-based analysis (Table 2).

Combination of CE-MRCA with MPI/LGE

In the 46 patients, 23.2% (171/736) was positive on MPI/LGE. The diagnostic performance for the combination of CE-MRCA and MPI/LGE compared to MPI/LGE are given in Table 2. Compared to MPI/LGE alone, adding CE-MRCA showed higher sensitivity (100% vs. 76.5%, $p < 0.01$) and similar specificity (58.3% vs. 66.7%, $p = 0.6$). Overall accuracy was improved from 73.9% to 89.1% on per-patient basis (Fig. 4). ROC analysis showed that there was no significant difference between the combined CE-MRCA and MPI/LGE (AUC = 0.79; 95% CI, 0.65–0.90), compared with MPI/LGE (AUC = 0.72; 95% CI, 0.56–0.84) ($p = 0.17$). AUC was improved on per-vessel basis (0.84 [95% CI, 0.77–0.90] vs. 0.75 [95% CI, 0.67–0.82], $p = 0.01$) (Fig. 5).

It should be pointed out that these results were the same as that of MPI/LGE compared to MPI alone. A positive diagnosis is obtained when either of MPI or LGE is positive. Positive LGE in comparison to negative MPI may result from small subendocardial infarcts. Apparently it was not the case in this patient population.

Discussion

To our knowledge, this is the first study to evaluate the additive value of 3D whole-heart CE MRCA to conventional CMR MPI and LGE for detecting CAD on a 3 T CMR system. We demonstrated that the integration of CE-MRCA into a comprehensive stress-rest MPI and LGE protocol significantly improved sensitivity and diagnostic accuracy. These results conflict with the previous

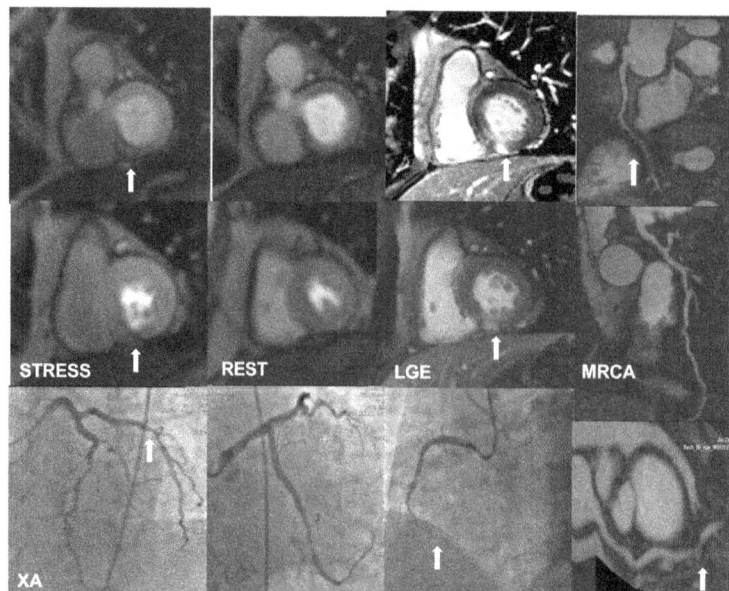

Fig. 4 One case illustrating myocardial perfusion imaging (MPI), late gadolinium enhancement (LGE), CE-MRCA and x-ray angiography (XA) angiographic findings in patient with coronary artery disease (CAD), Male/60 yrs. MPI (+) + MRCA (+) = combination (+). LGE (+) + MRCA (+) = combination (+). MPI/LGE (+) + MRCA (+) = combination (+). Corresponding XA shows significant RCA and LCX stenoses

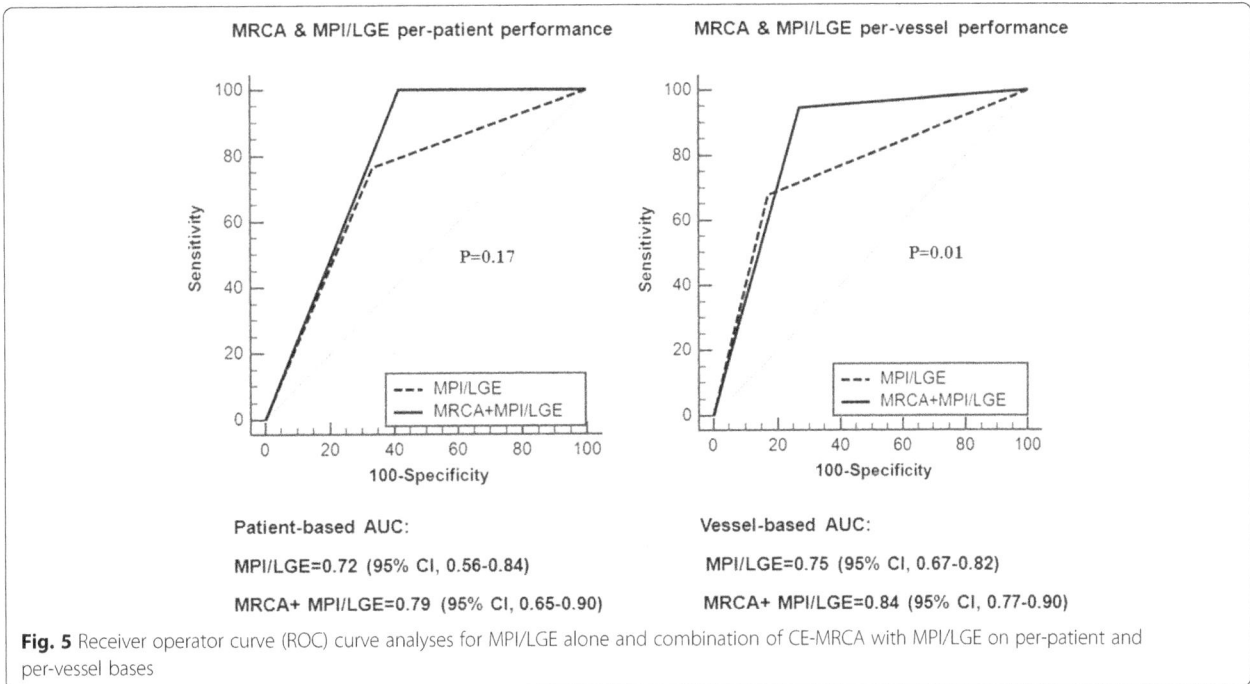

Fig. 5 Receiver operator curve (ROC) curve analyses for MPI/LGE alone and combination of CE-MRCA with MPI/LGE on per-patient and per-vessel bases

study at 1.5 T [15], in which MRCA did not increase the overall diagnostic accuracy. Possible reasons include the enhanced contrast between blood and background and increased image quality due to contrast enhanced imaging and shorter scan time on 3 T as compared to non-contrast-enhanced imaging at 1.5 T. CE-MRCA

increased the number of assessable coronary artery segments in comparison to unenhanced MRCA [16], especially distal segments [17]. Sommer et al. [18] and Bi et al. [19] demonstrated a significant increase in SNR from 1.5 to 3.0 T. Liu et al. [20] and Prompona et al. [21] found significant increase in contrast-to-noise ratio at 3.

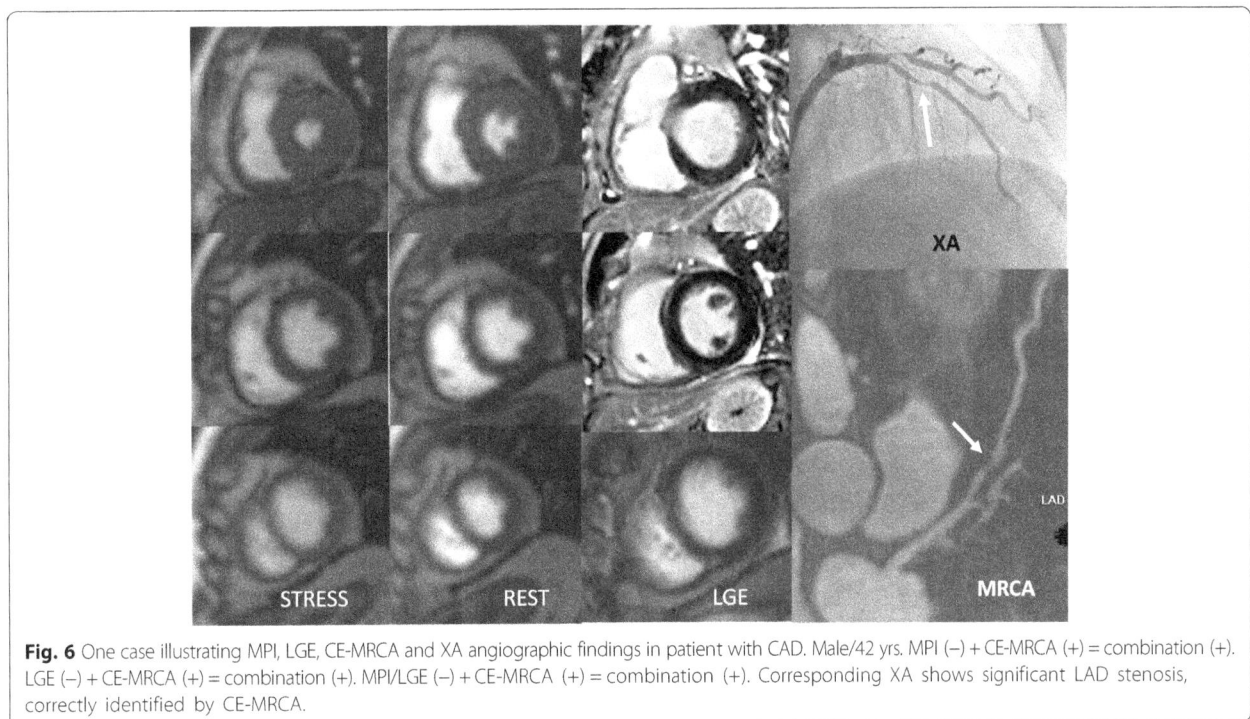

Fig. 6 One case illustrating MPI, LGE, CE-MRCA and XA angiographic findings in patient with CAD. Male/42 yrs. MPI (−) + CE-MRCA (+) = combination (+). LGE (−) + CE-MRCA (+) = combination (+). MPI/LGE (−) + CE-MRCA (+) = combination (+). Corresponding XA shows significant LAD stenosis, correctly identified by CE-MRCA.

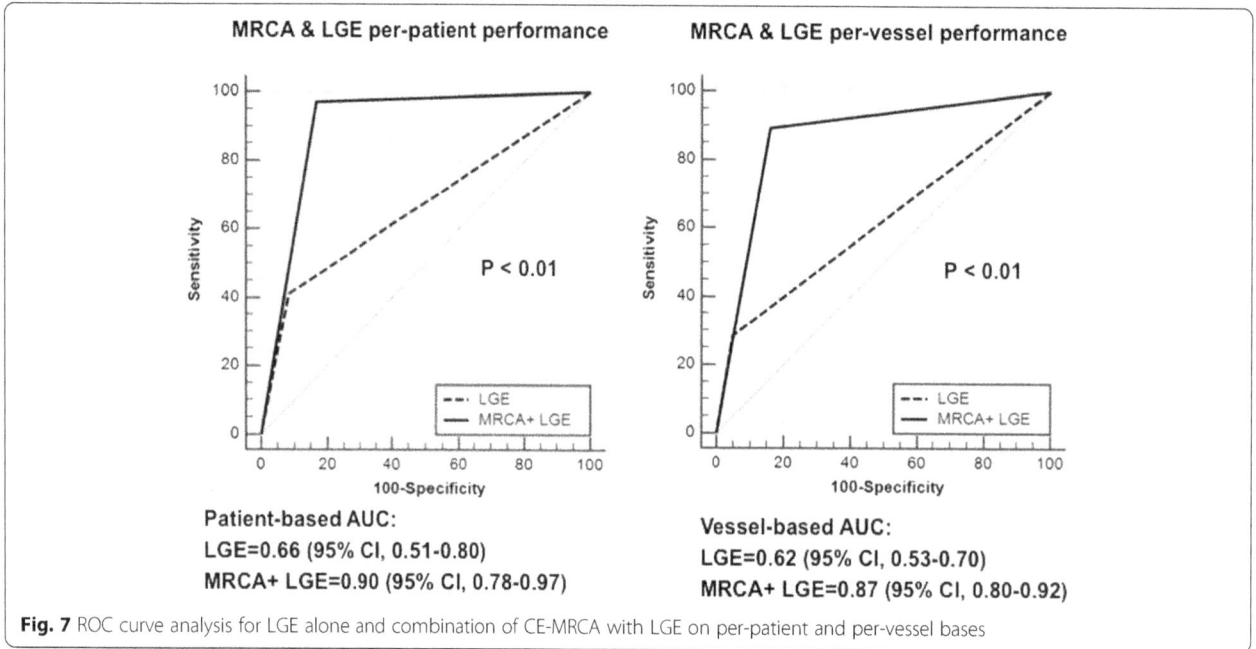

Fig. 7 ROC curve analysis for LGE alone and combination of CE-MRCA with LGE on per-patient and per-vessel bases

0 T as compared to 1.5 T. Indeed, 19% of MRCA at 1. 5 T had poor image quality [15] as compared to 3.6% in this study at 3 T.

Another difference between this study and the previous studies at 1.5 T is the definition of significant stenosis. In this study, significant stenosis was defined as luminal narrowing of ≥50% as determined on XA, while in previous studies, significant stenosis was defined as luminal narrowing of ≥90% stenosis or fractional flow reserve (FFR) ≤ 0.80 by Bettencourt N et al. [15]; or luminal narrowing of ≥70% by Ripley DR et al. [22].

In this study, adding CE-MRCA to MPI and LGE reduced the incidents of false negative (from 8 to 0). These 8 false negative patients were confirmed by coronary angiography as having 50–70% stenosis ($n = 4$), 70–80% stenosis ($n = 2$), chronic total occlusion with good collateral circulation ($n = 2$). CE-MRCA accurately identified these stenoses without myocardial ischemia or infarction, thereby reducing false negatives and improving the sensitivity of diagnosis. By adding CE-MRCA to LGE, 19 of the 20 false negatives were correctly depicted by CE-MRCA.

In this study, there were 4 false-positives using MPI. Among the four patients, three had microvascular coronary dysfunction patients, showing extensive annular ischemia in the endocardium but no coronary artery stenosis on XA.

Therefore, although the detection of the morphologically significant coronary stenosis and that of hemodynamically significant coronary stenosis are clinically different, but this study shows that CE-MRCA can detect the morphologically significant coronary stenosis in patients without hemodynamic significant stenosis, so as

to avoid the omission of severe stenosis, so that patients can get the corresponding clinical treatment as early as possible; and CE-MRCA can screened out the patients without three main coronary artery morphologically stenosis but with hemodynamic stenosis, so that these patients can avoid invasive examination.

Study limitations

In this study, 10% patients excluded due to CE-MRCA imaging issues, 3/51 patients were not able to complete CE-MRCA due to low respiratory gating efficiency and 2/51 patients had severe motion artifacts. They were not included in data analysis. 26% of CE-MRCA segments were not analysable for small diameter (161/690) and severe image artifacts and poor signal and contrast (19/690). This is a single center study with very small patient numbers. A prospective, multicenter study with a larger sample size is needed to further confirm the findings of the study.

Conclusion

On 3 T, integration of successful 3D whole-heart CE-MRCA into a comprehensive stress-rest myocardial perfusion or LGE protocol significantly improved sensitivity and diagnostic accuracy for detection of CAD.

Abbreviations

AHA: American Heart Association; AUC: The area under the ROC curves; CAD: Coronary artery disease; CE-MRCA: Contrast-enhanced magnetic resonance coronary angiography; CMR: Cardiovascular magnetic resonance; ECG: Electrocardiogram; FFR: Fractional flow reserve; FN: False negative; FP: False positive; HR: Heart rate; ImQ: Image quality; LAD: Left anterior descending coronary artery; LCX: Left circumflex coronary artery; LGE: Late gadolinium enhancement; LV: Left ventricle/left ventricular; MPI: Stress/rest myocardial perfusion imaging; RCA: Right coronary artery.; ROC: Receiver operating characteristic; TI: Inversion time; TN: True negative; TP: True positive; XA: X-ray coronary angiography

Acknowledgements
We thank Xiantao Song and his team for their assistance. We are particularly grateful for the assistance given by Debiao Li.

Authors' contributions
LZ made substantial contributions to the acquisition and interpretation of data for the work and to drafting the manuscript. ZF and DL made substantial contributions to the conception and design of the work, the acquisition, analysis, and interpretation of data for the work and to drafting the work and revising it critically for important intellectual content. XS, JL, RD and LD made substantial contributions to the acquisition and interpretation of data for the work and to revising it critically for important intellectual content. JA made substantial contributions to the design and improvement of MR scanning sequences. All authors provided final approval of the version to be published.

Competing interests
The authors declare that they have no competing interests.

Author details
[1]Department of Radiology, Beijing Anzhen Hospital, Capital Medical University, Anzhenli Avenue, Chao Yang District, Beijing 100029, China. [2]Department of Cardiology, Beijing Anzhen Hospital, Capital Medical University, Beijing, China. [3]Siemens Shenzhen Magnetic Resonance Ltd, Guangdong Shenzhen, China. [4]Biomedical Imaging Research Institute, Cedars-Sinai Medical Center, University of California, Los Angeles, USA.

References
1. Murray CJ, Lopez AD. Global mortality, disability, and the contribution of risk factors: global burden of disease study. Lancet. 1997;349(9063):1436–42.
2. Lozano R, Naghavi M, Foreman K, Lim S, Shibuya K, Aboyans V, et al. Global and regional mortality from 235 causes of death for 20 age groups in 1990 and 2010: a systematic analysis for the global burden of disease study 2010. Lancet. 2012;380(9859):2095–128.
3. Pakkal M, Raj V, Mccann GP. Non-invasive imaging in coronary artery disease including anatomical and functional evaluation of ischaemia and viability assessment. Br J Radiol. 2011;84(Spec Iss 3):S280–95.
4. Rocha-Filho JA, Blankstein R, Shturman LD, Bezerra HG, Okada DR, Rogers IS, et al. Incremental value of adenosine induced stress myocardial perfusion imaging with dual-source ct at cardiac ct angiography. Radiology. 2010;254(2):410–9.
5. Pontone G, Andreini D, Baggiano A, Bertella E, Mushtaq S, Conte E, et al. Functional relevance of coronary artery disease by cardiac magnetic resonance and cardiac computed tomography: myocardial perfusion and fractional flow reserve. Biomed Res Int. 2015;2015:297696.
6. Pilz G, Patel PA, Fell U, Ladapo JA, Rizzo JA, Fang H, et al. Adenosine-stress cardiac magnetic resonance imaging in suspected coronary artery disease: a net cost analysis and reimbursement implications. Int J Cardiovasc Imaging. 2011;27:113–21.
7. He Y, Pang J, Dai Q, Fan Z, An J, Li D. Diagnostic performance of self-navigated whole-heart contrast-enhanced coronary 3-T MR angiography. Radiology. 2016;281(2):401–8.
8. Sakuma H, Ichikawa Y, Chino S, Hirano T, Makino K, Takeda K. Detection of coronary artery. stenosis with whole-heart coronary magnetic resonance angiography. J Am Coll Cardiol. 2006;48(10):1946–50.
9. Kato S, Kitagawa K, Ishida N, Ishida M, Nagata M, Ichikawa Y, et al. Assessment of coronary artery disease using magnetic resonance coronary angiography: a national multicenter trial. J Am Coll Cardiol. 2010;56(12):983–91.
10. Yang Q, Li K, Liu X, Bi X, Liu Z, An J, et al. Contrast-enhanced whole-heart coronary magnetic resonance angiography at 3.0-T: a comparative study with X-ray angiography in a single center. J Am Coll Cardiol. 2009;54(1):69–76.
11. Nagata M, Kato S, Kitagawa K, Ishida N, Nakajima H, Nakamori S, et al. Diagnostic accuracy of 1.5-T unenhanced whole-heart coronary MR angiography performed with 32-channel cardiac coils: initial single-center experience. Radiology. 2011;259(2):384–92.
12. Heer T, Reiter S, Höfling B, Pilz G. Diagnostic performance of non-contrast-enhanced whole-heart magnetic resonance coronary angiography in combination with adenosine stress perfusion cardiac magnetic resonance imaging. Am Heart J. 2013;166(6):999–1009.
13. Klein C, Gebker R, Kokocinski T, Dreysse S, Schnackenburg B, Fleck E, et al. Combined magnetic resonance coronary artery imaging, myocardial perfusion and late gadolinium enhancement in patients with suspected coronary artery disease. J Cardiovasc Magn Reson. 2008;10:45.
14. Cerqueira MD, Weissman NJ, Dilsizian V, Jacobs AK, Kaul S, Laskey WK, et al. Standardized myocardial segmentation and nomenclature for tomographic imaging of the heart. A statement for healthcare professionals from the cardiac imaging Committee of the Council on clinical cardiology of the American Heart Association. Circulation. 2002;105(4):539–42.
15. Bettencourt N, Ferreira N, Chiribiri A, Schuster A, Sampaio F, Santos L, et al. Additive value of magnetic resonance coronary angiography in a comprehensive cardiacmagnetic resonance stress-rest protocol for detection of functionally significant coronary artery disease: a pilot study. Circ Cardiovasc Imaging. 2013;6(5):730–8.
16. Wagner M, Rösler R, Lembcke A, Butler C, Dewey M, Laule M, et al. Whole-heart coronary magnetic resonance angiography at 1.5 Tesla: does a blood-pool contrast agent improve diagnostic accuracy? Investig Radiol. 2011;46(3):152–9.
17. Yang Q, Li K, Liu X, Du X, Bi X, Huang F, et al. 3.0T whole-heart coronary magnetic resonance angiography performed with 32-channel cardiac coils: a single-center experience. Circ Cardiovasc Imaging. 2012;5:573–9.
18. Sommer T, Hackenbroch M, Hofer U, Schmiedel A, Willinek W, Flacke S, et al. Coronary MR angiography at 3.0 T versus that at 1.5 T: initial results in patients suspected of having coronary artery disease. Radiology. 2005;234:718–25.
19. Bi X, Li D. Coronary arteries at 3.0 T: contrast-enhanced magnetization-prepared three-dimensional breathhold MR angiography. J Magn Reson Imaging. 2005;21:133–9.
20. Liu X, Bi X, Huang J, Jerecic R, Carr J, Li D. Contrast-enhanced whole-heart coronary magnetic resonance angiography at 3.0 T: comparison with steady-state free precession technique at 1.5 T. Investig Radiol. 2008;43:663–8.
21. Prompona M, Cyran C, Nikolaou K, Bauner K, Reiser M, Huber A. Contrast-enhanced whole-heart MR coronary angiography at 3.0 T using the intravascular contrast agent Gadofosveset. Investig Radiol. 2009;44(7):369–74.
22. Ripley DP, Motwani M, Brown JM, Nixon J, Everett CC, Bijsterveld P, et al. Individual component analysis of the multi-parametric cardiovascular magnetic resonance protocol in the CE-MARC trial. J Cardiovasc Magn Reson. 2015;17:59.

15

Breath-hold imaging of the coronary arteries using Quiescent-Interval Slice-Selective (QISS) magnetic resonance angiography

Robert R. Edelman[1,2*], S. Giri[3], A. Pursnani[1,4], M. P. F. Botelho[1], W. Li[1,4] and I. Koktzoglou[1,4]

Abstract

Background: Coronary magnetic resonance angiography (MRA) is usually obtained with a free-breathing navigator-gated 3D acquisition. Our aim was to develop an alternative breath-hold approach that would allow the coronary arteries to be evaluated in a much shorter time and without risk of degradation by respiratory motion artifacts. For this purpose, we implemented a breath-hold, non-contrast-enhanced, quiescent-interval slice-selective (QISS) 2D technique. Sequence performance was compared at 1.5 and 3 Tesla using both radial and Cartesian k-space trajectories.

Methods: The left coronary circulation was imaged in six healthy subjects and two patients with coronary artery disease. Breath-hold QISS was compared with T2-prepared 2D balanced steady-state free-precession (bSSFP) and free-breathing, navigator-gated 3D bSSFP.

Results: Approximately 10 2.1-mm thick slices were acquired in a single ~20-s breath-hold using two-shot QISS. QISS contrast-to-noise ratio (CNR) was 1.5-fold higher at 3 Tesla than at 1.5 Tesla. Cartesian QISS provided the best coronary-to-myocardium CNR, whereas radial QISS provided the sharpest coronary images. QISS image quality exceeded that of free-breathing 3D coronary MRA with few artifacts at either field strength. Compared with T2-prepared 2D bSSFP, multi-slice capability was not restricted by the specific absorption rate at 3 Tesla and pericardial fluid signal was better suppressed. In addition to depicting the coronary arteries, QISS could image intra-cardiac structures, pericardium, and the aortic root in arbitrary slice orientations.

Conclusions: Breath-hold QISS is a simple, versatile, and time-efficient method for coronary MRA that provides excellent image quality at both 1.5 and 3 Tesla. Image quality exceeded that of free-breathing, navigator-gated 3D MRA in a much shorter scan time. QISS also allowed rapid multi-slice bright-blood, diastolic phase imaging of the heart, which may have complementary value to multi-phase cine imaging. We conclude that, with further clinical validation, QISS might provide an efficient alternative to commonly used free-breathing coronary MRA techniques.

Keywords: Quiescent-interval slice-selective (QISS), Coronary artery, Magnetic resonance angiography, Breath-holding, Navigator, Free-breathing

* Correspondence: Redelman999@gmail.com
[1]Department of Radiology, NorthShore University HealthSystem, 2650 Ridge Avenue, Evanston, IL 60201, USA
[2]Feinberg School of Medicine, Northwestern University, Chicago, USA
Full list of author information is available at the end of the article

Background

Cardiovascular magnetic resonance is an excellent test for evaluating anatomy, function, and blood flow in the heart [1]. It is a valuable adjunct to echocardiography and is routinely used to evaluate a variety of disorders including masses, congenital heart disease, valve abnormalities, inflammatory conditions, and cardiomyopathies. Aside from the recent introduction of quantitative T1 and T2 mapping sequences, cardiac imaging protocols in routine clinical use have remained largely stable over the last decade. Typical imaging protocols consist of a combination of bright blood cine balanced steady-state free precession (bSSFP), 2D phase contrast, dark blood turbo spin-echo, and late gadolinium enhancement scans using inversion recovery-prepared gradient-echo. When coronary artery evaluation is needed, a free-breathing, navigator-gated 3D acquisition is applied [2]. However, a drawback of currently available free-breathing coronary imaging techniques is their dependence on the patient's respiratory pattern, which can result in inconsistent image quality and unpredictably long scan times.

Quiescent-interval slice-selective (QISS) is a non-contrast-enhanced, bright blood sequential 2D imaging technique that was originally developed for the evaluation of peripheral arterial disease [3, 4]. The original method had temporal resolution on the order of 300 ms, too slow to be applicable for cardiac applications such as coronary MRA. We therefore implemented multi-shot versions of QISS offering higher temporal resolution and compared them with breath-hold T2-prepared 2D bSSFP and standard-of-care free-breathing, navigator-gated 3D bSSFP for imaging of the coronary arteries. In addition, since bSSFP-based imaging techniques can be problematic at high field due to increased specific absorption rate (SAR), B0 and B1 inhomogeneities [5], we also evaluated the performance of these three imaging techniques at both 1.5 Tesla and 3 Tesla.

Methods

The study was approved by the Institutional Review Board and used written, informed consent. Imaging was performed using a six-element cardiac phased array coil at 1.5 Tesla (MAGNETOM Avanto, Siemens Healthcare, Erlangen, Germany) and 3 Tesla (MAGNETOM Verio, Siemens Healthcare, Erlangen, Germany) with peak gradients and slew rates of 45 mT/m and 200 T/m/s. The prototype QISS pulse sequence was evaluated for imaging of the proximal and mid left coronary circulation of healthy subjects (six male, age range 23–35 years). No pre-medication was administered. In addition, two subjects (both male, ages 39 and 57 years) who had undergone coronary CT angiography for the evaluation of suspected coronary artery disease (CAD) were imaged.

The differences between the QISS imaging parameters typically used for peripheral artery MRA and coronary MRA are summarized in Table 1. For this pilot study, nearly identical QISS pulse sequence parameters were used for coronary MRA at 1.5 Tesla and 3 Tesla. The pulse sequence diagrams for QISS and 2D T2-prepared bSSFP are given in Fig. 1. An in-plane frequency offset corrected inversion (FOCI) pulse [6] (pulse duration 10.24 ms, $\mu = 12$, $\beta = 900$, gradient factor of 2.0) having double the imaging slice thickness was applied immediately after the R-wave to suppress background signal, followed by a quiescent interval to allow inflow of unsaturated arterial spins. Based on empirical experience, the longest quiescent interval that could be accommodated within the RR interval was used. A fat saturation radio-frequency (RF) pulse was applied, followed by an alpha/2 catalyzation, after which data were collected using a 2D bSSFP readout. Sampling bandwidth was 820 or 1008 Hz/pixel resulting in an inter-view repetition time of 4.0 ms or 3.7 ms, respectively.

Breath-hold coronal and axial scout images were acquired using single-shot or two-shot radial QISS. Using the coronal scout images to visualize the proximal LAD, single oblique, tilted axial images were obtained for long-axis evaluation of the LAD. The axial scout images were used to center the field of view (FOV) on the heart and, for small FOV radial imaging, to exclude lung tissue in order to ensure an optimal shim (since shimming is only performed on tissue within the selected FOV). For the formal sequence comparisons, breath-hold scans (QISS and T2-prepared bSSFP) were acquired using two shots of 48 views each (total of 96 views), with the shots acquired over two success heartbeats. For Cartesian QISS, the matrix size was 256 × 170, FOV 358-mm × 237-mm, parallel acceleration (ipat) factor of 2. For radial QISS, the matrix was 160 and FOV was 225-mm. A small equidistant azimuthal radial view angle increment ≈ 10–20° was applied since prior experience indicated that this resulted in fewer artifacts than linear or golden angle trajectories [7]. For both k-space trajectories, ten slices were typically acquired in each breath-hold. In-plane spatial resolution was 1.4-mm (0.7-mm after interpolation), with slice thicknesses of 2.1-mm for coronary MRA and 3.1-mm for imaging of the heart.

Table 1 Coronary QISS vs. peripheral QISS MRA

	Coronary QISS	Peripheral QISS
K-Space Trajectory	Radial or Cartesian	Cartesian
Readout Duration	~82–192 ms	~300 ms
Magnetization Preparation	FOCI inversion	Saturation
Fat Suppression	Yes	Yes
Venous Suppression	No	Yes
Fold Over Artifact with Small FOV	Cartesian only	Yes

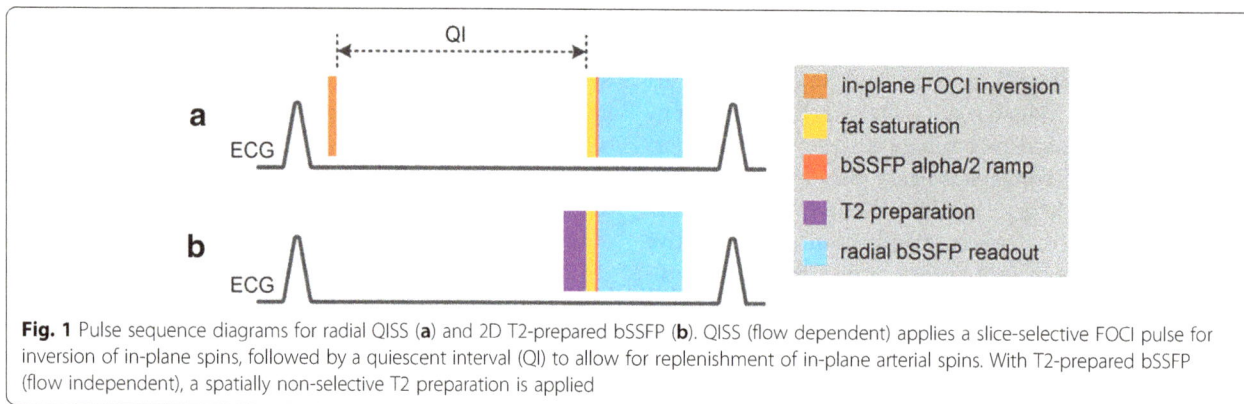

Fig. 1 Pulse sequence diagrams for radial QISS (**a**) and 2D T2-prepared bSSFP (**b**). QISS (flow dependent) applies a slice-selective FOCI pulse for inversion of in-plane spins, followed by a quiescent interval (QI) to allow for replenishment of in-plane arterial spins. With T2-prepared bSSFP (flow independent), a spatially non-selective T2 preparation is applied

QISS was compared with a breath-hold T2-prepared 2D bSSFP sequence (TE = 40 ms, identical to QISS except for the magnetization preparation) in order to distinguish the impact of the magnetization preparation from the impact of breath-holding. Additionally, QISS was compared with a free-breathing, navigator-gated fat-suppressed, T2-prepared (TE = 53 ms) 3D bSSFP pulse sequence. For the latter technique, a cross-pair navigator was placed over the right hemi-diaphragm using a ±2.5-mm acceptance window with slice following and adaptive correction; typically 24 slices were acquired using slice thickness, in-plane resolution, and sampling bandwidth identical to those used for QISS.

For quantitative analysis, the contrast-to-noise ratios (CNR) between the coronary arteries and the background tissues of myocardium, epicardial fat and lung were computed as the respective signal differences divided by noise, with noise estimated as the standard deviation of signal within a homogeneous region of the lung tissue located adjacent to the heart. Coronary vessel sharpness was measured as the inverse of the distance between the 20th and 80th percentile points of a signal profile through the left anterior descending artery (LAD) [8]. A fellowship-trained cardiovascular radiologist (MPFB) scored image quality for the left main (LM), LAD and left circumflex (LCx) coronary arteries on a 4-point scale (1: non-diagnostic, 2: poor, 3: good; 4: excellent). Due to the length of time required to run all of the pulse sequence comparisons for the left coronary circulation, additional scan volumes directed to the right coronary artery were not routinely acquired. Consequently, this vessel was not included in the formal analysis.

Differences in quantitative and qualitative scores were assessed using parametric student's t and non-parametric Wilcoxon tests, respectively; statistical tests were paired when comparing matched data. Statistical tests were performed using R software (version 3.2.1, R Foundation for Statistical Computing, Vienna) and P values less than 0.05 were considered to indicate significant differences.

Results and discussion

Cartesian vs. *radial QISS:* The mean RR interval was 1020 ms (range 720–1250 ms). QISS image quality was comparable for Cartesian and radial k-space trajectories (P = NS). Coronary sharpness, however, was significantly improved with radial as compared with Cartesian sampling (0.67 ± 0.12 mm^{-1} vs 0.57 ± 0.09 mm^{-1}, $P < 0.01$). The improved sharpness may be due to the motion insensitivity of radial k-space trajectories [9]. On the other hand, CNR between the coronaries and background myocardium, pericardial fat, and lung parenchyma was 49 % (37.0 ± 13.0 vs 24.8 ± 9.5), 42 % (50.7 ± 16.0 vs 35.7 ± 11.5) and 47 % (54.2 ± 17.9 vs 36.8 ± 12.4) higher with Cartesian sampling ($P < 0.001$); data expressed as mean ± standard deviation. Radial QISS showed mild streak artifacts due to undersampling. These artifacts were concentrated in the periphery of the image where they did not adversely impact coronary image quality.

1.5 Tesla vs. *3 Tesla:* QISS image quality was excellent at both 1.5 Tesla and 3 Tesla (mean scores of 3.86 and 3.91, respectively, P = NS) (Figs. 2 and 3). QISS images could be acquired in arbitrary planes so as to optimally demonstrate the coronary lumen, either within a single (Fig. 4) or multiple breath-holds (Fig. 5). In addition to the coronary arteries, QISS images provided excellent delineation of the aortic root, ventricular myocardium, pulmonary veins, and pericardium.

Coronary CNR with respect to the myocardium, fat and lung was 1.50-fold (34.1 ± 13.3 vs 22.7 ± 10.2), 1.49-fold (47.6 ± 17.0 vs 32.0 ± 10.9), and 1.50-fold (50.1 ± 19.0 vs 33.4 ± 12.7) higher at 3 Tesla ($P < 0.001$). Stripe artifacts due to off-resonance effects were generally limited to the region of the pulmonary vein ostia and transverse portion of the aortic arch; these artifacts were more prominent at 3 Tesla than at 1.5 Tesla. Coronary sharpness was slightly improved at 3 Tesla versus 1.5 Tesla (0.65 ± 0.12 mm^{-1} vs 0.59 ± 0.10 mm^{-1}, $P < 0.05$).

The flip angle for QISS at 1.5 Tesla was fixed at 120°; at 3 Tesla, the flip angle was subject-dependent due to SAR limitations and ranged from 75 to 90°. Whereas

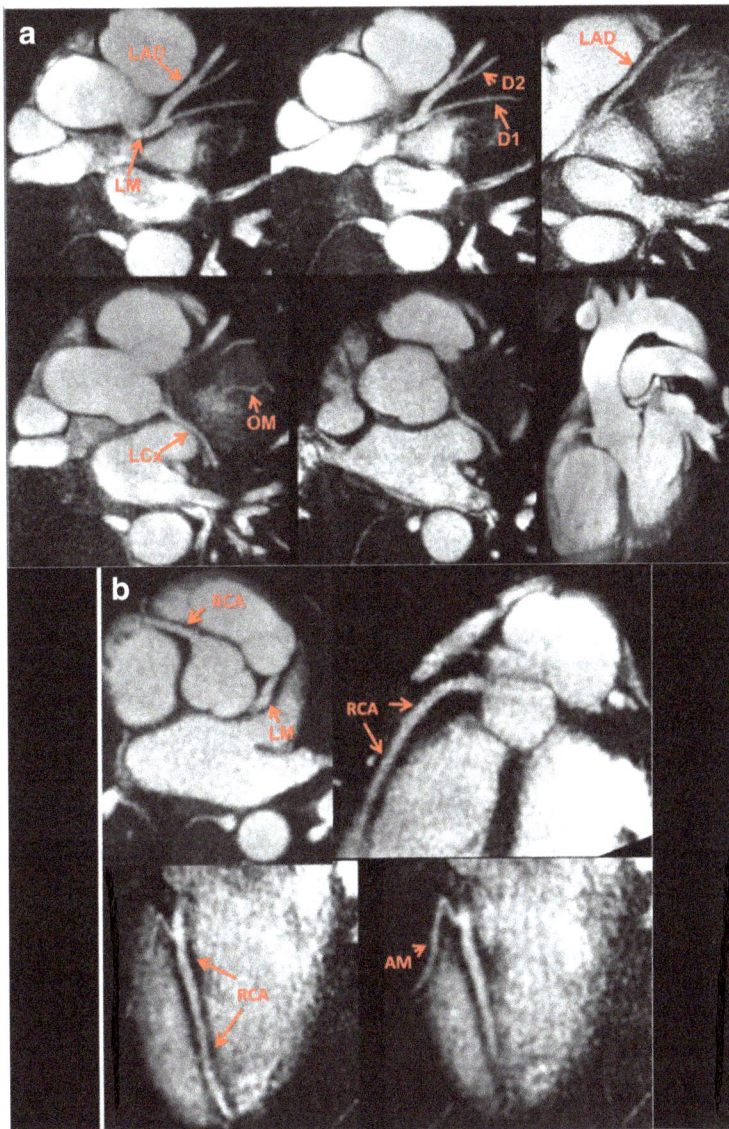

Fig. 2 Examples of thin (4 to 10-mm) maximum intensity projections reconstructed from single breath hold, radial QISS (10–12 slices per breath hold, slice thickness = 2.1-mm with 20-50 % slice overlap, in-plane spatial resolution of 0.4-mm to 0.5-mm after interpolation). Images were acquired at 3 Tesla using various scan orientations. **a** Aorta and left coronary circulation. LM = left main; LAD = left anterior descending; D1 = first diagonal branch; D2 = second diagonal branch; LCx = left circumflex; OM = obtuse marginal branch. **b** Right coronary circulation. RCA = right coronary artery; AM = acute marginal branch

QISS involves the application of a single FOCI magnetization preparation pulse, the T2-prepared bSSFP pulse sequence on our scanner applies four adiabatic 180-degree RF pulses during the magnetization preparation, which substantially increases the SAR. At 3 Tesla, due to SAR limitations resulting from the T2-weighted magnetization preparation, both breath-hold T2-prepared 2D bSSFP and navigator-gated 3D bSSFP could only be triggered to every second R-wave, whereas QISS was triggered to every R-wave. Thus, at 3 Tesla only 5 slices could be acquired per breath-hold due to the lower scan

efficiency of T2-prepared 2D bSSFP versus 10 slices with QISS.

Breath-hold QISS vs. *free-breathing 3D bSSFP:* Scan time for breath-hold QISS was on the order of 20 s for an RR interval of 1 s and 10 slices. Scan time for free-breathing 3D bSSFP ranged from 1 min 57 s to 4 min 3 s at 1.5 Tesla, and 3 min 25 s to 14 min 14 s at 3 Tesla. Breath-hold QISS depicted the left main, LAD including diagonal branches, and the LCx in all subjects without substantial motion artifacts. By comparison, the quality of free-breathing navigator-gated 3D bSSFP was

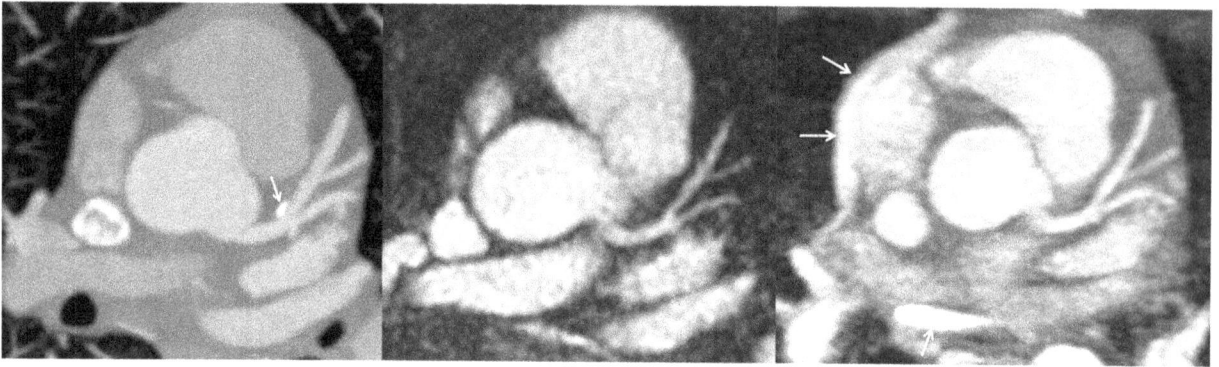

Fig. 3 39-year-old male evaluated for chest pain. *Left*: 5-mm MIP of coronary CT angiography shows mild narrowing of the proximal LAD and a punctate coronary calcification (arrow). Middle: MIP of breath-hold radial QISS MRA obtained at 1.5 Tesla demonstrates the left main and LAD coronary arteries, including the D1 and D2 branches. The appearances are similar to the coronary CT angiogram except that the wall calcification is not visible. *Right*: MIP from navigator-gated 3D bSSFP also demonstrates the left coronary anatomy comparably to the coronary CTA. Compared with QISS, there is increased pericardial fluid signal (arrows)

more variable, with image degradation due to respiratory motion in 50 % (6/12) of scans. Fluid in the pericardial recesses appeared brighter on both breath-hold 2D (Fig. 6) and free-breathing 3D T2-prepared bSSFP than with QISS. In no subject did the free-breathing technique outperform QISS with respect to image quality. Averaged over both main magnetic field strengths, mean image quality scores for the left main/LAD/LCx using breath-hold radial QISS and free-breathing navigator-gated 3D coronary MRA were, respectively, 3.91/3.91/3.82 and 3.33/3.46/3.17 ($P < 0.05$ at all three locations). In the LAD, CNR values for radial QISS [navigator-gated coronary MRA] were 26.6 ± 12.0 [26.7 ± 9.83] with respect to myocardium, 36 ± 12.5 [33.7 ± 7.99] with

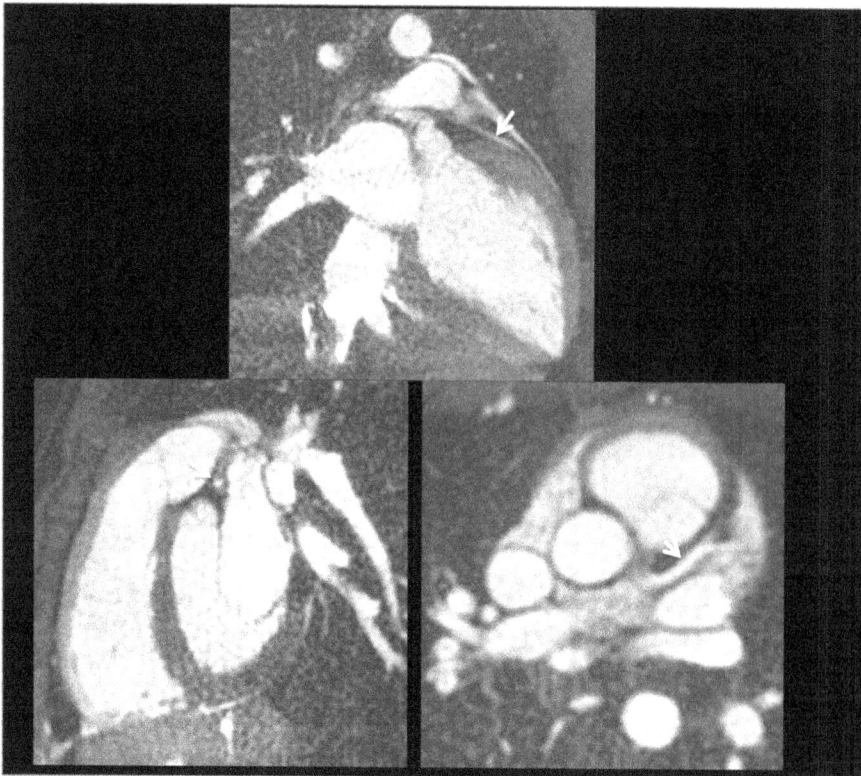

Fig. 4 Radial QISS images acquired in three orthogonal planes within a single breath-hold show the LAD (arrow) in long and short axes. Left and right ventricular myocardium, pulmonary veins, and mitral valve leaflets are also well depicted

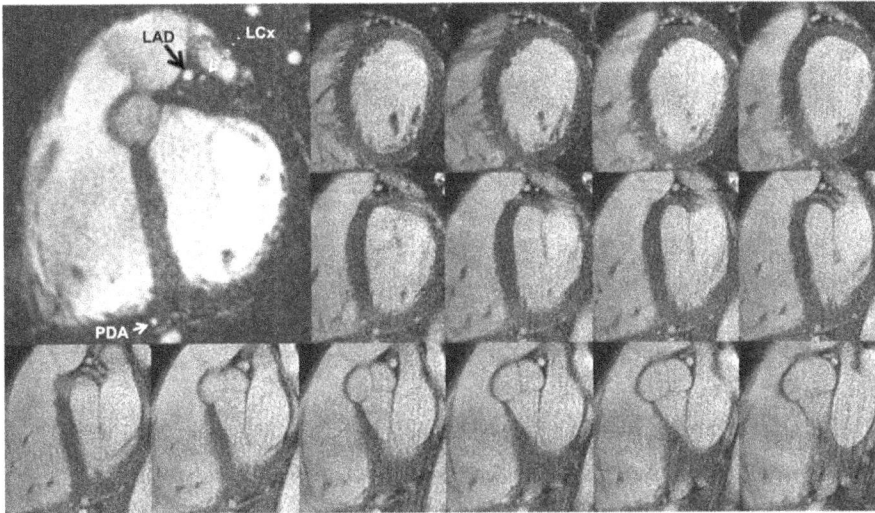

Fig. 5 Montage of radial QISS images that were oriented orthogonally to the long axis of the LAD. Images were acquired at 1.5 Tesla in two breath-holds (14 images shown out of 18 acquired). The LAD and LCx, including their takeoffs from the left main coronary artery, are well seen. Magnified view (inset) shows the LAD, left circumflex, and posterior descending branch of the right coronary artery (PDA)

respect to fat, and 37.5 ± 14.4 [39.8 ± 15.0] with respect to lung at 1.5 Tesla. At 3 Tesla, CNR values were 38.8 ± 11.8 [33.5 ± 11.8], 52.4 ± 15.1 [44.4 ± 21.5], and 55.6 ± 17.6 [51.9 ± 20.9] with respect to myocardium, fat and lung, respectively. Compared with free-breathing 3D bSSFP, coronary sharpness was significantly improved with breath-hold coronary QISS (0.62 ± 0.11 mm^{-1} vs 0.43 ± 0.14 mm^{-1}, $P < 0.001$).

Breath-hold QISS vs. breath-hold T2-prepared bSSFP: Coronary sharpness was significantly better with QISS (0.66 ± 0.09 mm^{-1} with QISS vs 0.55 ± 0.12 mm^{-1} with T2-prep bSSFP, $P < 0.01$). QISS image quality was better for the LCx (mean values of 3.98 vs 3.29, $P < 0.05$), but not significantly different for the left main (3.92 vs 3.54) or LAD (4.00 vs 3.73). Coronary-to-myocardium CNR values were 1.6-fold better for QISS than T2-prepared

bSSFP (26.8 ± 10.7 vs 16.6 ± 5.2, $P < 0.05$). Corresponding values for coronary-to-fat CNR were 36.3 ± 11.8 vs 25.5 ± 6.4 ($P < 0.01$) and for coronary-to-lung CNR were 37.5 ± 13.2 vs 26.7 ± 6.61 ($P < 0.01$).

Differences in flow dependence between QISS and T2-prepared bSSFP techniques were anecdotally demonstrated in a patient study (Fig. 7). Breath-hold T2-prepared 2D bSSFP and navigator-gated T2-prepared 3D bSSFP, both of which are substantially flow-independent, suggested a severe LAD stenosis as was prospectively reported on the coronary CTA. However, radial QISS, which is flow-dependent, showed a vessel cut-off indicating an LAD occlusion that was confirmed on subsequent x-ray coronary catheterization.

For more than two decades, attempts have been made to use breath-hold 2D and 3D MRA techniques to image

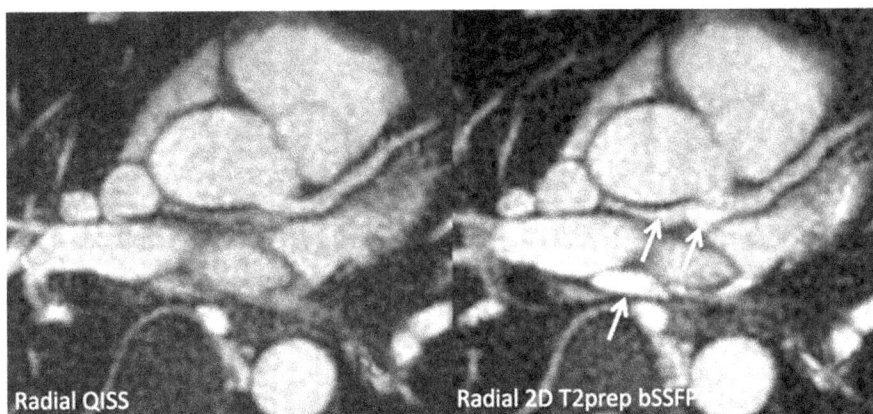

Fig. 6 Comparison of source images from breath-hold radial QISS (*left*) and T2-prepared radial 2D bSSFP (*right*) in a healthy volunteer at 1.5 Tesla. Compared with QISS, pericardial fluid signal (arrows) is substantially increased with T2-prepared bSSFP

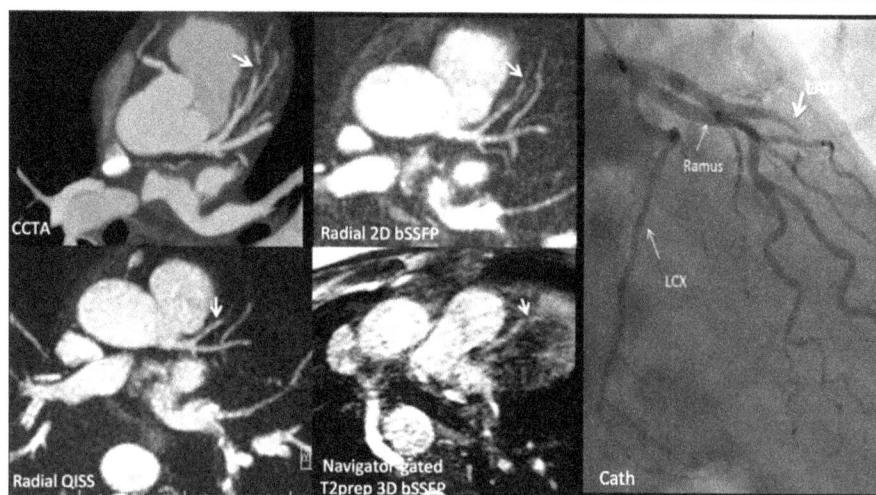

Fig. 7 57-year-old patient with hyperlipidemia and chest pain. Breath-hold 2D T2-prepared bSSFP and free-breathing 3D T2-prepared bSSFP showed similar findings to the coronary CTA, which was prospectively interpreted as showing a severe LAD stenosis (arrow). However, radial QISS indicated an LAD occlusion, which was confirmed by subsequent x-ray coronary catheterization

the coronary arteries [10–13]. To date, suboptimal image quality (e.g., due to low spatial resolution, poor flow contrast and/or motion artifact) along with a lack of robustness has impeded the widespread adoption of breath-hold coronary MRA techniques into clinical practice. This pilot study demonstrated that multi-shot QISS MRA has the potential to overcome many of the limitations of previously described breath-hold MRA techniques, enabling consistent, artifact-free imaging of the coronary arteries at both 1.5 Tesla and 3 Tesla.

The QISS technique, as originally described for peripheral nonenhanced MRA, is a flow-dependent, cardiac-gated 2D single-shot acquisition. Arterial flow contrast is maximized by the combination of in-plane and fat saturation RF pulses to suppress signal from stationary spins, along with a quiescent interval of a few hundred milliseconds in order to allow full replenishment of saturated in-plane arterial spins. For coronary MRA, the temporal resolution of the bSSFP readout needs to be improved, which is accomplished by using a multi-shot acquisition. Moreover, the quiescent interval is substantially lengthened, which maximizes replenishment of in-plane arterial spins when the coronary artery is viewed in long axis. Given the lengthy quiescent interval, optimal suppression of myocardial signal is obtained using in-plane inversion with a FOCI RF pulse instead of the saturation pulse typically used for peripheral MRA.

Coronary QISS bears some similarities to flow-dependent inversion-prepared 3D MRA techniques in widespread use for renal MRA [14]. However, there are substantial differences as well. For instance, free-breathing renal MRA requires respiratory gating. Although breath holding is theoretically possible with a 3D acquisition, efficiency is limited by the non-rectangular slab profile when small numbers of slices are acquired. Compared with QISS, flow contrast is inferior since there is much less replenishment of saturated arterial spins between sequence repetitions using a thick-slab 3D acquisition compared with a thin-slice 2D QISS acquisition. It should also be noted that, unlike the case of a thick-slab 3D acquisition, the sequential acquisition of thin 2D slices with QISS causes negligible signal saturation of the aorta and cardiac chambers irrespective of slice orientation.

In comparing Cartesian and radial k-space trajectories for QISS, we found that CNR was better with Cartesian QISS while coronary sharpness was better with radial QISS. From theory, it can be predicted that radial images should have about 87 % of the signal-to-noise ratio of a corresponding Cartesian image [15]. Nonetheless, we found that a radial k-space trajectory has several benefits that make it the preferred approach. Compared with Cartesian, radial k-space trajectories are less sensitive to motion artifacts and provide more flexibility in trading off spatial and temporal resolution, which is helpful for coronary MRA given the range of vessel sizes and heart rates that may be encountered. Radial QISS is immune from fold over artifacts, which allows the use of much smaller FOV than is practical using Cartesian imaging. With radial QISS, the high degree of background suppression from the combination of in-plane tissue inversion and fat suppression minimizes streak artifacts, which facilitates the use of high undersampling factors.

QISS is a flow-dependent MRA technique whereas T2-prepared bSSFP techniques are substantially flow-independent. This difference is anecdotally illustrated by

Fig. 7 in which QISS accurately depicted an LAD occlusion, whereas flow-independent techniques (T2-prepared 2D and 3D bSSFP as well as coronary CTA) incorrectly suggested a severe stenosis due to retrograde filling of the distal LAD segment from collaterals. However, our clinical experience with CAD is very limited. In some circumstances the flow dependence of QISS might prove to be a limitation, in which case the additional acquisition of a flow-independent T2-prepared 2D bSSFP MRA could be helpful.

Free-breathing T2-prepared 3D bSSFP is the current mainstay for coronary MRA [16]. However, in our study, SAR limitations at 3 Tesla arising from the four adiabatic 180° RF pulses in the T2-weighted magnetization preparation necessitated triggering to every second R-wave, whereas SAR was not a significant impediment for QISS. Another limitation of the T2-prepared approaches was bright signal from pericardial fluid. In some subjects, high signal from fluid within the inferior aortic recess [17] obscured the proximal portion of the left main coronary artery in thin MIPs, which did not occur with QISS. Alternatively, one could use a low SAR, inversion-prepared 3D spoiled gradient-echo technique [18]. However, unlike non-contrast-enhanced QISS, it requires the slow infusion of a relatively high dose of gadolinium-based contrast agent.

The performance of commercially available free-breathing techniques is predicated on the patient's respiratory pattern. Consequently, image quality can be unpredictably degraded and scan times inordinately lengthened when the respiratory pattern is irregular [19]. By comparison, image quality with QISS should be consistent so long as the subject is able to sustain a breath hold. Breath-hold times can be reduced as needed, although at the expense of multi-slice capability. The combination of short scan times and immediate image reconstruction should be helpful in providing rapid feedback about image quality and parameter optimization, as well as in determining the need for additional scan planes.

Whole-heart coverage is achievable with free-breathing 3D coronary MRA [20]. By comparison, a drawback of QISS is that it provides substantially less volume coverage in each breath-hold scan. For instance, a QISS scan with ten 2.1-mm thick contiguous, non-overlapping slices only spans a 21-mm thick volume. Nonetheless, QISS allows extensive lengths of a coronary artery to be imaged in each single breath-hold. In our study, coronary arteries were well depicted in all subjects including routine visualization of small LAD branch vessels. Another drawback of QISS compared with free-breathing 3D techniques is the inability to image with isotropic spatial resolution. However, slices can be overlapped as needed to improve the delineation of particular vessel segments or to enhance

the quality of 3D multi-planar reformats. A potential advantage of QISS compared with free-breathing techniques may be its ability to simultaneously image a coronary stenosis in both long-axis and short-axis views within a single breath-hold. Moreover, the spatial resolution of a cross-sectional QISS image can be increased as desired to better evaluate the severity of a stenosis. Signal averaging can be performed to compensate for signal-to-noise loss with the smaller pixel, although at the expense of multi-slice capability. While theoretically possible to image a coronary artery in multiple slice orientations and with arbitrary spatial resolutions using free-breathing 3D techniques, scan time constraints make it impractical to do so in clinical practice.

Despite the much shorter scan time of QISS, coronary CNR values were comparable between free-breathing 3D bSSFP and breath-hold QISS scans at 1.5 Tesla. Although the lengthier free-breathing scan benefits from the intrinsic signal averaging of a 3D acquisition, this benefit may be offset by the much greater inflow of un-saturated spins with the 2D acquisition and elimination of noise from respiratory motion artifact by breath-holding [21]. At 3 Tesla, coronary CNR was significantly better for QISS than free-breathing 3D, which may in part be due to the SAR-dependent decrease in efficiency for the latter technique. Respiratory motion artifacts degraded coronary artery image quality in half the free-breathing 3D bSSFP scans but none of the breath-hold QISS scans. In no subject did a free-breathing scan outperform breath-hold QISS. However, our results may not be generalizable to other MRI systems, since free-breathing 3D techniques are highly system and vendor dependent. More advanced approaches under development, such as continuous scanning golden angle MRA [22], will likely provide more consistent image quality with reduced scan time.

The QISS data acquisition was restricted to the diastolic phase of the cardiac cycle for this study. This was done in order to minimize cardiac motion and to ensure that the in-plane FOCI pulse (applied immediately after the R-wave) was coincident with the imaging slice at the time of data acquisition. Since the FOCI pulse has twice the thickness of the imaging slice, image contrast should not be altered if the imaging slice moves by just a few millimeters. However, for a systolic acquisition the myocardium will move to a substantially different position than the one to which the FOCI pulse was applied, which would result in increased background signal. This limitation is not encountered when a spatially non-selective T2-weighted magnetization preparation is used.

Further improvements in QISS image quality should be readily achievable. Our studies were performed on older generation 1.5 Tesla and 3 Tesla MRI systems. Newer generation systems provide a substantial boost in

SNR (up to 50 %) through improved phased array coil designs and RF electronics. Compressed sensing techniques have the potential to greatly improve QISS image quality, particularly given the high degree of background signal suppression and resultant sparsity [23]. Multi-slice imaging efficiency can also be improved. It may be possible to at least double the number of slices per breath-hold through the use of simultaneous multi-slice imaging [24].

Temporal resolution is another important consideration, since the coronary arteries will appear blurred if temporal resolution is insufficient. For subjects with rapid heart rates, one can enhance temporal resolution by using fewer radial views or by acquiring more shots. Although the use of more shots in conjunction with a faster heart rate increases scan time, this effect is largely compensated by the proportionately shorter RR interval. An alternative approach might be to use a golden angle radial trajectory. One could then reconstruct QISS images from subsets of data providing arbitrarily high temporal resolution in order to minimize blurring from coronary motion [25]. Additionally, beta-blockers can be administered to slow the heart rate, as is routinely done for coronary CT angiography.

Aside from coronary MRA, QISS may have complementary value to cine bSSFP for evaluating cardiac morphology. While an excellent technique for measuring ventricular function, multi-phase cine bSSFP is inefficient for anatomic evaluation since only a few cine slices can be acquired in each breath-hold. By comparison, single-phase QISS allows the entire left ventricle to be imaged in just a few breath-holds. Unlike cine bSSFP, QISS permits the use of fat saturation to improve contrast between epicardial fat and the myocardium and coronary arteries. Other potential clinical applications include evaluation of the aortic root, pulmonary veins, intra-cardiac masses and pericardial disease.

A limitation of this pilot study is that imaging was performed in cooperative subjects. Free-breathing techniques will likely prove advantageous in sicker patients who are unable to breath-hold. Our study design involved comparisons of multiple pulse sequences, which did not allow time for formal evaluation of the right coronary artery. Parameter modifications, such as the use of more shots for higher temporal resolution and optimization of the quiescent interval so that data are collected during the period of least coronary artery motion, might be beneficial for imaging of the right coronary artery due to its greater mobility compared with the left coronary circulation. Another concern for QISS is that diaphragm drift may cause subtle changes in position for slices acquired late in the breath-hold compared with those acquired earlier. Potential solutions include shorter breath-holds, as well as prospective navigator-based slice correction [26].

Conclusions

Breath-hold QISS MRA provides a simple, versatile, and time-efficient alternative to free-breathing 3D techniques for evaluation of the coronary arteries at both 1.5 Tesla and 3 Tesla. Initial results suggest advantages for radial QISS, including improved image sharpness, relative insensitivity to flow and motion artifacts, and absence of fold over artifact with small FOV. The consistently short scan times and ease of use should facilitate incorporation into routine cardiac imaging protocols. Future efforts will be directed towards clinical validation in patients with CAD and other cardiovascular disorders.

Abbreviations

QISS: Quiescent-interval slice-selective; MRA: Magnetic resonance Angiography; LAD: Left anterior descending coronary artery; LCx: Left circumflex coronary artery; LM: Left main coronary artery; RCA: Right coronary artery; SNR: Signal-to-noise ratio; CNR: Contrast-to-noise ratio; bSSFP: Balanced steady-state free precession; RF: Radiofrequency; SAR: Specific absorption rate; FOCI: Frequency offset corrected inversion.

Competing interests

Dr. Edelman: Research support and invention licensing agreement, Siemens Healthcare. Dr. Giri: Employee, Siemens Healthcare.

Authors' contributions

RE: participated in all aspects of the study and is the guarantor of study integrity. SG: assisted with pulse sequence implementation and manuscript review. AP: assisted with protocol design, image analysis and manuscript review. MPFB: assisted with qualitative image analysis and manuscript review. WL: assisted with quantitative image analysis and manuscript review. IK: assisted with pulse sequence implementation, statistical analysis and manuscript review. All authors read and approved the final manuscript.

Acknowledgement

The authors would like to thank Kieran O' Brien (Siemens Ltd., Australia and New Zealand) for providing the optimized FOCI pulse used in this work.

Author details

[1]Department of Radiology, NorthShore University HealthSystem, 2650 Ridge Avenue, Evanston, IL 60201, USA. [2]Feinberg School of Medicine, Northwestern University, Chicago, USA. [3]Siemens Medical Solutions USA, Inc., Chicago, USA. [4]The University of Chicago Pritzker School of Medicine, Chicago, USA.

References

1. Pennell DJ. Cardiovascular magnetic resonance. Circulation. 2010;121:692–705. doi:10.1161/CIRCULATIONAHA.108.811547.
2. Kato S, Kitagawa K, Ishida N, et al. Assessment of coronary artery disease using magnetic resonance coronary angiography: a national multicenter trial. J Am Coll Cardiol. 2010;56(12):983–91. doi:10.1016/j.jacc.2010.01.071.
3. In the original publication (Magn Reson Med 2010;63:951–958), the QISS acronym stood for "quiescent-interval single shot". However, we have modified the acronym to stand for "quiescent-interval slice-selective" in order to more flexibly encompass more recent implementations of the technique for carotid and coronary MRA.
4. Hodnett PA, Koktzoglou I, Davarpanah AH, et al. Evaluation of peripheral arterial disease with nonenhanced quiescent-interval single-shot MR angiography. Radiology. 2011;260(1):282–93.
5. Oshinski JN, Delfino JG, Sharma P, Gharib AM, Pettigrew RI. Cardiovascular magnetic resonance at 3.0 T: current state of the art. J Cardiovasc Magn Reson. 2010;12:55. doi:10.1186/1532-429X-12-55.
6. Payne GS, Leach MO. Implementation and evaluation of frequency offset corrected inversion (FOCI) pulses on a clinical MR system. Magn Reson Med. 1997;38:828–33.

7.   Edelman RR, Giri S, Murphy IG, Flanagan O, Speier P, Koktzoglou I. Ungated radial quiescent-inflow single-shot (UnQISS) magnetic resonance angiography using optimized azimuthal equidistant projections. Magn Reson Med. 2014;72(6):1522–9. doi:10.1002/mrm.25477. Epub 2014 Sep 24.

8.   Li D, Carr JC, Shea SM, Zheng J, Deshpande VS, Wielopolski PA, et al. Coronary arteries: magnetization-prepared contrast-enhanced three-dimensional volume-targeted breath-hold MR angiography. Radiology. 2001;219(1):270–7.

9.   Bansmann PM, Priest AN, Muellerleile K, Stork A, Lund GK, Kaul MG, et al. MRI of the coronary vessel wall at 3 T: comparison of radial and Cartesian k-space sampling. AJR Am J Roentgenol. 2007;188(1):70–4.

10. Edelman RR, Manning WJ, Burstein D, Paulin S. Coronary arteries: breath hold MR angiography. Radiology. 1991;181:641–3.

11. Santos JM, Cunningham CH, Lustig M, Hargreaves BA, Hu BS, Nishimura DG, et al. Single breath-hold whole-heart MRA using variable-density spirals at 3 T. Magn Reson Med. 2006;55(2):371–9.

12. Soleimanifard S, Stuber M, Hays AG, Weiss RG, Schär M. Robust volume-targeted balanced steady-state free-precession coronary magnetic resonance angiography in a breathhold at 3.0 Tesla: a reproducibility study. J Cardiovasc Magn Reson. 2014;16:27. doi:10.1186/1532-429X-16-27.

13. Niendorf T, Hardy CJ, Giaquinto RO, Gross P, Cline HE, Zhu Y, et al. Toward single breath hold whole heart coverage coronary MRA using highly accelerated parallel imaging with a 32-channel MR system. Magn Reson Med. 2006;56:167–76.

14. Katoh M, Buecker A, Stuber M, Günther RW, Spuentrup E. Free-breathing renal MR angiography with steady-state free-precession (SSFP) and slab-selective spin inversion: initial results. Kidney Int. 2004;66(3):1272–8.

15. Lauzon ML, Rutt BK. Polar sampling in k-space: reconstruction effects. Magn Reson Med. 1998;40(5):769–82.

16. Botnar RM, Stuber M, Danias PG, Kissinger KV, Manning WJ. Improved coronary artery definition with T2-weighted, free-breathing, three-dimensional coronary MRA. Circulation. 1999;99(24):3139–48.

17. Groell R, Schaffler GJ, Rienmueller R. Pericardial sinuses and recesses: findings at electrocardiographically triggered electron-beam CT. Radiology. 1999;212(1):69–73.

18. Liu X, Bi X, Huang J, Jerecic R, Carr J, Li D. Contrast-enhanced whole-heart coronary magnetic resonance angiography at 3.0 T: comparison with steady-state free precession technique at 1.5 T. Invest Radiol. 2008;43(9):663–8. doi:10.1097/RLI.0b013e31817ed1ff.

19. Wang Y, Riederer SJ, Ehman RL. Respiratory motion of the heart: kinematics and the implications for the spatial resolution in coronary imaging. Magn Reson Med. 1995;33:713–9.

20. Sakuma H, Ichikawa Y, Suzawa N, Hirano T, Makino K, Koyama N, et al. Assessment of coronary arteries with total study time of less than 30 min by using whole-heart coronary MR angiography. Radiology. 2005;237(1): 316–21. doi:10.1148/radiol.2371040830.

21. Nezafat R, Herzka D, Stehning C, Peters DC, Nehrke K, Manning WJ. Inflow quantification in three-dimensional cardiovascular MR imaging. J Magn Reson Imaging. 2008;28(5):1273–9. doi:10.1002/jmri.21493.

22. Prieto C, Doneva M, Usman M, Henningsson M, Greil G, Schaeffter T, et al. Highly efficient respiratory motion compensated free-breathing coronary MRA using golden-step Cartesian acquisition. J Magn Reson Imaging. 2015; 41(3):738–46. doi:10.1002/jmri.24602. Epub 2014 Feb 27.

23. Lustig M, Donoho D, Sparse PJM, MRI. The application of compressed sensing for rapid MR imaging. Magn Reson Med. 2007;58(6):1182–95.

24. Yutzy SR, Seiberlich N, Duerk JL, Griswold MA. Improvements in Multislice Parallel Imaging Using Radial CAIPIRINHA. Magn Reson Med. 2011;65(6):1630–7.

25. Winkelmann S, Schaeffter T, Koehler T, Eggers H, Doessel O. An optimal radial profile order based on the Golden Ratio for time-resolved MRI. IEEE Trans Med Imaging. 2007;26(1):68–76.

26. McConnell MV, Khasgiwala VC, Savord EU, et al. Prospective adaptive navigator correction for breath hold MR coronary angiography. Magn Reson Med. 1997;37:148–52.

16

Feasibility study of electrocardiographic and respiratory gated, gadolinium enhanced magnetic resonance angiography of pulmonary veins and the impact of heart rate and rhythm on study quality

John D Groarke[1]*, Alfonso H Waller[1], Tomas S Vita[1], Gregory F Michaud[2], Marcelo F Di Carli[1], Ron Blankstein[1], Raymond Y Kwong[1] and Michael Steigner[1]

Abstract

Background: We aimed to assess the feasibility of 3 dimensional (3D) respiratory and ECG gated, gadolinium enhanced magnetic resonance angiography (MRA) on a 3 Tesla (3 T) scanner for imaging pulmonary veins (PV) and left atrium (LA). The impact of heart rate (HR) and rhythm irregularity associated with atrial fibrillation (AF) on image and segmentation qualities were also assessed.

Methods: 101 consecutive patients underwent respiratory and ECG gated (ventricular end systolic window) MRA for pre AF ablation imaging. Image quality (assessed by PV delineation) was scored as 1 = not visualized, 2 = poor, 3 = good and 4 = excellent. Segmentation quality was scored on a similar 4 point scale. Signal to noise ratios (SNRs) were calculated for the LA, LA appendage (LAA), and PV. Contrast to noise ratios (CNRs) were calculated between myocardium and LA, LAA and PV, respectively. Associations between HR/rhythm and quality metrics were assessed.

Results: 35 of 101 (34.7%) patients were in AF at time of MRA. 100 (99%) patients had diagnostic studies, and 91 (90.1%) were of good or excellent quality. Overall, mean ± standard deviation (SD) image quality score was 3.40 ± 0.69. Inter observer agreement for image quality scores was substantial, (kappa = 0.68; 95% confidence interval (CI): 0.46, 0.90). Neither HR adjusting for rhythm [odds ratio (OR) = 1.03, 95% CI = 0.98,1.09; p = 0.22] nor rhythm adjusting for HR [OR = 1.25, 95% CI = 0.20, 7.69; p = 0.81] demonstrated association with image quality. Similarly, SNRs and CNRs were largely independent of HR after adjusting for rhythm. Segmentation quality scores were good or excellent for 77.3% of patients: mean ± SD score = 2.91 ± 0.63, and scores did not significantly differ by baseline rhythm (p = 0.78).

Conclusions: 3D respiratory and ECG gated, gadolinium enhanced MRA of the PVs and LA on a 3 T system is feasible during ventricular end systole, achieving high image quality and high quality image segmentation when imported into electroanatomic mapping systems. Quality is independent of HR and heart rhythm for this free breathing, radiation free, alternative strategy to current MRA or CT based approaches, for pre AF ablation imaging of PVs and LA.

Keywords: Pulmonary vein imaging, Respiratory gated, ECG gated, Magnetic resonance angiography, 3 Tesla, Image segmentation, Electroanatomic mapping systems, Pre ablation imaging, End-systole

* Correspondence: jgroarke@partners.org
[1]Cardiovascular Imaging Program, Cardiovascular Division, Department of Medicine and Department of Radiology, Brigham and Women's Hospital, Harvard Medical School, Boston, MA, USA
Full list of author information is available at the end of the article

Background

Catheter ablation of atrial fibrillation (AF) is considered appropriate treatment for symptomatic AF, refractory or intolerant to at least one antiarrhythmic medication, and may be considered as first line treatment for certain patients [1]. The rate of catheter ablation in patients with AF, across all age groups, is increasing significantly over time [2]. Computerized tomography (CT) or cardiovascular magnetic resonance (CMR) evaluation of the left atrium (LA) and pulmonary vein (PV) anatomy prior to catheter ablation is considered appropriate [3]. Such imaging provides accurate visualization of highly variable PV and LA anatomy, facilitates image integration with electroanatomic mapping systems, and demonstrates the atrioesophageal relationship that is important for risk assessment of thermal esophageal injury. Integration of pre-acquired cardiac images with electroanatomic mapping to guide catheter ablations is feasible and inconsistently reported to improve procedural success, reduce procedure duration, fluoroscopy time and occurrence of PV stenosis, compared to conventional electroanatomic mapping alone [4-10]. For example, PV isolation guided by image integration was associated with reduced AF recurrence in comparison with PV isolation guided by three dimensional (3D) electroanatomical mapping alone based on registry data from 573 patients undergoing catheter ablation for paroxysmal AF [10]; however, randomized trials of AF ablation guided by 3D electroanatomical mapping alone versus with image integration have shown no difference in AF outcomes [8,9].

CT angiography (CTA) of the PVs and LA offers high spatial resolution and fast acquisition times. However, CTA requires the use of iodinated contrast agents and radiation exposure, which increases overall radiation exposure when added to fluoroscopy related exposure during catheter ablation. Therefore, for patients with no contraindication, CMR is increasingly preferred for pre ablation PV and LA imaging. There is no significant difference in registration accuracy during image integration into electroanatomic mapping systems with contrast enhanced CT imaging versus gadolinium enhanced CMR [4,11]. CMR sequences for PV and LA imaging without intravenous contrast agents are used clinically; however, contrast enhanced CT is reported to provide superior LA anatomy reconstruction compared to a non contrast CMR dataset [12]. Similarly, non-contrast CMR sequences have been shown to be of significantly inferior quality compared to contrast enhanced MR images [13,14]. In clinical practice, CMR of the PVs is most often performed by contrast enhanced MR angiography (MRA) during an expiratory breath-hold, without electrocardiographic (ECG) gating that would prolong breath-hold time. Free breathing, respiratory and ECG gated MRA of the LA and PVs may offer higher spatial resolution and less motion artifacts

through ECG gating than the conventional breath held MRA [14]. Furthermore, accurate registration during image integration into electroanatomical mapping systems is critical [1]. Patients are free breathing throughout catheter ablation procedures; respiratory related changes in LA and PV anatomy during breath held imaging techniques may predispose to registration errors during image integration [15]. Free breathing imaging techniques may be preferable to either breath hold MRA or CT techniques, resembling the breathing pattern during electroanatomic mapping at catheter ablation.

Small studies have demonstrated the feasibility of free breathing, respiratory gated CMR for LA and PV imaging, with and without contrast enhancement [14,16-19]. The impact of heart rate (HR) and rhythm on image quality and registration accuracy, outside of data from very small studies, are uncertain [20,21]. End-systolic imaging has been suggested to improve image quality during magnetic resonance coronary angiography compared to diastolic acquisitions in 14 subjects with heart rates exceeding 65 beats/minute using a 1.5 tesla (T) MR scanner [22], and among 10 volunteers imaged using a 3 T scanner [23]. However, the feasibility of ECG triggering at ventricular *end-systole*, the phase of the cardiac cycle least sensitive to increases in heart rate [24] and irregular rhythm, has not yet been described in a large number of patients undergoing MRA with variable heart rhythm and heart rates.

The purpose of this study was to determine the feasibility and diagnostic quality of free breathing, respiratory and end-systolic ECG gated, contrast enhanced MRA of the PV and LA anatomy on a 3 T scanner in an unselected cohort of consecutive patients referred for pre-ablation imaging. The impact of HR and rhythm at the time of image acquisition on image quality, and the quality of image segmentation obtained from these 3D MRA datasets using image integration software of an electroanatomic mapping system require investigation.

Methods

Study population

101 consecutive patients referred for pre-catheter ablation MR imaging of the PVs and LA over an eight month study period were included in this prospective study. The study was approved by the Institutional Review Board and was compliant with the Health Insurance Portability and Accountability Act. The requirement for informed consent was waived because of the nature of the study. Baseline demographics, including HR and rhythm, were recorded for all patients at the time of CMR.

Image acquisition

All patients were scanned on a commercial 3 T MRI scanner (TimTrio, Siemens, Erlangen, Germany). Electrocardiographic electrodes were positioned for optimal gating before the study. Conventional multiplanar scout images were obtained followed by a high resolution four chamber steady state free precession (SSFP) sequence (echo time : 1 ms, repetition time (TR): 24.24 ms; flip angle : 50 degree; field of view: 340 mm; readout bandwidth: 930 Hz/pixel; matrix size: 1.8 x 1.3 x 8.0 mm; slice thickness: 8 mm; parallel imaging with an acceleration factor of 3 was applied) was used to identify the cardiac phase corresponding to *end-systole* by visual assessment. The timing of this end-systolic phase was then entered as the trigger delay for acquisitions. The acquisition window duration was set at 100 ms for all patients, given that the end-systolic phase that lasts approximately 100–150 ms is more or less independent of heart rate and related RR interval [25]. Free breathing, contrast enhanced MRA using a ECG triggered, respiratory gated, inversion recovery prepared, 3D volume whole heart acquisition segmented gradient echo sequence (echo time: 1.4 ms, echo spacing: 3.22 ms, number of k space lines per cardiac cycle: 35, flip angle: 20 degrees, inversion time = 200 ms, readout bandwidth = 698 Hz/pixel, slice thickness: 1.2 mm, acquired voxel size: $1.3 \times 1.3 \times 1.2$ mm3, 88–120 slices) was obtained, starting 45 seconds after initiation of an intravenous infusion of 0.15 mmol/kg of gadobenate dimeglumine (MultiHance®; Bracco Imaging SpA, Milan, Italy) at a rate of 0.3 ml/sec using a power injector (MEDRAD Inc., Warrendale, PA, USA), followed by 20 ml saline at the same rate. Gadolinium dimeglumine with a higher T1 relaxivity relative to other gadolinium chelates [26], a dosing regimen similar to that used in a smaller study [16], and the infusion protocol were all selected in an effort to maintain maximum blood pool enhancement for the duration of MRA acquisition. The FOV was selected to include the entire LA, LA appendage (LAA) and proximal PVs. An axial slab and a coronal image taken at end-expiration were used to position the navigator beam on the dome of the right hemi diaphragm to track the end expiratory position of the diaphragm to achieve respiratory gating, with an acceptance window of 5 mm. The position of the navigator bands was adjusted on an axial image to a location lateral to the proximal right pulmonary veins prior to acquisition. A parallel imaging technique with an acceleration factor of two was used to shorten acquisition times. An axial T1 weighted, fat saturated 3D gradient echo sequence (echo time: 1.26 ms, TR: 3.51 ms, flip angle: 10 degrees, readout bandwidth = 500 Hz/pixel; slice thickness: 4.0 mm) was performed after completion of the MRA to demonstrate the course of the esophagus relative to the pulmonary veins (Figure 1).

Image analysis
Qualitative analysis
Image quality, as assessed by visibility and definition of pulmonary veins on the 3D volume acquisition

dataset from each study, was graded on a four point scale (Figure 2), similar to scales used in other studies [17,27]: 1: not visualized; 2: poorly defined with blurring such that stenosis or diameter could not be confidently evaluated; 3: well defined with mild blurring only; 4: excellent image quality without blurring. These analyses were performed by two readers blinded to each other, and to HR and rhythm at time of imaging. A third blinded reader scored cases where quality scores were discordant (n = 26). As such, a consensus quality score was determined for all cases, and these scores were used for quality scores included in analyses.

Quantitative analysis
The following data were calculated for each subject using QMass Enterprise Solution 7.4° (Medis Medical Imaging System, Inc., Leiden, Netherlands); formulae used were similar to those used in published studies [14,28]:

A) Signal to noise ratios (SNRs):
   A region of interest (ROI) with an area of at least 1.0 cm^2 was placed in the LA and the mean signal intensity (SI) and standard deviation (SD) was calculated. The SNR$_{LA}$ is calculated using the following formula: (mean SI in blood in LA/SD). A similar method using a ROI within the largest PV and within the LAA was used to calculate the SNR$_{PV}$ and SNR$_{LAA}$, respectively.
B) Contrast to noise ratios (CNRs):
   A ROI with an area of at least 1.0 cm^2 was placed in the LA and also in the myocardium (basal anteroseptum) and the mean SI and SD for each site was calculated. The CNR$_{LA/myocardium}$ was calculated using the following formula: (mean SI in blood - mean SI in myocardium)/(0.5 x [SD in blood + SD in myocardium]). A similar method using a ROI within the largest PV and within the LAA was used to calculate CNR$_{PV/myocardium}$ and CNR$_{LAA/myocardium}$, respectively.

Image segmentation analyses
MRA datasets were imported into an electroanatomic mapping system (CartoMerge Image Integration Module, Biosense Webster Inc., Diamond Bar, CA USA). Using CartoMerge semi automated image integration software, a technician with over 10 years of experience, blinded to other results, segmented the LA and PVs. Segmentation quality was then assessed according to a 4 point score, similar to that used by Wagner et al. [14]: 1- poor segmentation quality due to inability to separate LA and PVs from adjacent structures; 2- moderate segmentation quality with incomplete separation of LA and PVs from adjacent structures; 3- good segmentation

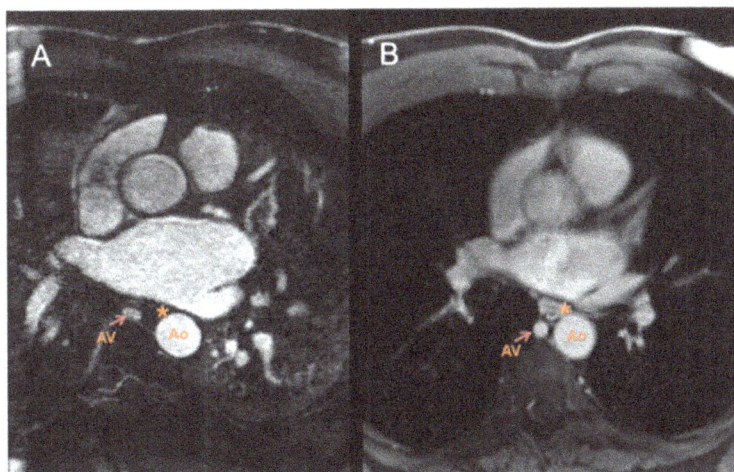

Figure 1 Anatomical relationship of the pulmonary veins to the esophagus. A- Axial slice from a 3D respiratory- and ECG-gated gadolinium-enhanced MRA demonstrating that the esophagus (labeled *) can be difficult to identify on this sequence. **B**- Axial T1- weighted, fat-saturated 3D-gradient echo sequence from the same patient at a similar level clearly demonstrating the esophagus and its anatomical relations. [Key: AV = azygos vein, Ao = descending thoracic aorta, * = esophagus].

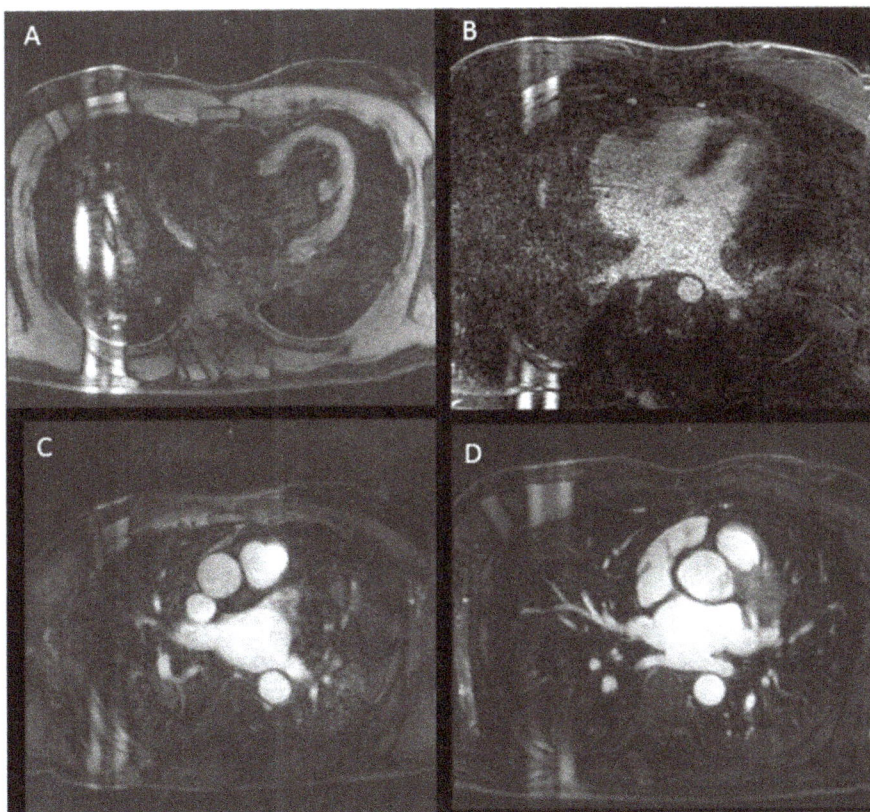

Figure 2 Qualitative analysis of image quality. A- Image quality grade 1: pulmonary veins not visualized; **B**- Grade 2: pulmonary veins poorly defined with significant blurring of vessels; **C**- Grade 3: pulmonary veins well defined with mild blurring of vessels; **D**- Grade 4: excellent pulmonary vein definition without blurring.

quality with near complete separation of LA and PVs, and 4- excellent segmentation quality with complete separation of LA and PVs achieved (Figure 3).

Patient follow up

Complications related to catheter ablation of AF were defined as per consensus guidelines [29] and recorded with interval from procedure for all patients. Patients were followed with clinic evaluations, 12 lead electrocardiogram, and/or 24 hour Holter monitor to detect recurrent atrial arrhythmias. Atrial arrhythmias (including documented AF, atrial flutter, or atrial tachycardias) after a 3 month blanking period following ablation were defined as recurrences.

Statistical analyses

Continuous, normally distributed data are presented as mean ± SD. Continuous, non-normal data are presented as median with interquartile range (IQR). Categorical data are presented as percentages. Data are presented for entire patient cohort, patients in normal sinus rhythm (NSR) and patients in AF at the time of imaging. Continuous variables and binary variables are compared between NSR and AF patient cohorts using a two tailed Student's t test and Fisher's exact test, respectively. The Mantel Haenszel Chi Square test is used to test for group comparisons of image quality and segmentation quality scores. The image quality scores of readers 1 and 2 are compared using a paired t test, dichotomized as poor (quality score =1 or 2) or good (quality score = 3 or 4), and inter observer agreement for dichotomized quality scores between readers is determined by calculating the kappa statistic.

The crude relationship between dichotomized consensus image quality (score ≥3 good versus score ≤2 poor) and heart rhythm is presented as an unadjusted odds ratio (OR), with associated 95% confidence intervals (CI). To adjust for the effect of HR at the time of CMR, a logistic regression model with dichotomized consensus image quality as the dependent variable and HR and heart rhythm at time of CMR as predictor variables is used.

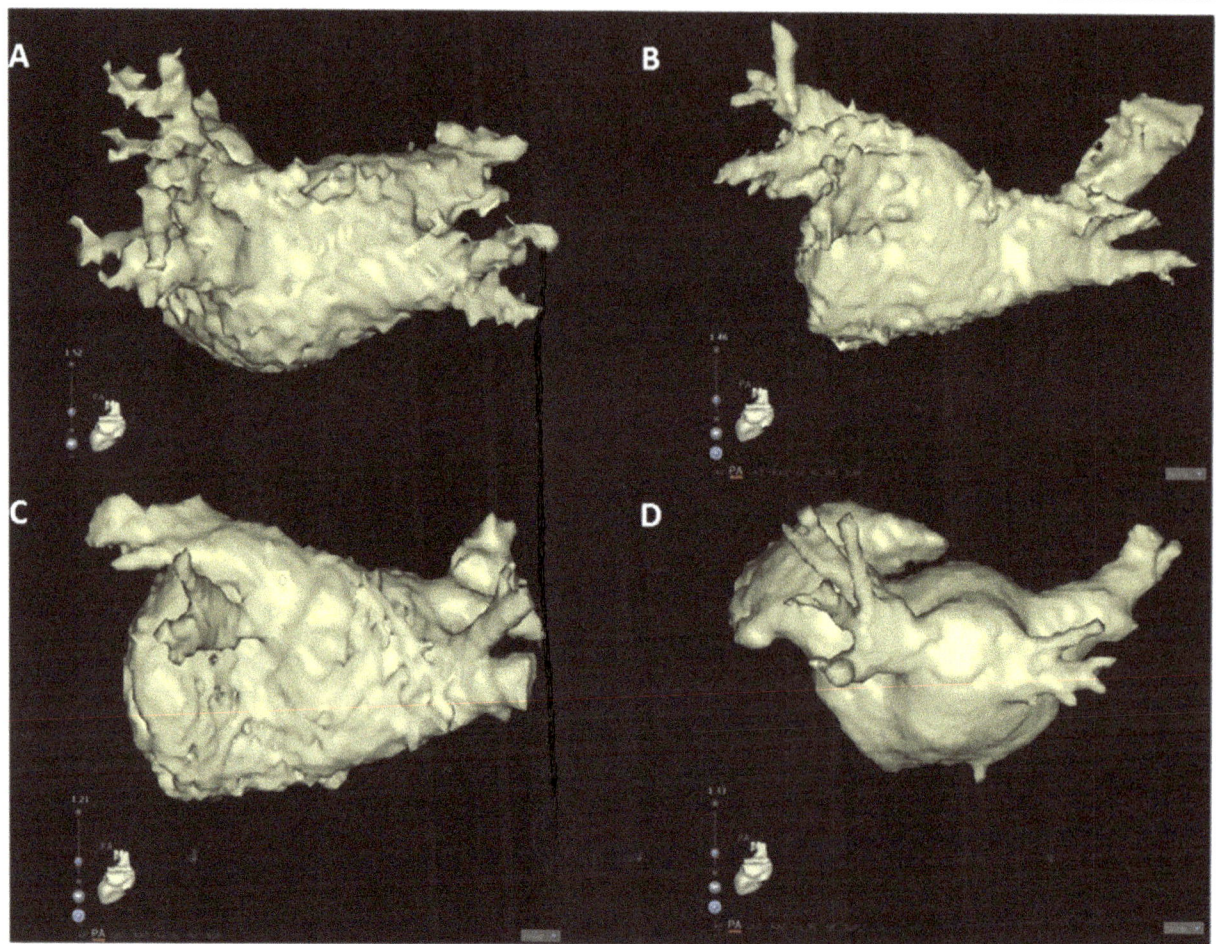

Figure 3 Image segmentation scoring: A- Grade 1: poor segmentation due to inability to separate LA and PVs from adjacent structures; B- Grade 2: moderate segmentation with incomplete separation of LA and PVs from adjacent structures; C- Grade 3: good segmentation with near complete separation of LA and PVs; D- excellent segmentation with complete separation of LA and PV.

Effect modification by HR on the association between heart rhythm and image quality is investigated using the same model with the inclusion of an interaction variable. To assess for non linear associations with HR, HR was tested in four formats: (i) continuous linear relationship, (ii) categorical relationship [3 categories: HR ≤ 55 bpm (n = 21), 55 < HR ≤ 90 bpm (n = 66), and HR > 90 bpm (n = 14)], (iii) log transformation of HR, and (iv) quadratic relationship. Multiple linear regression models were used to assess the relationship between categorical HR and rhythm with each of the SNRs and CNRs. A p value of <0.05 was considered significant. Analyses were performed using SAS 9.3® (SAS Institute Inc., Cary, NC, USA).

Results
Patient characteristics
101 patients were included in this study. All patients had a history of persistent or paroxysmal AF. 35 (34.7%) patients were in AF at the time of CMR. Baseline characteristics for entire patient cohort, as well as by AF status at time of imaging are outlined in Table 1. Patients in AF at time of CMR had a significantly higher mean HR and lower mean systolic BP (SBP) at the time of imaging, lower mean left ventricular ejection fraction (LVEF) and larger mean LA diameter, as measured on a 3 chamber SSFP sequence at end-systole, than patients in NSR.

Image quality
The mean ± SD acquisition time and acceptance rate were 7:51 ± 2:58 minutes and 54.4 ± 11.8%, respectively.

The mean ± SD dose of gadobenate dimeglumine delivered was 29.8 ± 8.5 mls, over a mean ± SD infusion duration of 1:39 ± 0:28 minutes. 100 (99%) patients' studies were considered diagnostic (consensus quality score > 1), and 91 (90.1%) were of good or excellent quality. Overall, mean ± SD consensus quality score was 3.40 ± 0.69. Among patients in NSR and AF, there were no significant differences in mean acquisition times, acceptance rates, quality scores, SNRs or CNRs, Table 2 and Figure 4.

The mean ± SD quality scores for reader 1 and 2 were 3.34 ± 0.70 and 3.31 ± 0.73, respectively (pooled t test p value = 0.57); the overall inter observer agreement for dichotomized quality scores assigned by these readers was substantial [30], (k = 0.68; 95% CI: 0.46, 0.90).

Impact of heart rate and heart rhythm on image quality
Heart rhythm was not significantly associated with dichotomized consensus image quality (crude OR = 0.44, 95% CI: 0.08, 2.19; p = 0.49). By logistic regression, neither HR adjusting for rhythm [OR = 1.03, 95% CI = 0.98,1.09; p = 0.22] nor rhythm adjusting for HR [OR = 1.25, 95% CI: 0.20, 7.69; p = 0.81] demonstrated significant association with dichotomized image quality. Further adjusting for LA diameter, LVEF, and SBP did not significantly alter results. Similarly, models fitted to allow for effect modification or non-linear associations with HR did not yield different results. Multiple linear regression models demonstrated that SNRs and CNRs were largely independent of categorical HR after adjusting for heart rhythm and vice versa; with the exceptions

Table 1 Baseline characteristics presented by entire cohort and by AF status

	Overall group	NSR cohort	AF cohort	p-value
n	101	66	35	-
Male sex	73 (72.3%)	48 (65.8%)	18 (64.3%)	1.00*
Age, years	58.9 ± 10.9	58.8 ± 11.1	59.1 ± 10.6	0.89
Body surface area, m²	2.07 ± 0.23	2.04 ± 0.22	2.11 ± 0.26	0.16
Hypertension	39 (38.6%)	25 (37.9%)	14 (40.0%)	0.83*
Beta blocker	46 (45.5%)	26 (39.4%)	20 (57.1%)	0.10*
Digoxin	5 (5.0%)	2 (3.0%)	3 (8.6%)	0.34*
Anti arrhythmic agent	39 (38.6%)	29 (43.9%)	10 (28.6%)	0.14*
HR at time of CMR	69 ± 17	61 ± 9	84 ± 20	<0.0001
HR range, bpm	37-121	37-76	44-121	
SBP, mmHg	129 ± 16	132 ± 16	124 ± 15	0.02
DBP, mmHg	73 ± 11	73 ± 10	74 ± 13	0.45
LVEF, %	56.4 ± 11.1	59.5 ± 9.4	49.7 ± 11.6	<0.0001
LVEDVI, ml/m²	76.7 ± 15.4	78.1 ± 15.9	72.7 ± 13.7	0.16
LVESVI, ml/m²	33.5 ± 13.5	32.3 ± 13.7	37.0 ± 12.6	0.17
LA diameter, cm	3.9 ± 0.9	3.7 ± 0.7	4.4 ± 0.9	0.0001

*Fisher's exact test.
[Key: SBP- systolic blood pressure; DBP- diastolic blood pressure; LVEF- left ventricular ejection fraction; LVEDVI- left ventricular end-diastolic volume indexed to body surface area; LVESVI- left ventricular end-systolic volume indexed to body surface area; LA- left atrium].

Table 2 Quantitative and qualitative CMR measures presented for entire patient cohort and by AF status

	Overall group	NSR cohort	AF cohort	p-value[*]
n	101	66	35	-
Mean ± SD acquisition time, mins	7:51 ± 2:58	8:14 ± 3:10	7:08 ± 2:25	0.08
Mean ± SD acceptance rate	54.4 ± 11.8%	53.8 ± 12.3%	55.5 ± 10.8%	0.50
Mean ± SD dose of MultiHance (mL)	29.8 ± 8.5	29.0 ± 7.8	31.4 ± 9.7	0.18
Mean ± SD consensus quality score	3.4 ± 0.7	3.4 ± 0.7	3.3 ± 0.7	0.58
Quality, n (%)				0.58[#]
Uninterpretable	1 (1.0%)	0 (0%)	1 (2.9%)	
Poor	9 (8.9%)	8 (12.1%)	1 (2.9%)	
Good	40 (39.6%)	22 (33.3%)	18 (51.4%)	
Excellent	51 (50.5%)	36 (54.6%)	15 (42.8%)	

[*]Two tailed Student t test, unless otherwise specified; [#]Mantel Haenszel Chi Square test.

of SNR_{PV} and $CNR_{PV/Myocardium}$ which demonstrate a negative association with HR < 55 bpm compared to a reference HR category ($55 < HR \leq 90$ bpm), Table 3. Although mean $CNR_{LA/myocardium}$ was higher than mean values of both $CNR_{PV/myocardium}$ (p < 0.0001) and $CNR_{LAA/myocardium}$ (p < 0.0001), mean values of $CNR_{PV/myocardium}$ and $CNR_{LAA/myocardium}$ were similar, (p = 0.51).

Image segmentation quality

97 (96%) patients' MRA datasets were segmented using CartoMerge semiautomated image integration software. Segmentation quality scores were good or excellent for 75 (77.3%) patients, with a mean ± SD score of 2.91 (+/− 0.63). There were no significant differences in segmentation quality scores between NSR and AF patient cohorts, Table 4.

Patient outcomes

94 of 101 (93.1%) patients included in this study proceeded to catheter ablation of AF. Three complications occurred in 2 (2.1%) patients: right phrenic nerve injury and heart block requiring permanent pacemaker insertion occurred at time of procedure in the same patient, and atrioesophageal fistula presented in another patient 17 days after ablation. Follow up data for recurrent arrhythmia were available for 91 of 94 (96.8%); 76 (83.5%) remained in NSR after median (IQR) follow up of 308 (87, 385) days following ablation. The median (IQR) interval from ablation to recurrence of atrial arrhythmias in 15 patients (16.5%) was 348 (191, 414) days.

Discussion

In our study, we found that free breathing 3D respiratory and ECG gated gadolinium enhanced MRA of the LA and PVs on a 3 T system is both feasible and reproducible, achieving diagnostic images in almost all patients (99%) and good or excellent diagnostic quality images in 90% of patients. Image quality is independent of HR or heart rhythm at the time of imaging. Furthermore, the quality of image segmentation obtained from these 3D MRA datasets

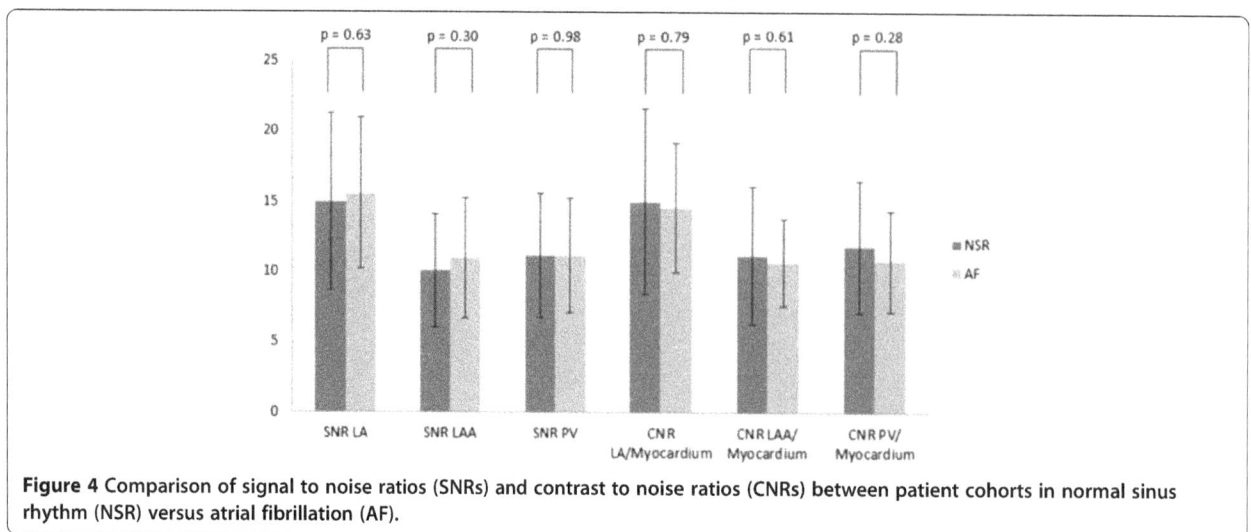

Figure 4 Comparison of signal to noise ratios (SNRs) and contrast to noise ratios (CNRs) between patient cohorts in normal sinus rhythm (NSR) versus atrial fibrillation (AF).

Table 3 Association of heart rate with signal to noise and contrast to noise ratios

	Heart rate ≤ 55 bpm (n = 21)			Heart rate > 90 bpm (n = 14)		
	β coefficient	95% CI	p value	β coefficient	95% CI	p value
SNR left atrium	−2.32	−5.30, 0.66	0.13	0.21	−3.93, 4.34	0.92
SNR LAA	−1.41	−3.62, 0.80	0.21	−0.33	−3.29, 2.63	0.83
SNR PV	−2.29	−4.42,-0.17	0.03	−1.06	−4.01, 1.88	0.48
CNR LA/Myocardium	−2.19	−5.16, 0.78	0.15	−0.23	−4.35, 3.90	0.91
CNR LAA/Myocardium	−1.77	−4.12, 0.58	0.14	−0.52	−3.67, 2.63	0.75
CNR PV/Myocardium	−2.26	−4.38,-0.14	0.04	−1.10	−4.04, 1.85	0.46

Legend: Beta coefficients from multiple linear regression models with the respective SNR or CNR as the dependent variable, and heart rhythm and categorical HR as predictor variables. Results for HR categories presented in this table are compared to the following 'reference' HR category: 55 < HR ≤ 90 bpm (n = 66), and adjusted for heart rhythm.

using image integration software of an electroanatomic mapping system is high.

Fast heart rates and irregular rhythm, common among patients undergoing pre ablation LA and PV imaging, can compromise quality and increase radiation dose of gated CT imaging [31,32]. However, image quality achieved with this MRA technique is independent of HR or rhythm at the time of imaging. Thus, this MRA technique is particularly suited for ECG gated imaging of this patient cohort. The likely explanation for this independent association between image quality and either HR or rhythm is that acquisitions were gated to coincide with relatively quiescent ventricular end-systole. At higher heart rates, the reduction in end-systolic duration is less than the reduction in diastolic duration [24], rendering this phase of the cardiac cycle less sensitive to faster rates and arrhythmia. This is the largest report of respiratory gated MRA of LA and PVs acquired during ventricular end-systole, and the robust quality achieved during this phase of the cardiac cycle, despite HR or rhythm, raises the suggestion that ventricular end-systole may be a suitable target for ECG gating during late gadolinium enhancement (LGE) CMR sequences for detection of atrial fibrosis in select patients with lower heart rates that provide sufficient opportunity for required inversion times. Studies reporting left atrial scarring on 3D LGE CMR are restricted to the mid-diastolic window

[33,34], and comparative studies of alternative strategies would be informative.

Although still practical, the overall mean acquisition time for this 3D respiratory and ECG gated MRA sequence of 7:51 ± 2:58 minutes is longer than acquisition times reported for commonly employed contrast enhanced MRA in expiratory breath hold, without ECG gating (5:45 ± 1:53 minutes) [13]. Furthermore, although the acquisition window is usually shorter for end-systolic compared to mid-diastolic imaging, mean acquisition time in this study was shorter than that reported in two smaller studies of 3D respiratory and ECG gated MRA of pulmonary veins where mid-diastolic ECG gating was used [13,16]. This increase in acquisition times compared to breath held, ungated MRAs may, in part, be offset by reductions in cardiac motion artifact associated through ECG gating and higher spatial resolution. While this study establishes the feasibility and high quality of 3D respiratory and ECG gated MRA, direct comparison with conventional breath held, ungated MRA was not performed in this study, and so conclusions about superiority of one technique over another cannot be made. Whether this technique reduces registration errors during image integration into electroanatomic mapping systems requires investigation.

The 3D dataset produced by free breathing respiratory and ECG gated MRA offers the potential to obtain a

Table 4 Segmentation quality scores for entire patient cohort and by AF status

	Overall group	NSR cohort	AF cohort	p-value
n	97	63	34	-
Mean ± SD segmentation score	2.91 ± 0.63	2.92 ± 0.58	2.88 ± 0.73	0.86*
Segmentation quality score, n (%)				0.78#
Poor	1 (1.0%)	0 (0%)	1 (2.9%)	
Moderate	21 (21.7%)	13 (20.6%)	8 (23.5%)	
Good	61 (62.9%)	42 (66.7%)	19 (55.9%)	
Excellent	14 (14.4%)	8 (12.7%)	6 (17.7%)	

*Student's t-test; #Mantel-Haenszel Chi-Square test.

range of important data using a single test prior to catheter ablation of AF:

(i) High image quality facilitates PV anatomy delineation.

(ii) Using post processing software, the 3D dataset facilitates accurate measurements of PV diameters with orthogonal planes and the double oblique technique.

(iii) LA volume can be quantified using 3D chamber reconstruction technique using similar software; LA volumes have been shown to predict AF recurrence post ablation [35,36].

(iv) Anatomical relationship of the pulmonary veins to esophagus and descending thoracic aorta can be reviewed. A simple and quick axial T1 weighted, fat saturated 3D gradient echo sequence is helpful in demonstrating these anatomical relationships in our experience (Figure 1).

(v) High quality PV segmentation using image integration software of an electroanatomic mapping system as shown in this study, facilitating intra procedural image guidance.

(vi) The SNRs and CNRs for the LA and LAA were similar in this study. Contrast opacification of the LA and LAA is generally good with this technique. No LA or LAA thrombi were identified within this patient cohort. Further studies to determine if intra atrial or appendage thrombus can be reliably detected using this technique, with comparisons to transesophageal echocardiography, would be interesting.

Furthermore, these data can be provided for a wide range of patients as HR, heart rhythm and ability to breath hold do not render patients ineligible for this imaging technique. These data could be further supplemented with an estimation of LV systolic function by acquiring additional images at the time of CMR; LV systolic dysfunction is another predictor of post ablation AF recurrence [37]. Similarly, to increase the diagnostic yield from gadolinium administration, quantification of atrial and PV antral fibrosis related to either AF or previous ablation procedures using high spatial resolution 3D LGE CMR could be performed at the same examination; such fibrosis is associated with LAA thrombus formation, AF recurrence post ablation and clinical outcomes [33,38-40]. There is the potential to provide a comprehensive pre-procedure report with this range of complementary data derived from this technique that could optimize electrophysiologists' assessment of likelihood of sustained procedural success as well as procedural risk.

Study limitations

Direct comparison of this 3D respiratory and ECG gated MRA sequence for imaging pulmonary veins to conventional contrast enhanced, breath held, ungated MRA is necessary, and is a major limitation of this study. While this study establishes the feasibility and high quality of 3D respiratory and ECG gated MRA for imaging pulmonary veins, the lack of a direct comparison precludes conclusions regarding superiority of one technique over another. Superiority over breath-held, ungated MRA will need to be investigated in future studies in order to justify longer acquisition times associated with 3D respiratory and ECG gated MRA. In addition, direct comparison to CTA would be informative. Such comparisons should include an assessment of registration errors during image integration into electroanatomic mapping systems. Certain patients, such as those with claustrophobia, may not tolerate longer acquisition times, but patient tolerance may be improved by the free breathing nature of this respiratory gated technique. Changes in LA and PV anatomy that occur during breath held imaging techniques may predispose to registration errors during image integration into electroanatomic mapping systems [15]; whether imaging in the free breathing state, in its similarity to the breathing pattern during electroanatomic mapping at catheter ablation, offers any advantage in terms of improvement in clinical outcomes is uncertain.

Conclusions

Pre ablation imaging of the PVs and LA by end systolic 3D respiratory and ECG gated gadolinium enhanced MRA on a 3 T system is a feasible technique that achieves high quality images, reproducible image interpretation, and high quality image segmentation when imported into electroanatomic mapping systems. Image quality is independent of HR and heart rhythm for this free breathing, radiation free strategy. This technique offers an alternative strategy for pre-ablation imaging of PVs and LA to current CMR or CT based approaches, and comparative effectiveness studies are necessary to determine the optimal approach.

Abbreviations

3D: Three dimensional; 3 T: Three tesla; AF: Atrial fibrillation; CI: Confidence interval; CMR: Cardiovascular magnetic resonance imaging; CNR: Contrast to noise ratio; CT: Computerized tomography; CTA: CT angiography; ECG: Electrocardiogram; FA: Flip angle; FOV: Field of view; HR: Heart rate; LA: Left atrium; LAA: Left atrial appendage; LGE: Late gadolinium enhancement; LVEF: Left ventricular ejection fraction; MR: Magnetic resonance; MRA: Magnetic resonance angiography; MRI: Magnetic resonance imaging; NSR: Normal sinus rhythm; OR: Odds ratio; PV: Pulmonary vein; ROI: Region of interest; SBP: Systolic blood pressure; SD: Standard deviation; SNR: Signal to noise ratio; SSFP: Steady state free precession; TE: Echo time; TR: Repetition time; TI: Inversion time; TSA: Total surface area.

Competing interests

The authors declare that they have no competing interests.

Authors' contributions

All authors (JDG, AHW, TSV, GFM, MFDC, RB, RYK, MS) made substantial contributions to the conception, design, drafting, and critical revision of the manuscript. All authors read and approved the final manuscript.

Acknowledgement

Tim Campbell of Biosense Webster Inc. contributed to image segmentation and reconstruction artifact analyses.

Author details

[1]Cardiovascular Imaging Program, Cardiovascular Division, Department of Medicine and Department of Radiology, Brigham and Women's Hospital, Harvard Medical School, Boston, MA, USA. [2]Cardiovascular Division, Department of Medicine, Brigham and Women's Hospital, Harvard Medical School, Boston, MA, USA.

References

1. Kottkamp H, Kumagai K, Lindsay BD, Mansour M, Marchlinski FE, McCarthy PM, Mont JL, Morady F, Nademanee K, Nakagawa H, Natale A, Nattel S, Packer DL, Pappone C, Prystowsky E, Raviele A, Reddy K, Ellenbogen MD, Ezekowitz DE, Haines M, Haissaguerre G, Hindricks Y, Iesaka W, Jackman J, Jalife P, Jais J, Kalman D, Keane YH, Kim P, Kirchhof G, et al. 2012 HRS/EHRA/ECAS expert consensus statement on catheter and surgical ablation of atrial fibrillation: recommendations for patient selection, procedural techniques, patient management and follow-up, definitions, endpoints, and research trial design. J Interv Card Electrophysiol. 2012; 33:171–257.
2. Kneeland PP, Fang MC. Trends in catheter ablation for atrial fibrillation in the United States. J Hosp Med. 2009; 4:E1–5.
3. Hendel RC, Patel MR, Kramer CM, Poon M, Hendel RC, Carr JC, Gerstad NA, Gillam LD, Hodgson JM, Kim RJ, Kramer CM, Lesser JR, Martin ET, Messer JV, Redberg RF, Rubin GD, Rumsfeld JS, Taylor AJ, Weigold WG, Woodard PK, Brindis RG, Hendel RC, Douglas PS, Peterson ED, Wolk MJ, Allen JM, Patel MR. ACCF/ACR/SCCT/SCMR/ASNC/NASCI/SCAI/SIR 2006 appropriateness criteria for cardiac computed tomography and cardiac magnetic resonance imaging: a report of the American College of Cardiology Foundation Quality Strategic Directions Committee Appropriateness Criteria Working Group, American College of Radiology, Society of Cardiovascular Computed Tomography, Society for Cardiovascular Magnetic Resonance, American Society of Nuclear Cardiology, North American Society for Cardiac Imaging, Society for Cardiovascular Angiography and Interventions, and Society of Interventional Radiology. J Am Coll Cardiol. 2006; 48:1475–97.
4. Dong J, Dickfeld T, Dalal D, Cheema A, Vasamreddy CR, Henrikson CA, Marine JE, Halperin HR, Berger RD, Lima JA, Bluemke DA, Calkins H. Initial experience in the use of integrated electroanatomic mapping with three-dimensional MR/CT images to guide catheter ablation of atrial fibrillation. J Cardiovasc Electrophysiol. 2006; 17:459–66.
5. Malchano ZJ, Neuzil P, Cury RC, Holmvang G, Weichet J, Schmidt EJ, Ruskin JN, Reddy VY. Integration of cardiac CT/MR imaging with three-dimensional electroanatomical mapping to guide catheter manipulation in the left atrium: implications for catheter ablation of atrial fibrillation. J Cardiovasc Electrophysiol. 2006; 17:1221–9.
6. Kistler PM, Rajappan K, Jahngir M, Earley MJ, Harris S, Abrams D, Gupta D, Liew R, Ellis S, Sporton SC, Schilling RJ. The impact of CT image integration into an electroanatomic mapping system on clinical outcomes of catheter ablation of atrial fibrillation. J Cardiovasc Electrophysiol. 2006; 17:1093–101.
7. Martinek M, Nesser HJ, Aichinger J, Boehm G, Purerfellner H. Impact of integration of multislice computed tomography imaging into three-dimensional electroanatomic mapping on clinical outcomes, safety, and efficacy using radiofrequency ablation for atrial fibrillation. Pacing Clin Electrophysiol. 2007; 30:1215–23.
8. Caponi D, Corleto A, Scaglione M, Blandino A, Biasco L, Cristoforetti Y, Cerrato N, Toso E, Morello M, Gaita F. Ablation of atrial fibrillation: does the addition of three-dimensional magnetic resonance imaging of the left atrium to electroanatomic mapping improve the clinical outcome?: a randomized comparison of Carto-Merge vs Carto-XP three-dimensional mapping ablation in patients with paroxysmal and persistent atrial fibrillation. Europace. 2010; 12:1098–104.
9. Kistler PM, Rajappan K, Harris S, Earley MJ, Richmond L, Sporton SC, Schilling RJ. The impact of image integration on catheter ablation of atrial fibrillation using electroanatomic mapping: a prospective randomized study. Eur Heart J. 2008; 29:3029–36.
10. Bertaglia E, Bella PD, Tondo C, Proclemer A, Bottoni N, De Ponti R, Landolina M, Bongiorni MG, Coro L, Stabile G, Dello Russo A, Verlato R, Mantica M, Zoppo F. Image integration increases efficacy of paroxysmal atrial fibrillation catheter ablation: results from the CartoMerge Italian Registry. Europace. 2009; 11:1004–10.
11. Heist EK, Chevalier J, Holmvang G, Singh JP, Ellinor PT, Milan DJ, D'Avila A, Mela T, Ruskin JN, Mansour M. Factors affecting error in integration of electroanatomic mapping with CT and MR imaging during catheter ablation of atrial fibrillation. J Interv Card Electrophysiol. 2006; 17:21–7.
12. Kettering K, Greil GF, Fenchel M, Kramer U, Weig HJ, Busch M, Miller S, Sieverding L, Laszlo R, Schreieck J. Catheter ablation of atrial fibrillation using the Navx-/Ensite-system and a CT-/MRI-guided approach. Clin Res Cardiol. 2009; 98:285–96.
13. Allgayer C, Zellweger MJ, Sticherling C, Haller S, Weber O, Buser PT, Bremerich J. Optimization of imaging before pulmonary vein isolation by radiofrequency ablation: breath-held ungated versus ECG/breath-gated MRA. Eur Radiol. 2008; 18:2879–84.
14. Wagner M, Rief M, Asbach P, Vogtmann T, Huppertz A, Beling M, Butler C, Laule M, Warmuth C, Taupitz M, Hamm B, Lembcke A. Gadofosveset trisodium-enhanced magnetic resonance angiography of the left atrium–a feasibility study. Eur J Radiol. 2010; 75:166–72.
15. Tops LF, Schalij MJ, den Uijl DW, Abraham TP, Calkins H, Bax JJ. Image integration in catheter ablation of atrial fibrillation. Europace. 2008; 10(Suppl 3):iii48–56.
16. Fodi E, McAreavey D, Abd-Elmoniem KZ, Ohayon J, Saba M, Elagha A, Pettigrew RI, Gharib AM. Pulmonary vein morphology by free-breathing whole heart magnetic resonance imaging at 3 tesla versus breathhold multi-detector computed tomography. J Magn Reson Imaging. 2012; 2012:2012.
17. Krishnam MS, Tomasian A, Malik S, Singhal A, Sassani A, Laub G, Finn JP, Ruehm S. Three-dimensional imaging of pulmonary veins by a novel steady-state free-precession magnetic resonance angiography technique without the use of intravenous contrast agent: initial experience. Invest Radiol. 2009; 44:447–53.
18. Fahlenkamp UL, Lembcke A, Roesler R, Schwenke C, Huppertz A, Streitparth F, Taupitz M, Hamm B, Wagner M. ECG-gated imaging of the left atrium and pulmonary veins: Intra-individual comparison of CTA and MRA. Clin Radiol. 2013; 68:1059–64.
19. Francois CJ, Tuite D, Deshpande V, Jerecic R, Weale P, Carr JC. Pulmonary vein imaging with unenhanced three-dimensional balanced steady-state free precession MR angiography: initial clinical evaluation. Radiology. 2009; 250:932–9.
20. Martinek M, Nesser HJ, Aichinger J, Boehm G, Purerfellner H. Accuracy of integration of multislice computed tomography imaging into three-dimensional electroanatomic mapping for real-time guided radiofrequency ablation of left atrial fibrillation-influence of heart rhythm and radiofrequency lesions. J Interv Card Electrophysiol. 2006; 17:85–92.
21. Dong J, Dalal D, Scherr D, Cheema A, Nazarian S, Bilchick K, Almasry I, Cheng A, Henrikson CA, Spragg D, Marine JE, Berger RD, Calkins H. Impact of heart rhythm status on registration accuracy of the left atrium for catheter ablation of atrial fibrillation. J Cardiovasc Electrophysiol. 2007; 18:1269–76.
22. Wu YW, Tadamura E, Yamamuro M, Kanao S, Nakayama K, Togashi K. Evaluation of three-dimensional navigator-gated whole heart MR coronary angiography: the importance of systolic imaging in subjects with high heart rates. Eur J Radiol. 2007; 61:91–6.
23. Gharib AM, Herzka DA, Ustun AO, Desai MY, Locklin J, Pettigrew RI, Stuber M. Coronary MR angiography at 3T during diastole and systole. J Magn Reson Imaging. 2007; 26:921–6.
24. Lu B, Mao SS, Zhuang N, Bakhsheshi H, Yamamoto H, Takasu J, Liu SC, Budoff MJ. Coronary artery motion during the cardiac cycle and optimal ECG triggering for coronary artery imaging. Invest Radiol. 2001; 36:250–6.
25. Ohnesorge BM FT, Becker CR, Knez A, Reiser MF. Multi-slice and dual-source CT in Cardiac Imaging: Principles - Protocols - Indications - Outlook. Secondth ed.: Springer Berlin Heidelberg; 2007.
26. Anzalone N, Scotti R, Vezzulli P. High relaxivity contrast agents in MR angiography of the carotid arteries. Eur Radiol. 2006; 16(Suppl 7):M27–34.
27. Schonberger M, Usman A, Galizia M, Popescu A, Collins J, Carr JC. Time-resolved MR venography of the pulmonary veins precatheter-based ablation for atrial fibrillation. J Magn Reson Imaging. 2013; 37:127–37.

28. Botnar RM, Stuber M, Danias PG, Kissinger KV, Manning WJ. Improved coronary artery definition with T2-weighted, free-breathing, three-dimensional coronary MRA. *Circulation.* 1999; **99**:3139–48.

29. Kottkamp H, Kumagai K, Lindsay BD, Mansour M, Marchlinski FE, McCarthy PM, Mont JL, Morady F, Nademanee K, Nakagawa H, Natale A, Nattel S, Packer DL, Pappone C, Prystowsky E, Raviele A, Reddy K, Ellenbogen MD, Ezekowitz DE, Haines M, Haissaguerre G, Hindricks Y, Iesaka W, Jackman J, Jalife P, Jais J, Kalman D, Keane YH, Kim P, Kirchhof G, et al. 2012 HRS/EHRA/ECAS expert consensus statement on catheter and surgical ablation of atrial fibrillation: recommendations for patient selection, procedural techniques, patient management and follow-up, definitions, endpoints, and research trial design: a report of the Heart Rhythm Society (HRS) Task Force on Catheter and Surgical Ablation of Atrial Fibrillation. Developed in partnership with the European Heart Rhythm Association (EHRA), a registered branch of the European Society of Cardiology (ESC) and the European Cardiac Arrhythmia Society (ECAS); and in collaboration with the American College of Cardiology (ACC), American Heart Association (AHA), the Asia Pacific Heart Rhythm Society (APHRS), and the Society of Thoracic Surgeons (STS). Endorsed by the governing bodies of the American College of Cardiology Foundation, the American Heart Association, the European Cardiac Arrhythmia Society, the European Heart Rhythm Association, the Society of Thoracic Surgeons, the Asia Pacific Heart Rhythm Society, and the Heart Rhythm Society. *Heart Rhythm.* 2012; **9**:632–696 e621.

30. Landis JR, Koch GG. The measurement of observer agreement for categorical data. *Biometrics.* 1977; **33**:159–74.

31. Zhang T, Bai J, Wang W, Wang D, Shen B. Preliminary study of prospective ECG-gated 320-detector CT coronary angiography in patients with ventricular premature beats. *PLoS One.* 2012; **7**:e38430.

32. Lee AM, Engel LC, Shah B, Liew G, Sidhu MS, Kalra M, Abbara S, Brady TJ, Hoffmann U, Ghoshhajra BB. Coronary computed tomography angiography during arrhythmia: Radiation dose reduction with prospectively ECG-triggered axial and retrospectively ECG-gated helical 128-slice dual-source CT. *J Cardiovasc Comput Tomogr.* 2012; **6**:172–183 e172.

33. Peters DC, Wylie JV, Hauser TH, Nezafat R, Han Y, Woo JJ, Taclas J, Kissinger KV, Goddu B, Josephson ME, Manning WJ. Recurrence of atrial fibrillation correlates with the extent of post-procedural late gadolinium enhancement: a pilot study. *JACC Cardiovasc Imaging.* 2009; **2**:308–16.

34. Peters DC, Wylie JV, Hauser TH, Kissinger KV, Botnar RM, Essebag V, Josephson ME, Manning WJ. Detection of pulmonary vein and left atrial scar after catheter ablation with three-dimensional navigator-gated delayed enhancement MR imaging: initial experience. *Radiol.* 2007; **243**:690–5.

35. Sohns C, Sohns JM, Vollmann D, Luthje L, Bergau L, Dorenkamp M, Zwaka PA, Hasenfuss G, Lotz J, Zabel M. Left atrial volumetry from routine diagnostic work up prior to pulmonary vein ablation is a good predictor of freedom from atrial fibrillation. *Eur Heart J Cardiovasc Imaging.* 2013; **14**:684–91.

36. Hof I, Chilukuri K, Arbab-Zadeh A, Scherr D, Dalal D, Nazarian S, Henrikson C, Spragg D, Berger R, Marine J, Calkins H. Does left atrial volume and pulmonary venous anatomy predict the outcome of catheter ablation of atrial fibrillation? *J Cardiovasc Electrophysiol.* 2009; **20**:1005–10.

37. Cha YM, Wokhlu A, Asirvatham SJ, Shen WK, Friedman PA, Munger TM, Oh JK, Monahan KH, Haroldson JM, Hodge DO, Herges RM, Hammill SC, Packer DL. Success of ablation for atrial fibrillation in isolated left ventricular diastolic dysfunction: a comparison to systolic dysfunction and normal ventricular function. *Circ Arrhythm Electrophysiol.* 2011; **4**:724–32.

38. Akoum N, Fernandez G, Wilson B, McGann C, Kholmovski E, Marrouche N. Association of Atrial Fibrosis Quantified Using LGE-MRI with Atrial Appendage Thrombus and Spontaneous Contrast on Transesophageal Echocardiography in Patients with Atrial Fibrillation. *J Cardiovasc Electrophysiol.* 2013; **24**:1104–9.

39. Badger TJ, Daccarett M, Akoum NW, Adjei-Poku YA, Burgon NS, Haslam TS, Kalvaitis S, Kuppahally S, Vergara G, McMullen L, Anderson PA, Kholmovski E, MacLeod RS, Marrouche NF. Evaluation of left atrial lesions after initial and repeat atrial fibrillation ablation: lessons learned from delayed-enhancement MRI in repeat ablation procedures. *Circ Arrhythm Electrophysiol.* 2010; **3**:249–59.

40. Daccarett M, McGann CJ, Akoum NW, MacLeod RS, Marrouche NF. MRI of the left atrium: predicting clinical outcomes in patients with atrial fibrillation. *Expert Rev Cardiovasc Ther.* 2011; **9**:105–11.

17

Use of oral gadobenate dimeglumine to visualise the oesophagus during magnetic resonance angiography in patients with atrial fibrillation prior to catheter ablation

Riccardo Faletti[1], Alessandro Rapellino[1*], Francesca Barisone[1], Matteo Anselmino[2], Federico Ferraris[2], Paolo Fonio[1], Fiorenzo Gaita[2] and Giovanni Gandini[1]

Abstract

Background: Atrio-oesophageal fistula was first reported as a fatal complication of surgical endocardial and percutaneous endocardial radiofrequency ablation for atrial fibrillation, with an incidence after catheter ablation between 0.03% and 0.5%. Magnetic resonance angiography (MRA) was usually performed to obtain pre-procedural 3D images, used to merging into an electro-anatomical map, guiding step-by-step ablation strategy of AF. Our aim was to find an easy, safe and cost-effective way to enhance the oesophagus during MRA.

Methods: In 105 consecutive patients, a right-left phase encoding, free breathing, 3D T1 MRA sequence was performed in the axial plane, >24 hours before catheter ablation, using an intravenous injection of gadobenate dimeglumine contrast medium. The oesophagus was enhanced using an oral gel solution of 0.7 mL gadobenate dimeglumine contrast medium mixed with approximately 40 mg thickened water gel, which was swallowed by the patients on the scanning table, immediately before the MRA sequence acquisition.

Results: The visualisation of the oesophagus was obtained in 104/105 patients and images were successfully merged, as left atrium and pulmonary veins, into an electro-anatomical map, during percutaneous endocardial radiofrequency ablation. All patients tolerated the study protocol and no immediate or late complication was observed with the oral contrast agent administration. The free-breathing MRA sequence used in our protocol took 7 seconds longer than MRA breath-hold conventional sequence.

Conclusion: Oesophagus visualization with oral gadobenate dimeglumine is feasible for integration of oesophagus anatomy images into the electro-anatomical map during AF ablation, without undesirable side effects and without significantly increasing cost or examination time.

Keywords: Atrial fibrillation, Percutaneous endocardial radiofrequency ablation, Magnetic resonance angiography, Atrio-esophageal fistula, Gadobenate dimeglumine oral administration

* Correspondence: alessandro.rapellino@fastwebnet.it
[1]Istituto di Radiologia dell'Università degli Studi di Torino, A.O. Città della Salute e della Scienza, Via Genova 3, 10126 Torino, Italy
Full list of author information is available at the end of the article

Background

Atrio-oesophageal fistulae were first reported as a fatal complication of endocardial surgical radiofrequency (RF) ablation for atrial fibrillation (AF) [1], and have since been reported after percutaneous endocardial RF catheter ablation (RFCA) [2,3]. The incidence of atrio-oesophageal fistula after catheter ablation was estimated at 0.03–0.5% [4,5] and associated with high mortality rates [6], even when the correct diagnosis was made relatively early in the clinical course. Atrio-oesophageal fistula after catheter ablation is caused by heat transfer to the oesophagus [7], which causes transmural tissue necrosis [8], mediastinitis, and a fistulous connection between the oesophageal lumen and the left atrial blood pool. Thus, prevention of the initial oesophageal injury during the ablation procedure is important if the development of atrio-oesophageal fistula is to be avoided.

Any strategy to limit or avoid RF energy delivery in close proximity to the oesophagus requires that the clinician have accurate information regarding the anatomy since the oesophagus is anatomically close to the left atrium (LA). However, the anatomical relationship between the oesophagus and the LA is highly variable [9,10]. In 15% of patients, minor oesophageal lesions have been detected as ulcerations by endoscopy [11]. Moreover, cardiac magnetic resonance angiography (MRA) or computed tomography (CT)-angiography (CTA) are often performed to obtain pre-procedural three-dimensional (3D) images of the anatomy of the LA and pulmonary veins (PVs) before the RFCA procedure. The electro-anatomical map was then integrated with 3D images of MRA or CTA to create a map that provides a step-by-step ablation strategy for AF.

The purpose of this study was to assess oesophageal anatomy and position prior to MRA using a technique that integrates an electro-anatomical map during the RFCA procedure.

Methods

This study included 105 consecutive patients with AF (92 males, 13 females, mean age 55.2 years) that were candidates for RFCA (Table 1). Three patients suffered from mild achalasia due to neurological complications. In all patients MRA was performed within 24 h before catheter ablation using gadobenate dimeglumine contrast medium (Gd-Bopta, Multihance, Bracco Altana

Pharma, Constance, Germany) for intravenous and oral administration. We collected informed consent for the MR examination and for oral administration of the contrast medium and our study design followed Declaration of Helsinki recommendations. After the MR examination, all patients were clinically monitored for 30 min before being returned to the cardiology department. Any adverse effects or anomalies were registered after RCFA prior to discharge.

MRA study protocol

We used a 1.5-Tesla Magnet (Philips Medical Systems, DA Best, Netherlands) with a cardiac coil volumetric phased array consisting of 32 elements from a rigid rear portion and a flexible front, each consisting of a 16-channel phased array. MRA was performed in the axial plane with a non-ECG-gated, breath-free sequence, Spoiled Gradient Eco 3D (TR 3–8 ms, TE 1–3 ms), with R-L phase encoding, using a FOV of 450 mm, 512×512 matrix with an isotropic voxel of 1.5 mm and flip angle of 20°. The mean sequence time was 25 s (range, 19–32 s). The acquisition was performed after intravenous infusion of gadobenate dimeglumine contrast agent (infusion rate = 2.5 ml/sec; 0,05 mmol*kg), followed by a 20-ml saline bolus. Bolus tracking was used to start the sequence at the exact moment at which the contrast intensified during the venous phase of pulmonary circulation to guarantee the maximum signal intensity in the PVs and into the LA.

The oesophagus was intensified by administration of a 0.7–0.8-ml gel solution of gadobenate dimeglumine contrast media mixed with ~40-mg thickened water gel (Nestlé Healthcare Nutrition SA, Barcelona, Spain), served with a disposable plastic spoon, while the patients were on the scanning table immediately before MRA sequence acquisition. The patients were previously instructed to swallow the bolus 2–3 s before starting the MRA sequence. A second-pass MRA sequence was acquired immediately after with the same first-pass settings to obtain suitable images in case of initial technical problems. During post-processing, LA volume and left appendage volume were calculated by locating the regions of interest, while 3D MIP and 3D volume rendering reconstruction was performed to assess the spatial position of the oesophagus and identify appendage morphology and any PV anatomical variations.

Results

Our technique was tested initially on a healthy volunteer to demonstrate feasibility and predict problems during the MR examination following gel administration. During the study, all patients tolerated the study protocol and no immediate or late complication was observed after administration of the oral contrast agent. The oesophagus was visualised and successfully merged

Table 1 Patients characteristics

	Men	Women
Number of Patients	92	13
Age (years)	58,5 (42 to 70)	52,6 (39 to 69)
Paroxistic Atrial Fibrillation	70 (76%)	9 (70%)
Persitent Atrial Fibrillation	22 (24%)	4 (30%)
Duration of Atrial Fibrillation (years)	6.4	6.1

into the electro-anatomical maps in 104/105 patients (Figure 1; Figure 2). One patient did not swallow the bolus because he did not hear our instruction to do so. We obtained a fully enhanced oesophagus in 100/104 patients (96%). In four patients, the oesophagus was not enhanced completely (Figure 3), due to peristaltic waves, but images were merged in an electro-anatomical map without difficulties. The breath-free MRA acquisition time, with double contrast agent administration using R-L phase encoding, was a mean of 7 s greater (range 5–12 s) than with the breath-hold MRA GRE-T1 breath-hold sequence without oral administration of contrast medium. No technical problems were encountered during first- or second-pass imaging.

Discussion

Oesophageal injury is a rare but serious complication of RFCA. The oesophagus is positioned relative to the LA, adjacent to the right antra and ostia PV, as well as the posterior LA between the right and left PVs, or the left PV antra and ostia [12-15]. However, the position of the oesophagus is variable. Thus, the oesophagus could be at risk of thermal injury during RF ablation from virtually anywhere at the posterior left atrial endocardium or within the PV near the ostia, depending on the anatomy of the individual patient.

CTA and MRA are now the standard reference imaging techniques for LA and PVs. Volume rendering images obtained by these methods are merged on an electro-anatomical map generated with Carto™ (Biosense Webster, Diamond Bar, CA, USA) or NavX™ (St. Jude Medical, Sylmar, CA, USA) to guide catheter ablation. A report by Bahnson categorised the imaging methods to define the oesophagus-atrium relationship into real-time methods, including trans-oesophageal ultrasounds, nasogastric tube and barium paste, that yield images during RF-energy delivery; and non-real-time methods, including CT and MR, that yield static images generated prior to RF energy delivery.

Ultrasound is the only real-time imaging modality that allows visualisation of the extent or thickness of the oesophagus wall. However, this is an invasive imaging technique that requires operator experience. Placement of a nasogastric tube to allow oesophageal location mapping is associated with some risk of trauma and bleeding, particularly for anti-coagulation. Barium paste can be used to visualise the true width of the lumen for a few seconds, although information regarding oesophageal wall thickness is difficult to infer as only the lumen is visualised [16].

Real-time methods are more reliable for identification of oesophageal anatomy during RFCA than non-real-time methods. Kobza et al. performed a CT study using a common gastric tube as a marker the day before RFCA, and reported that the position of the oesophagus relative to the LA was dynamic and did not correspond to the position reported in the pre-procedural study [17]. Further, when the oesophageal position was defined by a pre-procedure CT scan with barium paste or by post-processing tagging and compared with the intra-procedure position defined using an electro-anatomical mapping system, in 85% of cases the position of the oesophagus corresponded to that identified with the CT scan performed <48 h prior [18,19]. This could be explained by a thin gastric tube placed on the side of the oesophagus. Our study demonstrates that a bolus better represents the true anatomical shape and size of the oesophagus.

Pavone et al. first performed a MR scan with barium paste and the MR contrast agent, gadopentetate dimeglumine, to visualise the oesophageal lumen in patients with oesophageal stenosis [20]. MRA, besides providing detailed and complete imaging of the complex LA anatomy, does not expose the patient to ionising radiation [21]. Pollak et al. performed MRA with barium paste and gado-pentetate dimeglumine in four candidates for RFCA; in one patient, the contrast agent passed to the stomach without enabling visualisation of the oesophagus [22]. A MRA scan is usually of longer duration than CT, and swallowing a contrast medium bolus at the correct time during a long breath-hold period could be difficult for the patient. In this study, using R-L phase encoding the

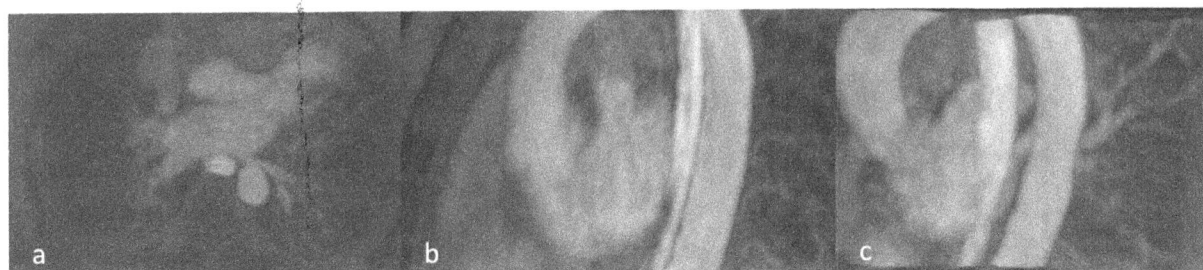

Figure 1 MRA of a 66 years old male with AF. MIP reconstruction in post-processing of MRA images acquired using both venous and oral Gadobenate Dimeglumine, 24 hr before percutaneous catheter ablation: **(a)** Axial MIP reconstruction **(b)** Left sagittal 3D MIP reconstruction **(c)** Left-Posterior 3D MIP reconstruction.

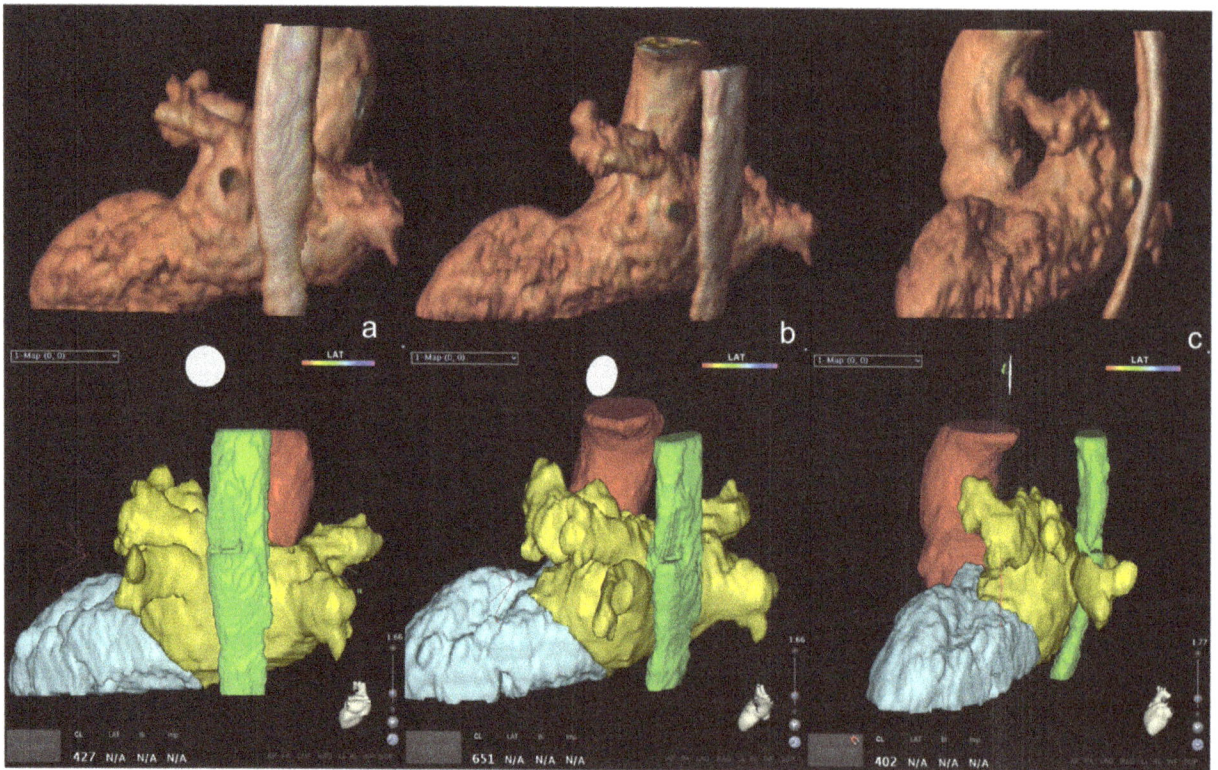

Figure 2 Same patient. MRA images and Electro-anatomical map 3D merging. On top line: 3D volume rendering from 3D GRE T1 scan; on bottom line: CARTO-MERGE^tm map using MRA examination data during RFCA procedure; **(a)** Posterior Coronal **(b)** Left-Posterior oblique **(c)** Left Sagittal.

patient could breathe freely and swallow the bolus during the MRA sequence without creating artefacts or affecting image quality. Although no technical problem was encountered with the first-pass MRA sequence, performing a second-pass immediately after the first MRA sequence could be useful for obtaining images suitable for anatomical assessment and calculating LA volume. With the second-pass MRA, we demonstrated that the contrast media and gel bolus rapidly pass through the oesophagus into the stomach, even in achalasic patients, without atrial

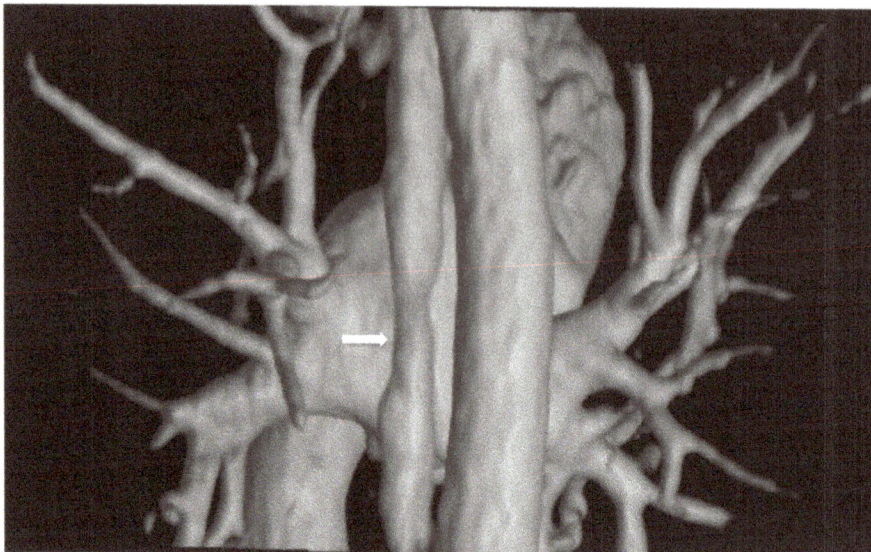

Figure 3 MRA of a 56 years old male, suffering AF. 3D volume rendering from 3D GRE T1 scan, showing the incomplete filling of the oesophagus (white arrow), due to a peristaltic wave.

wall artefacts, permitting fibrosis quantification associated with the likelihood of recurrent arrhythmia [23].

Allgayer *et al.* [24] reported that many MR protocols use atrial imaging to assess the anatomy and merge 3D images with an electro-anatomical map. However, only 3D-ECG-gated MRA allowed collection of the necessary anatomical information with optimal quality, although the acquisition time was >10 min. This study determined that the optimum solution for quality and patient tolerability was use of 3D MRA breath-hold non-ECG gated to assess the atrial anatomy necessary to merge the electro-anatomical map and 2D T2 axial images used to evaluate the theoretical position of the oesophagus. The MRA breath-free sequence used a comparable acquisition time to obtain 3D images of the atrium and oesophagus that could be merged into an electro-anatomical map.

Previous studies have reported that diluted gadolinium (Gd) complexes are safe for use as oral gastrointestinal contrast agents [25,26]. A Gd-BOPTA formulation was used in the present study because its signal intensity in T1-weighted images is greater than that of gadopentetate dimeglumine with increasing T1 relaxation times and dose. In human plasma, gadobenate dimeglumine is more effective in terms of shortening T1 relaxation times [27].

MR colonography is used in the gastrointestinal tract for faecal tagging because it is partly excreted in bile. Furthermore, the C-functionalised compound gadobenate dimeglumine exhibits high transmetallation towards metallic ions, such as Zn^{2+}, and a long half-life dissociation in a strong hydrochloric acid (pH = 1) [28]. In addition, a study demonstrated that 99.2% of orally administered gadolinium contrast medium was excreted in the faeces and not absorbed [29]. In our study, we reported that the novel use of gadolinium-based contrast agent without barium paste allowed oesophageal enhancement during MRA. Furthermore, thickened gel water, which is often used when feeding weak and critical patients [30], could be used safely in patients suffering from a swallowing dysfunction and airway problems. Moreover, unlike barium, it is gluten, lactose, sugar and allergy free. Barium sulphate is also more costly than thickened water gel (2.18 € *vs.* ~0.60 € per patient), and at our institution, 1 ml of gadopentetate dimeglumine is priced similarly to gadobenate dimeglumine (5.7€ *vs.* 5.9€) [31].

Conclusions

Oesophagus visualisation with oral administration of gadobenate dimeglumine MRA is a feasible technique without side effects and without significant increase in cost or examination time. Three-dimensional images obtained can be successfully merged during RFCA to characterise LA, PVs and oesophageal anatomy. Integration of oesophageal images into the electro-anatomical LA map could help to prevent RFCA injury to the oesophagus.

Competing interest
The authors declare that they have no competing interests.

Authors' contributions
AR, RF, FB: development of the technique and MRA imaging post-processing. MA, FF, FG: Interventional Cardiologists performing RFCA procedures and developing of electro-anatomical map integration. PF, GG, FG: Radiology and Cardiology Department Chiefs revising the manuscript. All authors read and approved the final manuscript.

Acknowledgements
We would like to express our very great appreciation to Dr. Daniele Petrone and Dr. Davide Zamorani for their technical support and collaboration in this Study.

Author details
[1]Istituto di Radiologia dell'Università degli Studi di Torino, A.O. Città della Salute e della Scienza, Via Genova 3, 10126 Torino, Italy. [2]Istituto di Cardiologia dell'Università degli Studi di Torino, A.O. Città della Salute e della Scienza, Corso Dogliotti 14, 10126 Torino, Italy.

References
1. Gillinov AM, Pettersson G, Rice TW. Esophageal injury during radiofrequency ablation for atrial fibrillation. *J Thorac Cardiovasc Surg.* 2001; **122**:1239–40.
2. Scanavacca MI, D'avila A, Parga J, Sosa E. Left atrial-esophageal fistula following radiofrequency catheter ablation of atrial fibrillation. *J Cardiovasc Electrophysiol.* 2004; **15**:960–62.
3. Pappone C, Oral H, Santinelli V, Vicedomini G, Lang CC, Manguso F, Torracca L, Benussi S, Alfieri O, Hong R, Lau W, Hirata K, Shikuma N, Hall B, Morady F. Atrio-esophageal fistula as a complication of percutaneous transcatheter ablation of atrial fibrillation. *Circulation.* 2004; **109**:2724–26.
4. Ghia KK, Chugh A, Good E, Pelosi F, Jongnarangsin K, Bogun F, Morady F, Oral H. A nationwide survey on the prevalence of atriesophageal fistula after left atrial catheter ablation. *Circulation.* 2005; **112**:II-392–II-393.
5. Cummings JE, Schweikert RA, Saliba WI, Burkhardt JD, Kilikaslan F, Saad E, Natale A. Brief communication: Atrial-esophageal fistulas after radiofrequency ablation. *Ann Intern Med.* 2006; **144**:572–74.
6. Schmidt M, Nolker G, Marschang H, Gutleben KJ, Schibgilla V, Rittger H, Sinha AM, Ritscher G, Mayer D, Brachmann J, Marrouche NF. Incidence of esophageal wall injury post-pulmonary vein antrum isolation for treatment of patients with atrial fibrillation. *Europace.* 2008; **10**:205–09.
7. Teplitsky L, Hegland DD, Bahnson TD. Catheter based cryoablation and radiofrequency ablation for atrial fibrillation results in conduc- tive heat transfer from and to the esophagus. *Heart Rhythm.* 2006; **3**:S242-S242.
8. Berjano EJ, Hornero F. What affects esophageal injury during radiofrequency ablation of the left atrium? An engineering study based on finite-element analysis. *Physiol Meas.* 2005; **26**:837–48.
9. Cummings J, Schweikert R, Saliba W, Burkhardt D, Brachmann J, Gunther J, Schibgilla V, Verma A, Dery M, Drago JL, Kilicaslan F, Natale A. Assessment of temperature, proximity, and course of the esophagus during radiofrequency ablation of atrial fibrillation. *Circulation.* 2005; **112**:459–64.
10. Kottkamp H, Piorkowski C, Tanner H, Kobza R, Dorszewski A, Schirdewahn P, Gerds-Li JH, Hindricks G. Topographic variability of the esophageal left atrial relation influencing ablation lines in patients with atrial fibrillation. *J Cardiovasc Electrophysiol.* 2005; **16**:146–50.
11. Ripley KL, Gage AA, Olsen DB, Van Vleet JF, Lau CP, Tse HF. Time course of esophageal lesions after catheter ablation with cryothermal and radiofrequency ablation: Implication for atrio-esophageal fistula formation after catheter ablation for atrial fibrillation. *J Car- diovasc Electrophysiol.* 2007; **18**:642–46.
12. Lemola K, Sneider M, Desjardins B, Case I, Han J, Good E, Tamirisa K, Tsemo A, Chugh A, Bogun F, Pelosi F Jr, Kazerooni E, Morady F, Oral H. Computed tomographic analysis of the anatomy of the left atrium and the esophagus: Implications for left atrial catheter ablation. *Circulation.* 2004; **110**:3655–60.
13. Tsao HM, Wu MH, Higa S, Lee KT, Tai CT, Hsu NW, Chang CY, Chen SA. Anatomic relationship of the esophagus and left atrium: Implication for catheter ablation of atrial fibrillation. *Chest.* 2005; **128**:2581–87.

14. Perzanowski C, Teplitsky L, Hranitzky PM, Bahnson TD. **Real-time monitoring of luminal esophageal temperature during left atrial radiofrequency catheter ablation for atrial fibrillation: Observations about esophageal heating during ablation at the pulmonary vein ostia and posterior left atrium.** *J Cardiovasc Electrophysiol.* 2006; **17**:166–70.

15. Hranitzky PM, Contrafatto I, Kim R, Ashar MS, Bahnson TD. **MRI identifies significant variability in the anatomic relationship between the esophagus and left atrium in patients undergoing catheter ablation for atrial fibrillation.** *Circulation.* 2004; **110**:III-418-III-418.

16. Bahnson TD. **Strategies to minimize the risk of esophageal injury during catheter ablation for atrial fibrillation.** *Pacing Clin Electrophysiol.* 2009; **32(2)**:248–60.

17. Kobza R, Schoenenberger AW, Erne P. **Esophagus imaging for catheter ablation of atrial fibrillation: comparison of two methods with showing of esophageal movement.** *J Interv Card Electrophysiol.* 2009; **26**:159–64.

18. Scazzuso FA, Rivera SH, Albina G, de la Paz Ricapito M, Gomez LA, Sanmartino V, Kamflofsky M, Laino R, Giniger A. **Three-dimensional esophagus reconstruction and monitoring during ablation of atrial fibrillation: Combination of two imaging techniques.** *International Journal of Cardiology.* 2013; **168**:2364–68.

19. Piorkowski C, Hindricks G, Schreiber D, Tanner H, Weise W, Koch A, Gerds-Li JH, Kottkamp H. **Electroanatomic reconstruction of the left atrium, pulmonary veins, and esophagus compared with the "true anatomy" on multislice computed tomography in patients under- going catheter ablation of atrial fibrillation.** *Heart Rhythm.* 2006; **3**:317–27.

20. Pavone P, Cardone GP, Cisternino S, Di Girolamo M, Aytan E, Passariello R. **Gadopentetate dimeglumine-barium paste for opacification of the esophageal lumen on MR images.** *AJR Am J Roentgenol.* 1992; **159(4)**:762–4.

21. Anselmino M, Blandino A, Beninati S, Rovera C, Boffano C, Belletti M, Caponi D, Scaglione M, Cesarani F, Gaita F. **Morphologic analysis of left atrial anatomy by magnetic resonance angiography in patients with atrial fibrillation: a large single center experience.** *J Cardiovasc Electrophysiol.* 2011; **22(1)**:1–7.

22. Pollak SJ, Monir G, Chernoby MS, Elenberger CD. **Novel imaging techniques of the esophagus enhancing safety of left atrial ablation.** *J Cardiovasc Electrophysiol.* 2005; **16(3)**:244–8.

23. Marrouche NF, Wilber D, Hindricks G, Jais P, Akoum N, Marchlinski F, Kholmovski E, Burgon N, Hu N, Mont L, Deneke T, Duytschaever M, Neumann T, Mansour M, Mahnkopf C, Herweg B, Daoud E, Wissner E, Bansmann P, Brachmann J. **Association of atrial tissue fibrosis identified by delayed enhancement MRI and atrial fibrillation catheter ablation: the DECAAF study.** *JAMA.* 2014; **311(5)**:498–506.

24. Allgayer C, Zellweger MJ, Sticherling C, Haller S, Weber O, Buser PT, Bremerich J. **Optimization of imaging before pulmonary vein isolation by radiofrequency ablation: breath-held ungated versus ECG/breath-gated MRA.** *Eur Radiol.* 2008; **18(12)**:2879–84.

25. Coppens E, Metens T, Winant C, Matos C. **Pineapple juice labeled with gadolinium: a convenient oral contrast for magnetic resonance cholangiopancreatography.** *Eur Radiol.* 2005; **15**:2122–29.

26. Rubin DL, Falk KL, Sperling MJ, Ross M, Saini S, Rothman B, Shellock F, Zerhouni E, Stark D, Outwater EK, Schmiedl U, Kirby LC, Chezmar J, Coates T, Chang M, Silverman JM, Rofsky N, Burnett K, Engel J, Young SW. **A multicenter clinical trial of gadolite oral suspension as a contrast agent for MRI.** *J Magn Reson Imaging.* 1997; **7**:865–72.

27. Bracco Diagnostics Inc. *MultiHance® (gadobenate dimeglumine injection) United States Package Insert.* Princeton, New Jersey: Bracco Diagnostics Inc; 2009.

28. Sophie L, Luce Vander E, Muller RN. **Comparative study of the physicochemical properties of six clinical low molecular weight gadolinium contrast agents.** *Contrast Med Mol Imaging.* 2006; **1**:128–37.

29. Weinmann H, Brasch R, Press W, Wesbey G. **Characteristics of gadolinium-DTPA complex: a potential NMR contrast agent.** *Am J Roentgenol.* 1984; **142**:619–24.

30. Hines S, McCrow J, Abbey J, Gledhill S. **Thickened fluids for people with dementia in residential aged care facilities.** *Int J Evid Based Healthc.* 2010; **8**:252–55.

31. Ministero della Salute della Repubblica Italiana. *AIFA.* Roma: Prontuario Farmaceutico Nazionale Italiano; 2013.

18

Prevalence and extent of infarct and microvascular obstruction following different reperfusion therapies in ST-elevation myocardial infarction

Jamal N Khan[1,2], Naveed Razvi[1,2], Sheraz A Nazir[1,2], Anvesha Singh[1,2], Nicholas GD Masca[1,2], Anthony H Gershlick[1,2], Iain Squire[1,2] and Gerry P McCann[1,2]*

Abstract

Background: Microvascular obstruction (MVO) describes suboptimal tissue perfusion despite restoration of infarct-related artery flow. There are scarce data on Infarct Size (IS) and MVO in relation to the mode and timing of reperfusion. We sought to characterise the prevalence and extent of microvascular injury and IS using Cardiovascular magnetic resonance (CMR), in relation to the mode of reperfusion following acute ST-Elevation Myocardial Infarction (STEMI).

Methods: CMR infarct characteristics were measured in 94 STEMI patients (age 61.0 ± 13.1 years) at 1.5 T. Seventy-three received reperfusion therapy: primary percutaneous coronary-intervention (PPCI, n = 47); thrombolysis (n = 12); rescue PCI (R-PCI, n = 8), late PCI (n = 6). Twenty-one patients presented late (>12 hours) and did not receive reperfusion therapy.

Results: IS was smaller in PPCI ($19.8 \pm 13.2\%$ of LV mass) and thrombolysis ($15.2 \pm 10.1\%$) groups compared to patients in the late PCI ($40.0 \pm 15.6\%$) and R-PCI ($34.2 \pm 18.9\%$) groups, p <0.001. The prevalence of MVO was similar across all groups and was seen at least as frequently in the non-reperfused group (15/21, [76%] v 33/59, [56%], p = 0.21) and to a similar magnitude (1.3 (0.0-2.8) v 0.4 [0.0-2.9]% LV mass, p = 0.36) compared to patients receiving early reperfusion therapy. In the 73 reperfused patients, time to reperfusion, ischaemia area at risk and TIMI grade post-PCI were the strongest independent predictors of IS and MVO.

Conclusions: In patients with acute STEMI, CMR-measured MVO is not exclusive to reperfusion therapy and is primarily related to ischaemic time. This finding has important implications for clinical trials that use CMR to assess the efficacy of therapies to reduce reperfusion injury in STEMI.

Keywords: Cardiovascular magnetic resonance, Myocardial infarction, Microvascular obstruction, Primary angioplasty, Thrombolysis, Reperfusion, Ischaemia-reperfusion injury, Reperfusion injury

Background

In the setting of acute ST-segment elevation myocardial infarction (STEMI), microvascular obstruction (MVO) describes suboptimal tissue perfusion despite restoration of flow in the infarct-related artery (IRA). MVO is generally thought to be related primarily to reperfusion injury [1-3]. Cardiovascular magnetic resonance (CMR) provides unique characterisation of myocardial injury post STEMI [4].

CMR-measured MVO correlates strongly with ST-segment resolution in patients undergoing primary percutaneous coronary intervention (PPCI) but relatively weakly with myocardial blush-grade and poorly with TIMI flow [5]. Larger infarcts on CMR are consistently associated with larger ventricular volumes, lower ejection fraction and greater MVO [6], which occurs in 40-60% of patients treated by primary percutaneous coronary intervention (PPCI). CMR-derived infarct size (IS) [4,7] and MVO [8,9]

* Correspondence: gerry.mccann@uhl-tr.nhs.uk
[1]Department of Cardiovascular Sciences, University of Leicester, Glenfield Hospital, Groby Road, Leicester LE3 9QP, UK
[2]NIHR Leicester Cardiovascular Biomedical Research Unit, Glenfield Hospital, Groby Road, Leicester LE3 9QP, UK

are powerful predictors of adverse remodelling and prognosis post STEMI.

The European Society of Cardiology (ESC) [10] advocates four reperfusion strategies for acute STEMI: PPCI, thrombolysis, rescue coronary angioplasty (R-PCI) and late PCI (>12 hours after symptoms). There is a paucity of data on the prevalence and extent of MVO following STEMI, with different reperfusion therapies [11,12], and in particular in patients who do not receive any reperfusion therapy.

This study aimed to characterise the prevalence and extent of microvascular injury (MVO) and IS using CMR, in relation to the mode of reperfusion following STEMI.

Methods
Subjects and reperfusion therapy
Ninety-seven patients presenting to a single regional cardiac centre with a first acute STEMI from Jan 2010 to April 2012 were included. Diagnosis of STEMI was made according to ACCF/AHA and ESC definitions [10]. Seventy-six patients who received one of the four advocated reperfusion strategies were recruited prospectively in a study assessing left ventricular (LV) remodeling (Figure 1). Three patients were excluded due to inability to complete CMR. The remaining 73 patients were treated as follows: PPCI (n = 47), thrombolysis (n = 12), R-PCI (n = 8), late PCI (n = 6). Reperfusion therapy was decided at the point of first medical contact according to local guidelines. Late PCI patients underwent PCI >12 hours after symptom onset (TTR) in the presence of electrocardiographic or clinical evidence of ongoing ischaemia. Twenty-one consecutive STEMI patients who presented late (>12 hours after symptom onset) and were symptom-free on arrival and did

not receive reperfusion therapy formed the non-reperfused cohort. These patients underwent clinical CMR to assess myocardial viability. The local research ethics committee approved the study and prospectively recruited patients provided written consent prior to participation.

'Early-reperfused' patients were defined as those undergoing successful initial reperfusion within 12 hours of symptoms (PPCI, successful thrombolysis). Thrombolysis was performed in patients presenting to non-PCI capable regional hospitals using tissue plasminogen-activator analogues. Successful thrombolysis was defined as symptom resolution and ≥50% resolution of ST-segment elevation within 90 minutes, and was followed by transfer to our centre for coronary angiography. Immediate transfer for R-PCI was undertaken for thrombolysis failure. Time to reperfusion (TTR) was measured as the time between symptom onset and successful restoration of IRA flow for PCI-related revascularisation, and time until administration of successful thrombolytic therapy for thrombolysed patients.

Angiographic assessment
The Thrombolysis in Myocardial Infarction (TIMI) scoring system was used to quantify angiographic IRA flow [13]. The degree of collateral flow to the IRA territory was quantified using the Rentrop Score (Grade 0: absent visible collateral flow; Grade 1: IRA side-branches only filled; Grade 2: partial filling of main IRA vessel; Grade 3: IRA completely filled by collaterals) [14].

CMR image acquisition
CMR was performed on all subjects during the index admission on a 1.5 T scanner (Siemens Avanto, Erlangen,

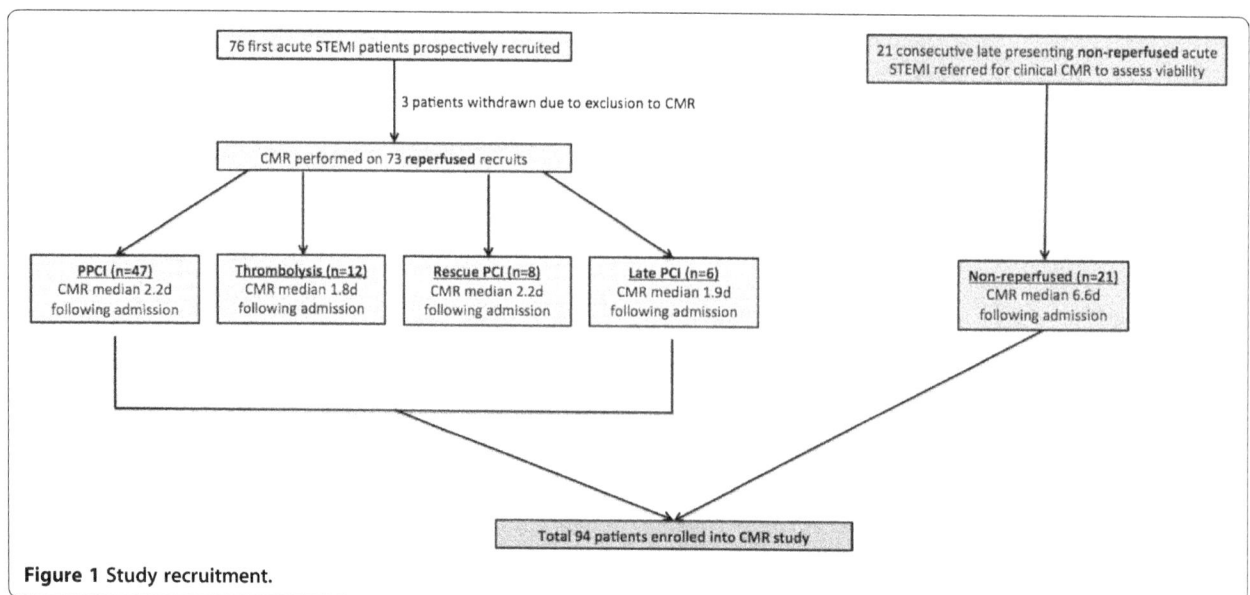

Figure 1 Study recruitment.

Germany) with retrospective electrocardiogram gating and a 6-channel phased-array cardiac receiver coil supervised by a cardiologist with a subspecialist interest in CMR (Figure 2). Cine imaging with steady-state free precession and Late Gadolinium Enhancement (LGE) imaging were performed in long-axis views and contiguous short-axis slices covering the entire LV. LGE images were acquired 10–15 minutes after contrast administration using a segmented inversion-recovery gradient-echo sequence. The inversion time was progressively adjusted to null unaffected myocardium. T2-weighted short-tau inversion recovery (T2w-STIR) imaging with coil signal intensity correction was performed on the 73 prospectively recruited reperfused subjects and not on the 21 non-reperfused patients since they underwent a routine clinical CMR protocol to assess for viability.

CMR image analysis

Analysis was performed offline blinded to patient details using QMass 7.1 (Medis, Leiden, Netherlands) by two experienced observers (JNK, NAR with 3 years CMR experience each). LV volumes and function were calculated as previously described [5]. Ischaemic area at risk ([AAR] oedema) was defined semi-automatically as areas of hyperenhancement ≥2 standard deviations above the signal intensity of unaffected myocardium. Infarct zone was defined semi-automatically on LGE imaging using the Full-Width Half-Maximum (FWHM) technique [15]. MVO was defined as areas of hypoenhancement within the infarct zone and was included in the assessed IS. AAR, IS and MVO were expressed as a percentage of LV end-diastolic mass (%LVM) and LV volumes were indexed by body-surface area.

Statistical analysis

Normality was assessed using the Kolmogorov-Smirnov test, histograms and Q-Q plots. Normally distributed data were expressed as mean ± standard deviation and analysed using ANOVA and independent t-tests. Non-normally distributed variables were expressed as median (25%-75% interquartile range) and analysed using Mann–Whitney U-tests. Chi-squared analysis was used to compare MVO prevalence between cohorts. The association between time from symptom onset to revascularisation (TTR), AAR, time to CMR after admission, left anterior descending artery infarct related artery (LAD IRA), TIMI flow pre and post-PCI and revascularisation method with IS and MVO were assessed for reperfused patients using univariate regression. Predictors with $p < 0.1$ underwent stepwise multivariate analysis. Since categorical and continuous variables were used, the strength of variables was expressed according to their p-value. CMR markers were corrected for TTR using ANCOVA. Reproducibility of CMR analysis was assessed using two-way mixed-effect intraclass correlation coefficient for absolute agreement (ICC) for a subset of 10 randomly chosen studies. Statistical tests were performed on SPSS version 20. $p < 0.05$ was considered significant.

Results

Baseline characteristics

Baseline demographics and angiography findings are summarised in Table 1. Diabetes was more prevalent in

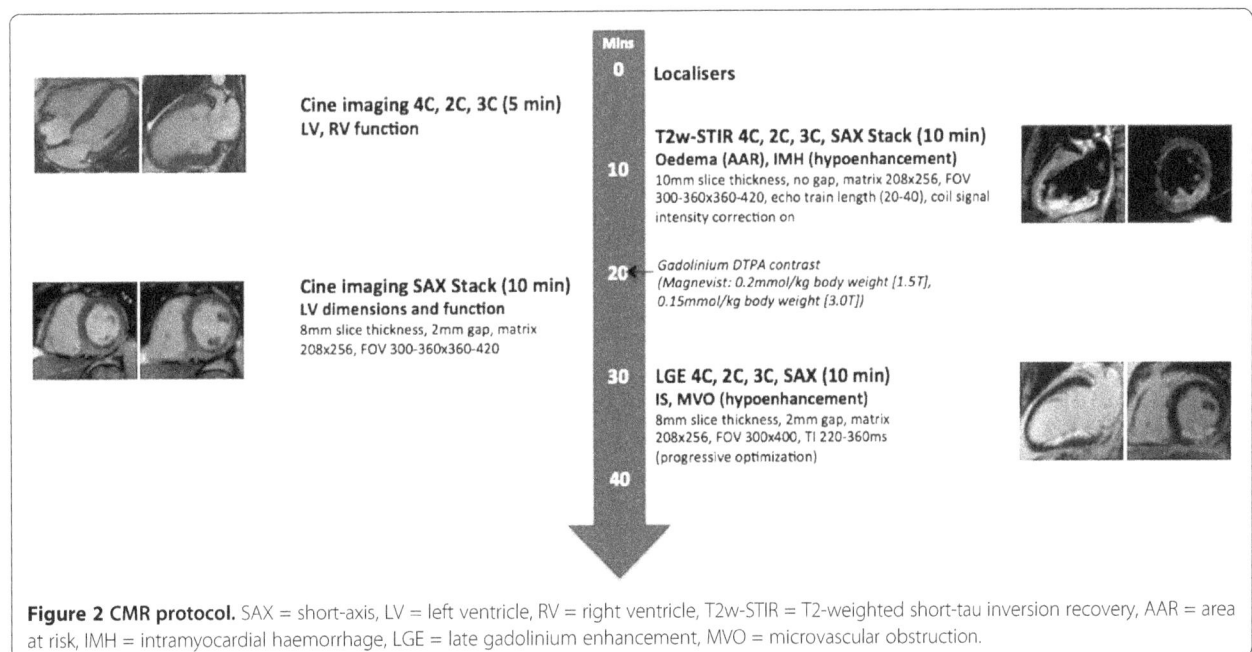

Figure 2 CMR protocol. SAX = short-axis, LV = left ventricle, RV = right ventricle, T2w-STIR = T2-weighted short-tau inversion recovery, AAR = area at risk, IMH = intramyocardial haemorrhage, LGE = late gadolinium enhancement, MVO = microvascular obstruction.

Table 1 Baseline demographics and angiographic data by reperfusion therapy

Variable	Group 1, n = 47 (PPCI)	Group 2, n = 12 (Thrombolysis)	Group 3, n = 8 (Rescue-PCI)	Group 4, n = 6 (Late PCI)	Group 5, n = 21 (Non-reperfused)	p
Age (years)	60.5 ± 12.3	59.3 ± 10.6	59.5 ± 12.5	54.7 ± 12.1	65.6 ± 16.2	0.37
Male sex (n,%)	42 (89.7)	11 (91.7)	8 (100)	5 (83.3)	16 (76.2)	0.21
Current smoking (n,%)	23 (48.9)	6 (50)	3 (37.5)	1 (16.7)	9 (42.9)	0.64
Diabetes (n,%)	2 (4.3)	1 (0)	0 (0)	0 (0)	6 (28.6)	0.01
Angina (n,%)	2 (4.3)	1 (8.3)	0 (0)	0 (0)	5 (23.8)	0.07
TTR (mins)	150 (120–240)	210 (75–300)	285 (211.25-345)	1113 (810–1342)	n/a	<0.001
Peak CK (iU/L)	875 (415.3-2061)	1034 (334.5-1384)	3002 (758–5045.5)	2633 (1073.3-5852)	1033 (87.8-2220.3)	0.88
Angiography					(n = 15)	
LAD IRA (n,%)	19 (40.4)	6 (50)	4 (50)	6 (100)	8 (53.3)	0.10
LCX IRA (n,%)	8 (17.0)	0 (0)	1 (12.5)	0 (0)	4 (26.7)	0.10
RCA IRA (n,%)	20 (42.6)	6 (50)	3 (37.5)	0 (0)	3 (20.0)	0.10
Multi-vessel disease (n,%)	16 (34)	4 (33.3)	1 (12.5)	0 (0)	5 (33.3)	0.38
Rentrop Score	0 (0–1)	0 (0–0)	0 (0–0)	0 (0-)	0 (0–0)	0.51
Rentrop B (Grd 2–3, n,%)	6 (13.3)	0 (0)	0 (0)	1 (16.7)	1 (6.7)	0.50
TIMI flow pre 0-II (n,%)	43 (95.6)	6 (83.3)	8 (100)	5 (83.3)	12 (80.0)	0.27
TIMI flow post III (n,%)	31 (68.9)	9 (58.3)	4 (50)	4 (66.7)	n/a	0.82
GPIIb/IIIa inhibitor use	18 (41.9)	0 (0)	3 (37.5)	2 (40)	n/a	0.39
Thrombectomy catheter?	20 (42.6)	0 (0)	5 (62.5)	1 (16.7)	n/a	0.01

Angiographic data available for 88/94 patients (angiography not performed in 6/21 non-reperfused patients).
TTR = time from symptom onset to revascularisation, PPCI = primary percutaneous coronary angioplasty, IRA = infarct-related artery, LAD = left anterior descending artery, LCX = left circumflex artery, RCA = right coronary artery, TIMI = thrombolysis in myocardial infarction, (pre) = TIMI score at start of coronary angiogram, (post) = TIMI score post-PCI, GPIIb/IIIa = glycoprotein IIb/IIIa inhibitor.

the non-reperfused group and TTR was longer in late PCI patients than the other groups. TIMI flow grade in successfully thrombolysed patients at the start of angiography was higher than in the other cohorts. Fifteen (71.4%) non-reperfused patients underwent coronary angiography (pre-CMR in 6 patients; post-CMR in 9). In 12 (80%) of these patients, TIMI flow-grade was abnormal (TIMI-0 in 6 patients, TIMI-1 in 4, TIMI-2 in 2).

CMR data
CMR data are shown in Table 2. The median time from admission to CMR was longer in the non-reperfused cohort compared with the other reperfusion strategies.

Volumes and function
LV volumes were higher and LV ejection fraction lower in the late-PCI, R-PCI groups and non-reperfused cohorts compared with the PPCI and thrombolysed patients. In reperfused patients, when corrected for TTR, the differences in LVESVI and LVEF were no longer significant (Table 2).

IS, AAR and MVO
IS differed across the five study cohorts, being higher in R-PCI and late PCI groups compared with PPCI and thrombolysed patients (late PCI vs PPCI p = 0.015, late

PCI vs thrombolysis p = 0.008, late PCI vs non-reperfused p = 0.014, R-PCI vs thrombolysis p = 0.06 on subgroup analysis). When corrected for TTR, the differences in IS in reperfused patients were no longer statistically significant (p = 0.33).

AAR was significantly larger in the late PCI group compared with those undergoing the 3 alternative reperfusion techniques (p < 0.01 compared with each strategy on subgroup analysis). When corrected for TTR, differences in AAR were only of borderline statistical significant (p = 0.054).

The prevalence of MVO was similar in the 5 cohorts. There was a trend towards the extent (% of LV mass) of MVO being greatest in the late PCI group, followed by non-reperfused and R-PCI patients. When corrected for TTR, the difference in MVO with the four reperfusion techniques was not statistically significant. Representative CMR and angiography images from patients in the 5 cohorts are shown in Figure 3.

Interobserver and intraobserver agreement of CMR analysis of infarct characteristics
Interobserver agreement for IS, MVO, AAR and MSI was excellent, with ICCs of 0.905, 0.958, 0.888 and 0.931 respectively. Intraobserver agreement was also excellent, with ICCs as follows: (a) observer 1: IS (0.980), MVO

Table 2 CMR data by reperfusion therapy

Variable	Group 1, n = 47 (PPCI)	Group 2, n = 12 (Thrombolysis)	Group 3, n = 8 (Rescue-PCI)	Group 4, n = 6 (Late PCI)	Group 5, n = 21 (Non-reperfused)	p	p (corrected for TTR)
Time admission-CMR (d)	1.8 (1.1-2.6)	2.2 (1.3-2.6)	1.9 (1.4-3.8)	1.9 (1.5-3.6)	6.6 (4.8-11.0)	*<0.001*	–
LVEDVI (ml/m2)	91.6 (84.9-102.7)	83.8 (76.1-107.6)	99.7 (88.5-116.6)	99.3 (83.7-106.7)	98.0 (88.1-125.0)	0.08[a]	0.44[a]
LVESVI (ml/m2)	51.3 (47.5-62.6)	55.1 (38.1-80.6)	63.1 (48.9-79.7)	64.1 (52.8-71.6)	61.1 (54.0-83.6)	*0.03[a]*	0.39[a]
LVMI (g/m2)	50.0 (47.4-55.7)	46.3 (42.8-67.3)	50.9 (43.2-56.7)	48.8(42.0-59.6)	58.0 (50.4-63.9)	0.24[a]	0.96[a]
LVEF (%)	42.0 ± 7.9	43.3 ± 7.5	36.5 ± 9.4	37.1 ± 10.0	35.0 ± 11.3	0.02	0.34
AAR (%LVM)	48.6 (35.9-66.5)	63.0 (49.7-65.3)	56.8 (37.6-67.7)	89.2 (77.2-98.1)	n/a	0.001	0.05
IS (%LVM)	25.4 ± 16.0	20.5 ± 12.5	39.8 ± 21.8	*47.4 ± 22.7*	23.8 ± 11.5	0.02[a]	0.33[a]
MVO presence (%)	26 (55.3%)	7 (58.3%)	5 (62.5%)	6 (100%)	15 (71.4%)	NS	–
MVO (%LVM)	0.5 (0.0-3.3)	0.2 (0.0-3.9)	1.2 (0.0-4.6)	6.4 (1.0-14.8)	1.3 (0.0-2.8)	0.08	0.37

PPCI = primary percutaneous coronary angioplasty, LVEDVI = left ventricular end-diastolic volume index, LVESVI = left ventricular end-systolic volume index, LVMI = left ventricular end-diastolic mass index, LVEF = left ventricular ejection-fraction, AAR = ischaemic area at risk (%LV mass), IS = infarct size (%LV mass), MSI = myocardial salvage index (%), MVO = microvascular obstruction (%LV mass).
[a]analysed using Log10 transformed data.

(0.984), AAR (0.946), MSI (0.937), and (b) observer 2: IS (0.991), MVO (0.991), AAR (0.948), MSI (0.982).

Predictors of IS and MVO in patients receiving reperfusion therapy

In reperfused patients (n = 73), univariate predictors of IS were TTR, AAR, LAD IRA, reperfusion method, TIMI grade post-PCI and time from admission to CMR. In a stepwise multivariate model including all of the above plus TIMI grade pre-PCI, independent predictors of IS were TTR, AAR and TIMI grade post-PCI (model R^2 = 0.41, Table 3).

Univariate predictors of MVO extent were TTR, AAR, reperfusion method and TIMI grade pre-PCI (Table 4). In a multivariate model including TTR, AAR, reperfusion method, TIMI-grade pre-PCI and TIMI-grade post-PCI, independent predictors of MVO were AAR, TIMI grade post-PCI and TTR (model R^2 = 0.23, Table 4).

IS and MVO in early v non-reperfused patients

The 59 patients receiving PPCI or successful lysis (<12 h) were grouped together as the 'early-reperfused' group for comparison with the non-reperfused group (n = 21) and results are shown in Table 5. LV volumes were higher and

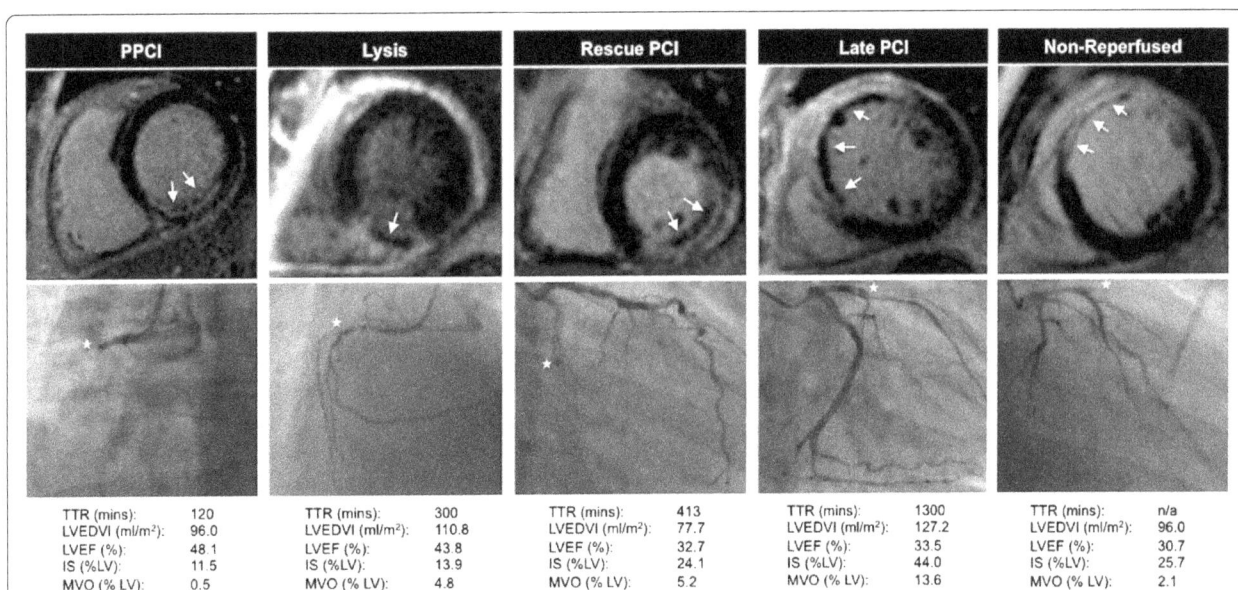

	PPCI		Lysis		Rescue PCI		Late PCI		Non-Reperfused	
TTR (mins):	120	TTR (mins):	300	TTR (mins):	413	TTR (mins):	1300	TTR (mins):	n/a
LVEDVI (ml/m²):	96.0	LVEDVI (ml/m²):	110.8	LVEDVI (ml/m²):	77.7	LVEDVI (ml/m²):	127.2	LVEDVI (ml/m²):	96.0
LVEF (%):	48.1	LVEF (%):	43.8	LVEF (%):	32.7	LVEF (%):	33.5	LVEF (%):	30.7
IS (%LV):	11.5	IS (%LV):	13.9	IS (%LV):	24.1	IS (%LV):	44.0	IS (%LV):	25.7
MVO (% LV):	0.5	MVO (% LV):	4.8	MVO (% LV):	5.2	MVO (% LV):	13.6	MVO (% LV):	2.1

Figure 3 Representative images of LGE CMR and coronary anatomy at the start of angiography in the cohorts. *Top row*: CMR late gadolinium images from a patient within each of the 5 study cohorts, demonstrating infarct (enhancement); microvascular obstruction (arrow) evident as hypointense areas within infarct. *Middle row*: coronary angiography images at the start of angiography in the same patients demonstrating infarct related artery; white star denotes culprit lesion (right coronary artery in PPCI and lysis patient, left circumflex in rescue-PCI patient, left anterior descending artery in late PCI and non-reperfused patient). *Bottom row*: Time from symptoms to revascularisation (TTR) and CMR data for the same patients.

Table 3 Predictors of Infarct Size (IS) in reperfused patients

Dependent variable for IS	r	R^2	B	p
Univariate				
TTR (mins)[a]	0.47	0.21	26.17	<0.001
AAR (%LVM)	0.46	0.20	0.39	<0.001
LAD IRA	0.39	0.15	–	0.001
Reperfusion method	0.39	0.15	–	0.003
TIMI grade post-PCI	0.32	0.09	−8.23	0.006
Time from admission to CMR (d)	0.29	0.07	4.62	0.01
TIMI grade pre-PCI	0.15	0.01	−2.74	0.22
Multivariate				
(Strongest model = TTR + AAR + LAD IRA + Reperfusion method + TIMI post + Time from admission to CMR):		0.41		
TTR (mins)[a]			17.72	0.02
AAR (%LVM)			0.23	0.02
TIMI grade post-PCI			−5.21	0.04
LAD IRA			6.49	0.10
Time from admission to CMR (d)			2.54	0.12
Lysis v PPCI			−8.60	0.08
R-PCI v PPCI			6.45	0.27
Late PCI v PPCI			−7.05	0.45

PCI = percutaneous coronary intervention, TTR = time from symptom onset to revascularisation, AAR = ischaemic area at risk (%LV mass), IRA = infarct-related artery, LAD = left anterior descending artery, TIMI = thrombolysis in myocardial infarction, R-PCI = rescue PCI.
[a]analysed using Log10 transformed data.

Table 4 Predictors of MVO extent in reperfused patients

Dependent variable for MVO	r	R^2	B	p
Univariate				
TTR (mins)[a]	0.37	0.13	0.27	0.001
AAR (%LVM)	0.39	0.14	0.004	0.001
Reperfusion method	0.40	0.13	–	0.008
TIMI grade pre-PCI	0.35	0.08	−0.32	0.03
TIMI grade post-PCI	0.32	0.06	−0.98	0.06
LAD IRA	0.16	0.01	–	0.18
Time from admission to CMR (d)	0.12	0.01	0.02	0.33
Multivariate				
(Strongest model = TTR + AAR + TIMI post)		0.23		
AAR (%LVM)			0.003	0.01
TIMI grade post-PCI			−0.08	0.03
TTR (mins)[a]			0.16	0.049

PCI = percutaneous coronary intervention, TTR = time from symptom onset to revascularisation, IRA = infarct-related artery, LAD = left anterior descending artery, TIMI = thrombolysis in myocardial infarction, AAR = ischaemic area at risk (%LV mass).
[a]analysed using Log10 transformed data.

Table 5 CMR data for early reperfused versus non-reperfused patients

Variable	Early reperfused (n = 59)	Non-reperfused (n = 21)	p
Age (y)	60.2 ± 11.9	65.6 ± 16.2	0.11
Male sex (%)	53 (89.8)	16 (76.2)	0.12
Time admission-CMR (d)	1.9 (1.2-2.6)	6.6 (4.8-11.0)	<0.001
LVEDVI (ml/m2)	90.7 (82.4-102.7)	98.0 (88.1-125.0)	0.005
LVESVI (ml/m2)	51.4 (45.4-62.6)	61.1 (54.0-83.6)	0.002
EF (%)	42.3 ± 7.8	35.0 ± 11.3	0.002
IS (%LVM)	24.4 ± 15.3	23.8 ± 11.5	0.87
MVO prevalence (n,%)	33 (55.9%)	15 (71.4%)	0.21
MVO (%LVM)	0.4 (0.0-2.9)	1.3 (0.0-2.8)	0.36

PPCI = primary percutaneous coronary angioplasty, LVEDVI = left ventricular end-diastolic volume-index, LVESVI = left ventricular end-systolic volume-index, LVEDMI = left ventricular end-diastolic mass, LVEF = left ventricular ejection fraction, IS = infarct size (%LV mass), MVO = microvascular obstruction (%LV mass).

LVEF lower in the non-reperfused group compared to the early-reperfused group. IS was similar in the two groups despite CMR being performed later in the non-reperfused group. The prevalence and extent of MVO was similar in the two groups. Representative CMR and angiographic images from patients within our 5 study groups are shown in Figure 3.

Discussion

Microvascular obstruction is widely regarded as a manifestation of reperfusion injury after STEMI [1-3,16,17]. Here, we demonstrate that MVO occurs frequently in all forms of reperfusion therapy for STEMI, but also in those presenting late, receiving no specific reperfusion therapy. Although IS and the extent of MVO appeared to be greatest in those receiving reperfusion late (R-PCI or late PCI]), this difference was not statistically significant when adjusted for TTR, an important determinant of IS [18,19] and prognosis [20] following PPCI. Indeed, there was a similar prevalence and trend towards increased extent of MVO in patients receiving no reperfusion therapy compared with those undergoing timely reperfusion. Our findings suggest that in real-life clinical patients presenting with STEMI, CMR-measured MVO is primarily an ischaemic injury rather than a reperfusion injury *per se*. This may have implications for currently planned and future trials in PPCI assessing therapies specifically designed to reduce reperfusion injury.

CMR-MVO and reperfusion injury

'No-reflow' was first demonstrated in canine myocardium in 1974 [3], and is characterized by ultrastructural changes secondary to severe microvascular injury [1,16]. MVO is generally assumed to be primarily related to reperfusion injury [1-3,16,17]. Animal studies have demonstrated infarct expansion and an almost three-fold increase in MVO extent in the first 48 hours post reperfusion, and a corresponding reduction in regional blood-flow to <45% of that pre-ischaemia, after 2 minutes of hyperaemia [21,22]. Reperfusion has been postulated to contribute to MVO through embolization of debris [23], release of vasoconstrictor and inflammatory substances (e.g. serotonin, thromboxane-B) [24] and mechanical damage to the capillary bed [16].

MVO is visualised on CMR by first-pass perfusion, early gadolinium imaging and LGE imaging as hypoenhanced areas within infarct cores [9] and is seen in up to 60% of PPCI patients post STEMI [25]. LGE-derived MVO ('late MVO') is felt to be the most important measure of MVO because of its strong correlation with ST-segment resolution, adverse ventricular remodeling [5] and major adverse cardiovascular events [9,26]. In both experimental models [27] and in patients treated by PPCI there is a strong correlation between MVO extent and IS on CMR [28,29].

Consistent with an extensive evidence base demonstrating correlation between the duration of ischaemia (TTR) and the extent of myocardial injury, our non-reperfused cohort had larger LV volumes and lower LVEF [18,19] compared with those promptly reperfused. CMR was performed later in the non-reperfused group. The extent of IS and MVO measured by CMR is known to decrease during the first week following treatment for STEMI (IS: reduction of ~21-30% in humans [30,31]; MVO: reduction of ~48% in humans [30], ~67% in animals [32]). It is therefore likely that had CMR been undertaken at a similar time-point after admission in non-reperfused and early-reperfused patients, the extent of IS and MVO may have been significantly greater in the non-reperfused cohort. Importantly, the FWHM technique requires minor operator input and results in extremely high intra- and interobserver agreement for quantification of MVO.

Our data suggest that CMR-measured MVO should not be used as a surrogate of subclinical angiographic 'no-reflow' or as a specific marker of reperfusion injury. Reperfusion injury is one component contributing to overall IS, [16,17] but in real-world patients presenting typically 2–3 hours after symptom onset with STEMI, the contribution of reperfusion to overall injury may be impossible to assess. Our data clearly show that CMR-measured MVO is extremely prevalent in non-reperfused patients and like IS, is strongly related to TTR and AAR in those receiving reperfusion therapy. This finding casts doubt on the selection of MVO, as opposed to IS or myocardial salvage index, as the primary CMR-based outcome in clinical trials that specifically aim to reduce reperfusion injury. As TTR is strongly related to IS and MVO, the potential to ameliorate true reperfusion injury will be greatest in those who have less ischaemic injury at the time of P-PCI, and short duration of symptoms, e.g. <3 hours from symptom onset may be where the benefit of effective treatments will be realised [20,27,28].

Myocardial and microvascular damage by revascularisation strategy

CMR characteristics were similar with PPCI and thrombolysis, consistent with Bodi who demonstrated no differences in LV volumes, LVEF, IS, MVO or myocardial salvage index (MSI) [11]. The small number of late-PCI and R-PCI patients make statistical comparisons difficult. Our observations are similar to Ruiz-Nodar who demonstrated only 9% MSI with R-PCI [33], and the MERLIN study demonstrated similar LV function at 30 days in R-PCI compared with conservatively treated patients [34]. The current evidence base demonstrates a lack of prognostic benefit with late PCI [35]. All late PCI patients in our study had LAD infarcts and tended to be younger, factors likely to influence the clinical decision to proceed to intervention. The LAD IRA is likely to account for their larger AAR. The effects of R-PCI and late PCI on reducing LV myocardial and microvascular damage in STEMI remain unclear.

Limitations

Patients were not randomized. The non-reperfused group were retrospectively identified and underwent CMR later than patients receiving reperfusion, however this difference should underestimate both the prevalence and extent of MVO in this group. The numbers of patients being treated with late PCI and R-PCI are small and no definitive conclusions can be drawn on the infarct characteristics.

Conclusions

CMR-derived MVO is highly prevalent in STEMI patients not receiving reperfusion therapy. CMR measured MVO is more closely related to ischaemic time than reperfusion therapy in STEMI and may not be a good surrogate marker of reperfusion injury.

Competing interests
The authors declare that they have no competing interests.

Authors' contributions
GPM, IBS and AHG conceived the idea for the study and developed the protocol. NR and GPM recruited patients and were present at study visits. JNK and NR performed the CMR analyses. JNK performed the angiographic analysis. JNK and NGDM performed the statistical analysis. JNK wrote the paper, which all authors critically reviewed for content. All authors read and approved the final manuscript.

Funding
GPM is supported by a National Institute for Health Research (NIHR) Postdoctoral Research Fellowship. This work is part of a project grant funded by the British Heart Foundation with support from the NIHR Leicester Cardiovascular Biomedical Research Unit.

References

1. Wu KC. Cmr of microvascular obstruction and hemorrhage in myocardial infarction. *JCMR*. 2012; **14**:68.
2. Eeckhout E, Kern MJ. The coronary no-reflow phenomenon: a review of mechanisms and therapies. *Eur Heart J*. 2001; **22**:729–39.
3. Kloner RA, Ganote CE, Jennings RB. The "no-reflow" phenomenon after temporary coronary occlusion in the dog. *J Clin Invest*. 1974; **54**:1496–508.
4. Klem I, Shah DJ, White RD, Pennell DJ, van Rossum AC, Regenfus M, Sechtem U, Schvartzman PR, Hunold P, Croisille P, Parker M, Judd RM, Kim RJ. Prognostic value of routine cardiac magnetic resonance assessment of left ventricular ejection fraction and myocardial damage: an international, multicenter study. *Circ Cardiovasc Imaging*. 2011; **4**:610–19.
5. Nijveldt R, Beek AM, Hirsch A, Stoel MG, Hofman MB, Umans VA, Algra PR, Twisk JW, van Rossum AC. Functional recovery after acute myocardial infarction: comparison between angiography, electrocardiography, and cardiovascular magnetic resonance measures of microvascular injury. *J Am Coll Cardiol*. 2008; **52**:181–89.
6. Hombach V, Grebe O, Merkle N, Waldenmaier S, Höher M, Kochs M, Wöhrle J, Kestler H. Sequelae of acute myocardial infarction regarding cardiac structure and function and their prognostic significance as assessed by magnetic resonance imaging. *Eur Heart J*. 2005; **26**:549–57.
7. Wu E, Ortiz JT, Tejedor P, Lee DC, Kansal P, Carr JC, Holly TA, Klocke FJ, Bonow RO. Infarct size by contrast enhanced cardiac magnetic resonance is a stronger predictor of outcomes than left ventricular ejection fraction or end-systolic volume index: prospective cohort study infarct size by contrast enhanced cardiac magnetic resonance i. *Heart*. 2008; **94**:730–36.
8. Klug G, Mayr A, Schenk S, Esterhammer R, Schocke M, Jaschke W, Pachinger O, Metzler B. Prognostic value at 5 years of microvascular obstruction after acute myocardial infarction assessed by cardiovascular magnetic resonance. *J Cardiovasc Magn Reson*. 2012; **14**:46.
9. de Waha S, Desch S, Eitel I, Fuernau G. Impact of early vs Late microvascular obstruction assessed by magnetic resonance imaging on longterm outcome after st-elevation myocardial infarction: a comparison with traditional prognostic markers. *Eur Heart J*. 2010; **31**:2660–68.
10. Steg PG, James SK, Atar D, Badano LP, Lundqvist CB, Borger MA, Di Mario C, Dickstein K, Ducrocq G, Fernandez-Aviles F, Gershlick AH, Giannuzzi P, Halvorsen S, Huber K, Juni P, Kastrati A, Knuuti J, Lenzen MJ, Mahaffey KW, Valgimigli M, Van't Hof A, Widimsky P, Zahger D, Bax JJ, Baumgartner H, Ceconi C, Dean V, Deaton C, Fagard R, Funck-Brentano C, et al. Esc guidelines for the management of acute myocardial infarction in patients presenting with st-segment elevation: the task force on the management of st-segment elevation acute myocardial infarction of the european society of cardiology (esc). *Eur Heart J*. 2012; **33**(20):2569–619.
11. Bodi V, Rumiz E, Merlos P, Nunez J, Lopez-Lereu MP, Monmeneu JV, Chaustre F, Moratal D, Trapero I, Blasco ML, Oltra R, Sanjuan R, Chorro FJ, Llacer A, Sanchis J. One-week and 6-month cardiovascular magnetic resonance outcome of the pharmacoinvasive strategy and primary angioplasty for the reperfusion of st-segment elevation myocardial infarction. *Rev Esp Cardiol*. 2011; **64**:111–20.
12. Thiele H, Eitel I, Meinberg C, Desch S, Leuschner A, Pfeiffer D, Hartmann A, Lotze U, Strauss W, Schuler G. Randomized comparison of pre-hospital-initiated facilitated percutaneous coronary intervention versus primary percutaneous coronary intervention in acute myocardial infarction very early after symptom onset: the lipsia-stemi trial (leipzig immediate preho). *JACC Cardiovasc Interv*. 2011; **4**:605–14.
13. TIMI-Collaborators. The thrombolysis in myocardial infarction (timi) trial. Phase i findings. Timi study group. *N Engl J Med*. 1985; **312**:932–36.
14. Rentrop KP, Cohen M, Blanke H, Phillips RA. Changes in collateral channel filling immediately after controlled coronary artery occlusion by an angioplasty balloon in human subjects. *J Am Coll Cardiol*. 1985; **5**:587–92.
15. Flett AS, Hasleton J, Cook C, Hausenloy D, Quarta G, Ariti C, Muthurangu V, Moon JC. Evaluation of techniques for the quantification of myocardial scar of differing etiology using cardiac magnetic resonance. *JACC Cardiovasc Imaging*. 2011; **4**:150–56.
16. Frohlich GM, Meier P, White SK, Yellon DM, Hausenloy DJ. Myocardial reperfusion injury: looking beyond primary pci. *Eur Heart J*. 2013; **34**:1714–22.
17. Yellon DM, Hausenloy DJ. Myocardial reperfusion injury. *N Engl J Med*. 2007; **357**:1121–35.
18. Francone M, Bucciarelli-Ducci C, Carbone I, Canali E, Scardala R, Calabrese F, Sardella G, Mancone M, Catalano C, Fedele F, Passariello R, Bogaert J, Agati L. Impact of primary coronary angioplasty delay on myocardial salvage, infarct size, and microvascular damage in patients with st-segment elevation myocardial infarction: insight from cardiovascular magnetic resonance. *J Am Coll Cardiol*. 2009; **54**:2145–53.
19. Hedström E, Engblom H, Frogner F, Åström-olsson K, Öhlin H, Jovinge S, Arheden H. Infarct evolution in man studied in patients with first-time coronary occlusion in comparison to different species - implications for assessment of myocardial salvage. *J Cardiovasc Magn Reson*. 2009; **10**:1–10.
20. Gersh BJ, Stone GW, White HD, Holmes DR Jr. Pharmacological facilitation of primary percutaneous coronary intervention for acute myocardial infarction: is the slope of the curve the shape of the future? *JAMA*. 2005; **293**:979–86.
21. Rochitte CE, Lima JAC, Bluemke DA, Reeder SB, Elliot R, Furuta T, Becker LC, Melin JA. Magnitude and time course of microvascular obstruction and tissue injury after acute myocadial infarction. *Circulation*. 1998; **98**:1006–14.
22. Reffelmann T, Kloner RA. Microvascular reperfusion injury: rapid expansion of anatomic no reflow during reperfusion in the rabbit. *Am J Physiol Heart Circ Physiol*. 2002; **283**:H1099–107.
23. Heusch G, Kleinbongard P, Bose D, Levkau B, Haude M, Schulz R, Erbel R. Coronary microembolization: from bedside to bench and back to bedside. *Circulation*. 2009; **120**:1822–36.
24. Kleinbongard P, Bose D, Baars T, Mohlenkamp S, Konorza T, Schoner S, Elter-Schulz M, Eggebrecht H, Degen H, Haude M, Levkau B, Schulz R, Erbel R, Heusch G. Vasoconstrictor potential of coronary aspirate from patients undergoing stenting of saphenous vein aortocoronary bypass grafts and its pharmacological attenuation. *Circ Res*. 2011; **108**:344–52.
25. Bogaert J, Kalantzi M, Rademakers FE, Dymarkowski S, Janssens S. Determinants and impact of microvascular obstruction in successfully reperfused st-segment elevation myocardial infarction. Assessment by magnetic resonance imaging. *Eur Radiol*. 2007; **17**:2572–80.
26. de Waha S, Desch S, Eitel I, Fuernau G, Lurz P, Leuschner A, Grothoff M, Gutberlet M, Schuler G, Thiele H. Relationship and prognostic value of microvascular obstruction and infarct size in st-elevation myocardial infarction as visualized by magnetic resonance imaging. *Clin Res Cardiol*. 2012; **101**(6):487–95.
27. Gerber BL, Rochitte CE, Melin JA, Mcveigh ER, Bluemke A, Wu KC, Becker LC, Lima JAC. Microvascular obstruction and left ventricular remodelling early after acute myocardial infarction. *Circulation*. 2000; **101**:2734–41.
28. Amabile N, Jacquier A, Gaudart J, Sarran A, Shuaib A, Panuel M, Moulin G, Bartoli J-m, Paganelli F. Value of a new multiparametric score for prediction of microvascular obstruction lesions in st-segment elevation myocardial infarction revascularized by percutaneous coronary intervention. *Arch Cardiovasc Dis*. 2010; **103**:512–21.
29. Ørn S, Manhenke C, Greve OJ, Larsen AI, Bonarjee VVS, Edvardsen T, Dickstein K. Microvascular obstruction is a major determinant of infarct healing and subsequent left ventricular remodelling following primary percutaneous coronary intervention. *Eur Heart J*. 2009; **30**:1978–85.
30. Mather AN, Fairbairn TA, Artis NJ, Greenwood JP. Timing of cardiovascular mr imaging after acute myocardial infarction: effect on estimates of infarct characteristics and prediction of late ventricular remodeling. *Radiology*. 2011; **261**:116–26.
31. Ibrahim T, Hackl T, Nekolla SG, Breuer M, Feldmair M, Schömig A. Acute myocardial infarction: serial cardiac mr imaging shows a decrease in delayed enhancement of the myocardium during the 1st week after reperfusion. *Radiology*. 2010; **254**:88–97.
32. Ghugre NR, Pop M, Barry J, Connelly KA, Wright GA. Quantitative magnetic resonance imaging can distinguish remodeling mechanisms after acute myocardial infarction based on the severity of ischemic insult. *Magn Reson Med*. 2013; **70**(4):1095–105.
33. Ruiz-Nodara J, Feliub E, Sánchez-Quiñonesa J, Valencia-Martína J, Garcíab J, Pinedaa J, Martínb P, Mainara V, Bordesa P, Herasa S, Quintanillaa MA, Sogor F. Minimum salvaged myocardium after rescue percutaneous coronary intervention: quantification by cardiac magnetic resonance. *Rev Esp Cardiol*. 2011; **64**:965–71.

19

Robust volume-targeted balanced steady-state free-precession coronary magnetic resonance angiography in a breathhold at 3.0 Tesla

Sahar Soleimanifard[1], Matthias Stuber[1,2,3], Allison G Hays[3,4], Robert G Weiss[3,4] and Michael Schär[3,5,6*]

Abstract

Background: Transient balanced steady-state free-precession (bSSFP) has shown substantial promise for noninvasive assessment of coronary arteries but its utilization at 3.0 T and above has been hampered by susceptibility to field inhomogeneities that degrade image quality. The purpose of this work was to refine, implement, and test a robust, practical single-breathhold bSSFP coronary MRA sequence at 3.0 T and to test the reproducibility of the technique.

Methods: A 3D, volume-targeted, high-resolution bSSFP sequence was implemented. Localized image-based shimming was performed to minimize inhomogeneities of both the static magnetic field and the radio frequency excitation field. Fifteen healthy volunteers and three patients with coronary artery disease underwent examination with the bSSFP sequence (scan time = 20.5 ± 2.0 seconds), and acquisitions were repeated in nine subjects. The images were quantitatively analyzed using a semi-automated software tool, and the repeatability and reproducibility of measurements were determined using regression analysis and intra-class correlation coefficient (ICC), in a blinded manner.

Results: The 3D bSSFP sequence provided uniform, high-quality depiction of coronary arteries (n = 20). The average visible vessel length of 100.5 ± 6.3 mm and sharpness of 55 ± 2% compared favorably with earlier reported navigator-gated bSSFP and gradient echo sequences at 3.0 T. Length measurements demonstrated a highly statistically significant degree of inter-observer (r = 0.994, ICC = 0.993), intra-observer (r = 0.894, ICC = 0.896), and inter-scan concordance (r = 0.980, ICC = 0.974). Furthermore, ICC values demonstrated excellent intra-observer, inter-observer, and inter-scan agreement for vessel diameter measurements (ICC = 0.987, 0.976, and 0.961, respectively), and vessel sharpness values (ICC = 0.989, 0.938, and 0.904, respectively).

Conclusions: The 3D bSSFP acquisition, using a state-of-the-art MR scanner equipped with recently available technologies such as multi-transmit, 32-channel cardiac coil, and localized B_0 and B_1+ shimming, allows accelerated and reproducible multi-segment assessment of the major coronary arteries at 3.0 T in a single breathhold. This rapid sequence may be especially useful for functional imaging of the coronaries where the acquisition time is limited by the stress duration and in cases where low navigator-gating efficiency prohibits acquisition of a free breathing scan in a reasonable time period.

Keywords: Coronary artery angiography, 3.0 T magnetic resonance imaging, Balanced steady-state free-precession, Reproducibility, Image-based shimming

* Correspondence: michael.schar@gmail.com
[3]Russell H. Morgan Department of Radiology and Radiological Science, Division of Magnetic Resonance Research, Johns Hopkins University, Baltimore, MD, USA
[5]Philips Healthcare, Cleveland, OH, USA
Full list of author information is available at the end of the article

Background

Coronary magnetic resonance angiography (CMRA), free of ionizing radiation, has provided a promising means for noninvasive assessment of coronary artery disease (CAD) [1]. Particularly, transient balanced steady-state free-precession (bSSFP) imaging [2] has shown substantial promise towards this goal. This sequence is often considered the method of choice for CMRA at 1.5 T [3-5] due to its high intrinsic blood signal intensity and blood-myocardium contrast requiring no exogenous contrast agent administration [6,7]. The increasing availability of MRI scanners with a static magnetic field (B$_0$) strength of 3.0 T and their ability to overcome some of the challenges of 1.5 T scanners have resulted in further efforts to develop 3.0 T CMRA techniques [8-10]. The increased magnetic field strength provides higher signal-to-noise ratio (SNR), which can be exchanged for faster imaging, improved spatial or temporal resolution. These improvements, however, often come with substantial drawbacks. High field strength results in more pronounced B$_0$ field inhomogeneities and radio frequency (RF) transmit field (B$_1$+) distortions [11,12], both of which degrade image quality and increase tissue energy absorption limiting application of certain sequences. The bSSFP acquisition is especially susceptible to high field artifacts [13,14] and its potential improvements in SNR and contrast-to-noise ratio are hampered by variable image quality at 3.0 T [15]. The bSSFP sequence is also reported to have inferior performance such as shorter arterial visible length, and higher inter-observer variability compared to conventional gradient echo techniques at 3.0 T, in contradiction to their relative performance at 1.5 T [16]. Modified bSSFP sequences have been recently developed for CMRA such as wideband bSSFP [17], which allow for high field off-resonance artifact suppression. However these modified implementations also come with notable drawbacks such as longer scan time and lower SNR compared with the conventional bSSFP [17]. Alternate acquisition techniques such as radial bSSFP [18] have been reported to achieve an improved image quality and vessel sharpness compared to Cartesian bSSFP. However, adoption of these navigator-gated techniques with 7–12 minutes of scan time [18] is still quite limited at 3.0 T. In fact, the challenging implementation of high field bSSFP has led to utilization of spoiled gradient echo techniques at 3.0 T, sometimes requiring the use of exogenous contrast agents [19].

Recent advances in hardware and software may nonetheless fill this gap and improve the previously mixed performance of bSSFP at 3.0 T. B$_0$ inhomogeneities linearly increase with field strength but can be sufficiently attenuated by localized second-order shimming and on-resonant frequency f$_0$ determination [20]. Parallel excitation with multi-channel RF transmit systems are reported to better

manage RF power deposition and provide a more homogeneous B$_1$+ field, facilitating the desired RF excitation angles in the heart [21,22]. A recent quantitative evaluation of B$_1$+ map before and after local RF shimming demonstrates that signal variations in cardiac bSSFP at 3.0 T are subject-specific. The study concludes that local RF shimming can significantly reduce such variations and improve the image quality of bSSFP at 3.0 T [23]. Additionally, the 32-channel phased-array coil provides an SNR increase of as much as 40% over conventional cardiac-optimized phased array coils, enhances image quality, and improves delineation of the coronary arteries [24]. Therefore, in this study, we aimed to utilize recently available advanced hardware and software to minimize the susceptibility off-resonance artifacts and improve the image quality at 3.0 T, and implement a robust and accelerated single-breathhold bSSFP coronary methodology. Subsequently, we sought to evaluate the performance of the developed sequence as well as its reproducibility in humans. To the best of our knowledge, the inter-scan reproducibility of bSSFP sequence for CMRA has not been previously investigated at 3.0 T. This rapid sequence should be important for functional imaging of the coronaries where the acquisition time is limited by the stress duration [25-27] and in cases where low navigator-gating efficiency prohibits acquisition of a free breathing scan in a reasonable time period [3].

Methods

Study population

Fifteen healthy adults with no history of cardiovascular disease and three patients with stable coronary artery disease (CAD), documented with at least one 50% lesion on clinically indicated cardiac catheterization within the prior six months, were enrolled in the study. All eighteen subjects underwent one CMRA examination. Additionally, eight volunteers and one patient underwent a second CMRA examination to study reproducibility of the bSSFP sequence. The subjects in the reproducibility sub-group were removed from the scanner after the first examination. They were returned to, and repositioned in, the scanner after a 15-minute rest period and the complete examination was repeated. The protocol was approved by the Johns Hopkins Institutional Review Board and written informed consent was obtained from all participants.

CMRA protocol and transient bSSFP sequence

All the studies were performed on a commercial whole body 3.0 T MR scanner (Achieva R3.2, Philips Healthcare, Best, The Netherlands) equipped with multi-transmit system, vector electrocardiography triggering [28], and a 32-channel cardiac phased-array coil. The imaging protocol began with a multi-slice segmented *k-space* gradient echo scout scan in transverse, sagittal, and coronal views to identify the heart and the lung-liver interface for navigator localization. Next, a B_1+ calibration scan [29] was acquired for localized B_1+ shimming and a more homogeneous transmit field in the heart in the subsequent scans. The calibration scan was followed by a sensitivity encoding (SENSE) reference scan [30]. Subsequently, an axial mid-ventricular bSSFP cine scan was obtained during free breathing to visually identify the period of minimal coronary motion. The beginning of this stationary period was chosen as trigger delay for subsequent scans in the protocol. The cine scan was followed by a quick low spatial resolution free breathing navigator-gated and corrected whole-heart three-dimensional (3D) coronary localizer scan in the transverse plane. The three-point plan tool [31] was utilized on this scout scan for planning the subsequent 3D acquisitions. Next, a fast B_0-map acquisition was performed allowing determination of localized second-order shim corrections and on-resonance f_0 frequency to improve B_0 field homogeneity and to reduce potential bSSFP off-resonance artifacts in the coronary arterial tree [20]. Three-dimensional CMRA acquisitions were then performed along the 3D track of the coronaries of interest using the volume-targeted bSSFP sequence with centric *k-space* profile ordering, and a half-Fourier-acquisition factor of 0.6. A half-alpha TR-half preparation pulse followed by 10 startup RF pulses were used to accelerate the approach to steady state [32]. A SENSE acceleration factor of 2.5 with an additional oversampling factor of 1.3 was used in the phase encoding direction. A spectrally selective saturation pulse preceded the data acquisition window for fat suppression. Scan parameters were the following: repetition/echo times were 3.9/1.9 ms, RF excitation angle 50°, standard Sinc-Gaussian RF pulse with time-bandwidth product of 6, field-of-view $300 \times 300 \times 20$ mm^3, acquired voxel size $1.0 \times 1.0 \times 2.0$ mm^3, reconstructed voxel size $0.8 \times 0.8 \times 1.0$ mm^3, acquisition window 105 ms. The data were acquired during one breathhold for respiratory motion suppression. The duration of each acquired scan was recorded, and the total examination time was measured accordingly.

Image analysis

The analysis of bSSFP scans was performed along the entire visualized course of each artery using Soap-Bubble, a previously reported interactive coronary visualization and analysis tool [33]. Using visually identified points throughout the 3D track of coronaries and multi-planar reformatting of the 3D CMRA images, vessel length as well as average vessel diameter and sharpness within the visualized course of each artery were measured on each dataset, as previously described [33].

To assess intra-observer variability, the first CMRA examinations in eighteen subjects were analyzed twice by observer 1 (SS) in a blinded manner. Additionally, blinded and independent analyses were performed in these scans by observer 2 (MS) to evaluate inter-observer variability.

Furthermore, scans obtained during the second successive examination in nine volunteers were analyzed by observer 1 to measure inter-scan variability (the scans in the first examination were considered the reference standard). Care was taken to ensure that the vessel diameter and sharpness measurements were performed at the same anatomical levels, and for example, observer 1 reported to observer 2 the distance from the ostium where the semi-automated measurements began.

Statistical analysis

All datasets were included in the analysis, and results reported as mean ± one standard error of mean. Intra-observer (observer 1 repeat measurements, n = 20) and inter-observer (observer 1 vs. observer 2 measurements, n = 20), and inter-scan (first scan vs. repeat scan observer 1 measurements, n = 9) agreements were assessed using Pearson's correlation coefficient, Bland-Altman analysis and intra-class correlation coefficient (ICC) [34], the proportion of total variability accounted for by the variability among observers. If the coefficient is high, it means only a small portion of the variability is due to variability in measurement on different occasions; hence, the reproducibility is high. A *p*-value < 0.05 was considered statistically significant in all analyses.

Results

All 18 subjects (age 21–75 years (mean ± SD: 38 ± 18); 8 women) including the 3 CAD patients (age 65–75 years (mean ± SD: 71 ± 5); 1 woman) successfully completed the CMRA examination. All subjects were in stable sinus rhythm and the average heart rate was 70 ± 12 beats per minute. A total of 20 coronary arteries (right coronary artery (RCA): n = 15; left anterior descending (LAD): n = 5) were imaged. Additionally, 9 subjects completed a repeated examination (8 healthy, age 21–51 years (mean ± SD: 30 ± 9); 1 patient, age 72 years) and their 9 coronary arteries (RCA: n = 7; LAD: n = 2) were successfully imaged twice. The total duration of each examination including the acquisition of scouts, reference, and calibration scans as well as geometry planning was 13 ± 3 minutes. The average duration of the low resolution scout MRA scan, acquired with respiratory navigator-gating, was 76 ± 15 sec (n = 18). The total duration of B_1 and B_0 calibration scans as well as the time required for local determination of on-resonant f_0 were 1–2 minutes. Localization of each coronary artery of interest took 2–3 minutes, and the duration of each bSSFP sequence was 20.5 ± 2.0 seconds. Figure 1 shows examples of multi-planar reformatted [33] images of RCA and LAD in (A) three volunteers and (B) one patient with a 50-70% lesion at the diagonal branch of the LAD, as identified on a diagnostic x-ray angiogram. Figure 2 illustrates an example of the proposed breath-hold acquisition and its navigator-gated and -corrected counterpart with the same spatial resolution and coverage

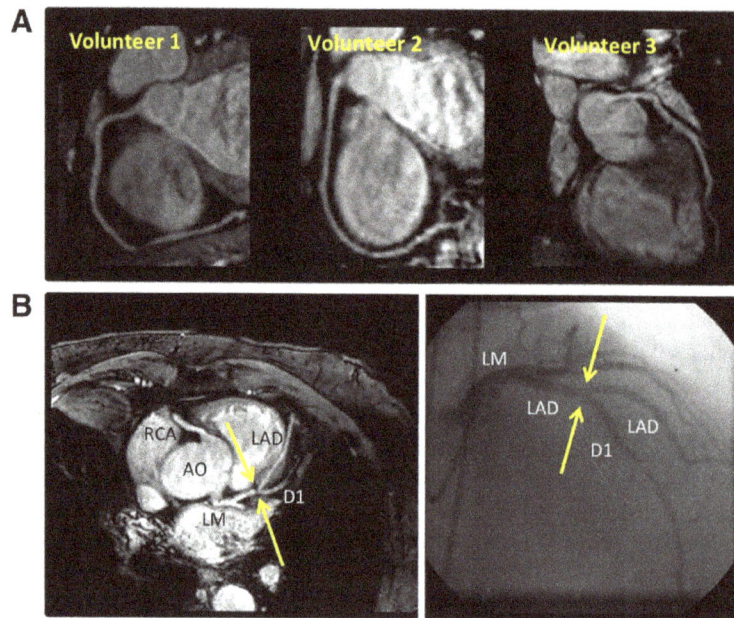

Figure 1 Double oblique single-breathhold 3D bSSFP coronary magnetic resonance angiograms of the right coronary artery and left anterior descending in three healthy volunteers (A) and in a 66-year-old patient (B) with 50-70% lesion at the diagonal branch of the LAD identified using diagnostic x-ray angiogram. AO: Aorta, RCA: Right Coronary Artery. LM: Left Main Artery. LAD: Left Anterior Descending Artery. D1: First Diagonal Branch. MRA Images were multi-planar reformatted.

in a 52-year-old healthy man. Using SENSE factor of 1.5 in the phase-encode direction and no half-Fourier acquisition, the free-breathing scan was completed in 3 minutes and 44 seconds (average navigator efficiency = 24%, gating window = 5 mm).

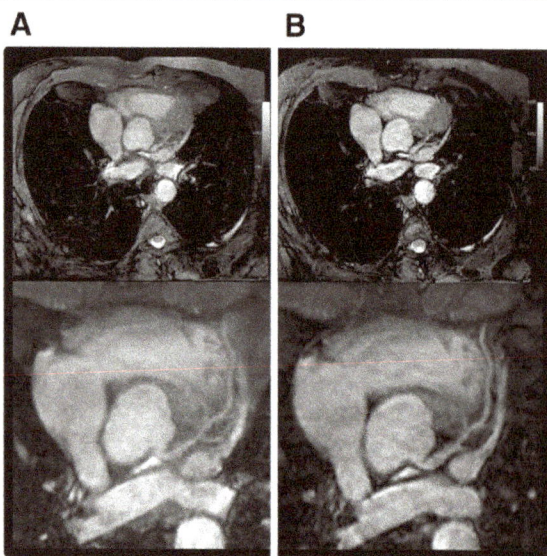

Figure 2 Volume-targeted bSSFP scans of the left anterior descending artery in a healthy volunteer, acquired during free breathing (A) and during one breathhold (B), with the same spatial coverage and resolution. Top: 2D slice from the 3D volume selected for demonstration. Bottom: multi-planar reformatted images of the artery.

The single breathhold approach achieved an average visualized vessel length of 100.5 ± 6.3 mm (n = 20), which was used for quantitative analysis of vessel sharpness and diameters as shown in Table 1. The mean vessel diameter was 2.8 ± 0.1 mm averaged over the visualized length of coronary arteries and 3.1 ± 0.1 mm for the proximal 4 cm segment. Mean vessel sharpness was $55 \pm 2\%$ over the visualized coronary length and $56 \pm 2\%$ in the proximal 4 cm segment (Table 1).

Figure 3 shows examples of multi-planar reformatted images of RCA and LAD obtained during separate scanning sessions in two healthy volunteers. The mean vessel length (original and repeat values) for the subjects who underwent the scans twice measured 95.7 ± 10.5 mm and 98.2 ± 9.5 mm, respectively (p = 0.298). In this subset of volunteers, the average diameter of coronary arteries was measured 2.7 ± 0.1 mm and 2.8 ± 0.1 mm in the original and repeat examinations, respectively (p = 0.609). Average vessel sharpness values from the two scans were also found in strong concordance (original: $55 \pm 3\%$, repeat: $54 \pm 3\%$; p = 0.269) between the reference and repeated analyses of observer 1 as well as the reference analysis of observer 1 and the analysis of observer 2 were excellent for vessel length, diameter and vessel sharpness measurements (Table 1). Using Pearson's correlation coefficient, there was a highly statistically significant intra-observer (r = 0.994, $R^2 = 98.9\%$, SE = 0.28), inter-observer (r = 0.894, $R^2 = 80.0\%$, SE = 1.36) and inter-scan (r = 0.980, $R^2 = 96.1\%$, SE = 0.60) agreement for vessel length measurements.

Table 1 Vessel length, diameter, and vessel sharpness averaged in 18 subjects (20 coronary arteries: RCA = 15, LAD = 5)

	Intra-observer (n = 20)			Inter-observer (n = 20)		Inter-scan (n = 9)		
	Reference analysis	Repeat analysis	ICC	Analysis	ICC	Reference analysis (subset)	Repeat scan analysis	ICC
Length [mm]	100.5 ± 6.3	101.6 ± 6.1	0.993	98.7 ± 6.6	0.896	95.7 ± 10.0	98.2 ± 9.5	0.974
Diameter [mm]								
Proximal 40 mm	3.1 ± 0.1	3.1 ± 0.1	0.986	3.1 ± 0.1	0.979	3.0 ± 0.1	3.0 ± 0.1	0.952
Full length	2.8 ± 0.1	2.8 ± 0.1	0.987	2.8 ± 0.1	0.976	2.7 ± 0.1	2.8 ± 0.1	0.961
Sharpness [%]								
Proximal 40 mm	56 ± 2	55 ± 2	0.979	56 ± 2	0.972	57 ± 2	55 ± 3	0.736
Full length	55 ± 2	54 ± 2	0.989	56 ± 1	0.938	55 ± 3	54 ± 3	0.905

Data are presented as mean ± standard error of mean. ICC = intra-class correlation coefficient.

The results of the Bland–Altman analysis demonstrating intra-observer, inter-observer, and inter- scan agreements are shown in Figure 4A, B and C. Additionally, ICC values demonstrated a high degree of intra-observer, inter-observer, and inter-scan concordance for length measurements (ICC = 0.993, 0.896, and 0.974, respectively). Similarly, a large degree of agreement was observed for mean vessel diameter measurements (intra-observer: r = 0.990, R^2 = 98.0%, SE = 0.05, ICC = 0.987; inter-observer: r = 0.977, R^2 = 95.5%, SE = 0.08, ICC = 0.976; intra-scan: r = 0.959, R^2 = 92.0%, SE = 0.14, ICC = 0.961). Figure 4D,E and F illustrate the Bland-Altman analysis

results for diameter measures. Lastly, vessel sharpness values revealed high degree of reproducibility as well (intra-observer: r = 0.993, R^2 = 98.7%, SE = 0.88, ICC = 0.989; inter-observer: r = 0.953, R^2 = 90.8%, SE = 2.00, ICC = 0.938; intra-scan: r = 0.932, R^2 = 86.9%, SE = 3.68, ICC = 0.905). Figure 4G, H and K summarize the results of Bland-Altman analysis for vessel sharpness measurements.

Discussion

Fat saturated, segmented bSSFP imaging has been widely used in cardiac MR imaging because it produces

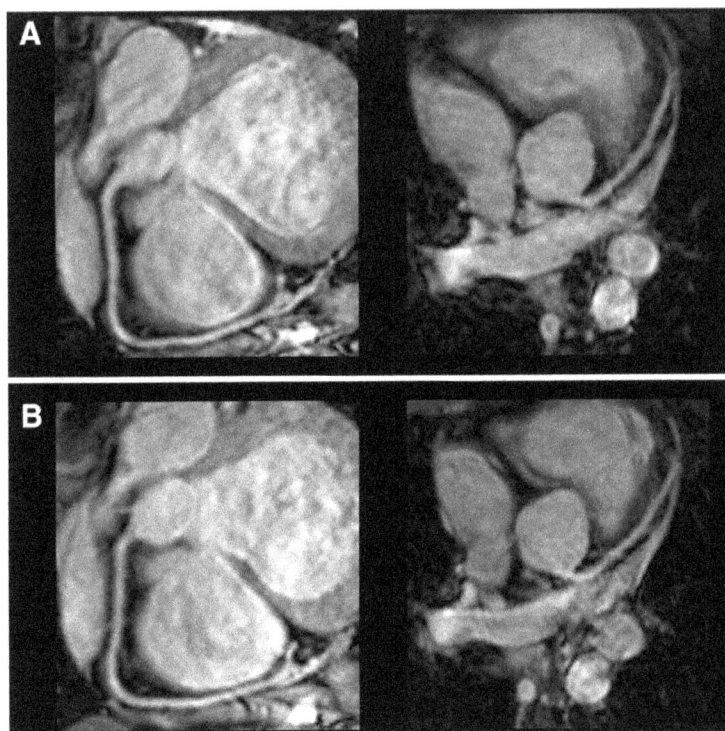

Figure 3 Double oblique single-breathhold 3D bSSFP coronary magnetic resonance angiograms of the right coronary artery and left anterior descending in two healthy volunteers obtained during two separate scanning sessions: reference (A), repeat (B). Images were multi-planar reformatted.

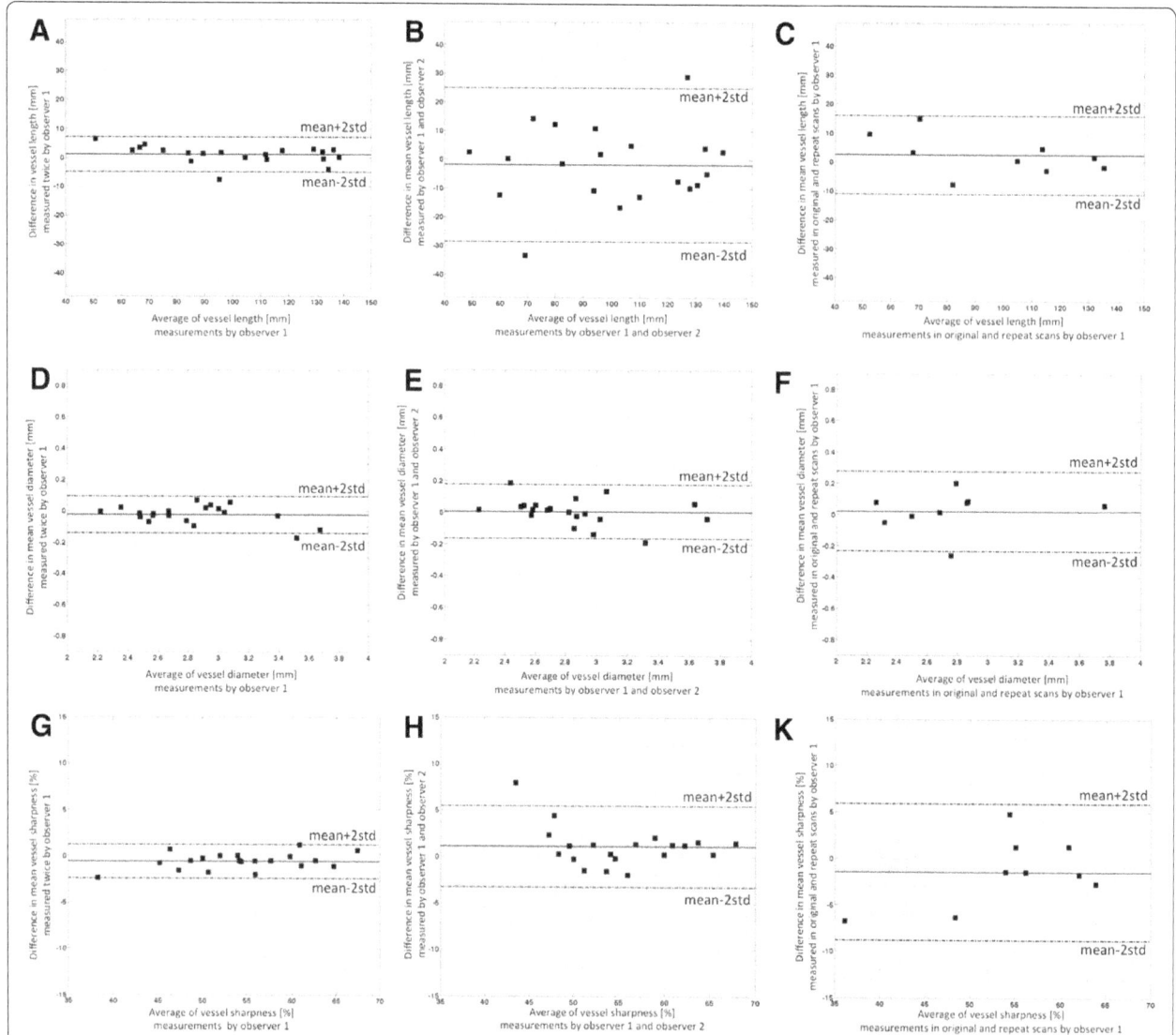

Figure 4 Repeatability and reproducibility of vessel length, mean diameter, mean sharpness measurements with bSSFP sequence. Bland-Altman plot shows good (**A**) intra-observer (r = 0.994), (**B**) inter-observer (r = 0.894), and (**C**) intra-class (r = 0.980) agreement between length measurements [mm] with low variability. Bland-Altman plot shows good (**D**) intra-observer (r = 0.990), (**E**) inter-observer (r = 0.977), and (**F**) intra-class (r = 0.959) agreement between mean diameter measurements [mm] with low variability. Bland-Altman plot shows good (**G**) intra-observer (r = 0.993), (**H**) inter-observer (r = 0.953), and (**K**) intra-class (r = 0.932) agreement between mean sharpness measurements [%] with low variability.

images with inherently higher signal and contrast than conventional gradient echo counterparts, and it does not require the administration of contrast agents to yield improved SNR and spatial resolution. bSSFP at 1.5 T has been evaluated in healthy and patient populations with X-ray angiographic correlation, and reported to noninvasively detect CAD with high sensitivity [4,5]. Higher field MR systems offer a theoretically higher SNR, which can be traded for higher spatial resolution or reduced imaging time and thereby reduced motion artifacts, all of which are especially important in coronary imaging. However, high field cardiac imaging entails some major restrictions such as increased RF power deposition and susceptibility-related field inhomogeneities. Because of these limitations, conventional bSSFP imaging in particular has inferior quality and higher variability at higher fields [15,16], which has led to readoption of conventional gradient echo sequences, often requiring administration of contrast agents for a sufficient blood-myocardium contrast [9,19,35].

This study demonstrates that advances in MR hardware and software can address the shortcomings of 3.0 T bSSFP imaging and provide a step forward to a more robust, reproducible, and fast technique with a high intrinsic contrast for 3D imaging of human coronary arteries at higher fields. The MR scanner, used in this study, equipped with a 32-channel phased-array coil and multi-transmit system allowed volume targeted acquisition of 3D images in a single breathhold. 32-channel phased-array coils are reported to have significantly improved SNR and geometry factor, which facilitate use of large parallel imaging acceleration factors [36]. Second-order shimming, reported to be considerably more effective than linear shimming [20], was applied for suppression of B_0 field inhomogeneities, and on-resonant frequency was determined at the level of the coronary arteries. Multi-transmit technology and localized RF shimming were integrated with higher order shimming and utilized to obtain proper knowledge of the B_1+-field and accurate estimation of SAR [22]. Although we did not perform a quantitative analysis of the B_1+-field, subject-specific B_1 shimming has been shown to significantly enhance the homogeneity of the local field and to achieve more accurate excitation angles [23]. These refinements have been reported to improve the quality of cardiac bSSFP imaging with respect to image homogeneity, diagnostic confidence, and off-resonance artifacts [22]. Combined with parallel imaging and half-Fourier-acquisition imaging of a $300 \times 300 \times 20$ mm^3 volume with acquired voxel size of $1.0 \times 1.0 \times 2.0$ mm^3 was supported. This spatial coverage and resolution compared equally or favorably with the prior volume-targeted implementations of bSSFP [15-17] and the common gradient echo sequences at 3.0 T [10,16], as well as with the well-tested volume-targeted implementations of bSSFP at 1.5 T [4,37,38]. The single-breathhold scan with an average duration of 20.5 seconds, was comfortably tolerated by all subjects and achieved with an acquisition window of 105 ms. This temporal resolution too compared favorably with the previously reported single-breathhold implementations of bSSFP with similar spatial resolution and coverage at 1.5 T as well as 3.0 T (acquisition window between 108-150 ms [4,15,17]).

The present implementation of the bSSFP sequence provided high-quality images of arterial lumen with enhanced contrast. The average vessel sharpness of $55 \pm 2\%$ compared favorably with bSSFP imaging at 1.5 T as well as gradient echo imaging at 3.0 T (average reported sharpness ranging between 40-46% [37,39]). Reproducible assessment of arterial lumen was provided within a long continuous segment of the vessels with an average visualized vessel length of 100.5 ± 6.3 mm, which too compared favorably with standard bSSFP sequences at 1.5 and 3.0 T (average visible length ranging between 50.0-95.0 mm [4,16]). The mean vessel diameter imaged by this technique was consistent with what has been published in literature for similar cohorts.

Although, the bSSFP sequence has been shown to be a highly reproducible technique for quantitative assessment of major coronary arteries at 1.5 T [37], to the best of our knowledge the reproducibility of this technique at higher fields has never been fully investigated. This study demonstrated that the present 3D bSSFP protocol has a very high degree of concordance in repeat measures of vessel length, diameter, and sharpness (Table 1) with no significant difference between the two observers or the two scans. A comparison of variability in diameter measures reveals that the intra-observer, inter-observer, and inter-scan ICC values from the current study (0.987, 0.976, and 0.961, respectively) are higher than the reported values from 3D bSSFP at 1.5 T (intra-observer, inter-observer, and inter-scan ICC values ranging between 0.89-0.98, 0.89-0.98, and 0.63-0.86, respectively [37]).

These results suggest that single-breathhold 3D bSSFP, successfully tested in healthy volunteers and CAD patients within a diverse age group (ranging between 21–75 years), provides a highly reproducible technique at 3.0 T, with a high spatial resolution and a well-defined time requirement. This rapid approach may facilitate functional 3D CMRA studies during stress conditions [25], which are currently conducted with 2D techniques. Furthermore, it can provide an appealing alternate in cases where the navigator-gated free-breathing counterparts, relying on breathing patterns and diaphragm position, result in prolonged and sometimes unpredictable scanning time. In the worst case, the low navigator efficiency may lead to unsuccessful imaging sessions [3]. In this study, the bSSFP sequence was tested in a targeted volume, which requires prescription of a separate 3D volume along each major coronary artery by a skilled operator. This usually adds about 2–3 minutes of planning per coronary artery to the imaging session. In comparison, whole-heart CMRA considerably improves both volumetric coverage and procedural ease-of-use and can be completed in 7–12 minutes of free-breathing scan time [18]. Nevertheless, volumetric-targeted CMRA continues to be a valuable alternate at higher fields [40]. Yet, it would be important in future work to determine whether the present single-breathhold bSSFP sequence could be adapted to a whole-heart approach. With higher volumetric coverage, scanning time naturally increases if the spatial and temporal resolution remain constant, but it offers the opportunity to exploit 2D rather than 1D SENSE [41]. The boundaries of this strategy remain to be explored in this context but provide a promising opportunity to extend this technique for enhanced volumetric coverage. Clinical evaluation of this current technique and assessment of its diagnostic accuracy also remain to be systematically investigated in a larger cohort of patients with coronary artery disease.

Limitations

One limitation to this study is that the imaging sequence was not evaluated in both the right and left coronary systems in every volunteer. The coronary artery that was best visualized on the whole-heart scout scan was selected for imaging and when visual image quality was equivalent for the RCA and the LAD, both arteries were selected for imaging.

Conclusions

This study demonstrates that a 3D bSSFP acquisition, using advances in 3.0 T MR such as multi-transmit system, 32-channel cardiac coil, and localized B_0 and B_1+ shimming, provides high-quality noninvasive imaging of the proximal to distal segments of the major coronary arteries in a single breathhold. This accelerated sequence enables highly reproducible assessment of coronary arterial tree in healthy subjects and patients with CAD.

Competing interests

Michael Schär is a full-time employee of Philips Healthcare, the manufacturer of equipment used in this study.

Authors' contributions

SS: made substantial contributions to design of study, acquisition, analysis and interpretation of data, and drafted the manuscript. MS: made substantial contributions to design of study, acquisition and interpretation of data, and revision of manuscript. AGH: made substantial contributions to acquisition of data. RGW: made substantial contributions to design of study, acquisition and interpretation of data, and revision of manuscript. MS: substantial contributions to design of study, acquisition, analysis and interpretation of data, and revision of manuscript. All authors read and approved the final manuscript.

Acknowledgements

This work was supported in part by NIH/NHLBI (R01HL084186, ARRA 3R01HL084186-04S1, R01HL061912), AHA (12PRE11510006), and Swiss National Science Foundation (320030_143923) research grants.

Author details

[1]Department of Electrical and Computer Engineering, Johns Hopkins University, Baltimore, MD, USA. [2]Department of Radiology, Centre Hospitalier Universitaire Vaudois, Center for Biomedical Imaging (CIBM) and University of Lausanne, Lausanne, Switzerland. [3]Russell H. Morgan Department of Radiology and Radiological Science, Division of Magnetic Resonance Research, Johns Hopkins University, Baltimore, MD, USA. [4]Department of Medicine, Division of Cardiology, Johns Hopkins University, Baltimore, MD, USA. [5]Philips Healthcare, Cleveland, OH, USA. [6]Barrow Neurological Institute, Keller Center for Imaging Innovation, 350 W. Thomas Rd, Phoenix, AZ 85013, USA.

References

1.   Kim WY, Danias PG, Stuber M, Flamm SD, Plein S, Nagel E, Langerak SE, Weber OM, Pedersen EM, Schmidt M, Botnar RM, Manning WJ. Coronary Magnetic Resonance Angiography for the Detection of Coronary Stenoses. New Engl J Med. 2001; 345:1863–9.
2.   Oppelt A, Graumann R, Barfuss H, Fischer H, Hartl W, Schajor W. FISP—a new fast MRI sequence. Electromedica. 1986; 54:15–8.
3.   Sakuma H, Ichikawa Y, Chino S, Hirano T, Makino K, Takeda K. Detection of Coronary Artery Stenosis With Whole-Heart Coronary Magnetic Resonance Angiography. J Am Coll Cardiol. 2006; 48:1946–50.
4.   McCarthy RM, Deshpande VS, Beohar N, Meyers SN, Shea SM, Green JD, Liu X, Bi X, Pereles FS, Finn JP, Kobayashi Y, Sakuma H. Three-Dimensional Breathhold Magnetization-Prepared TrueFISP: A Pilot Study for Magnetic Resonance Imaging of the Coronary Artery Disease. Invest Radiol. 2007; 42:665–70.
5.   Kato S, Kitagawa K, Ishida N, Ishida M, Nagata M, Ichikawa Y, Katahira K, Matsumoto Y, Seo K, Ochiai R, Kobayashi Y, Sakuma H. Assessment of Coronary Artery Disease Using Magnetic Resonance Coronary Angiography: A National Multicenter Trial. J Am Coll Cardiol. 2010; 56:983–91.
6.   Spuentrup E, Bornert P, Botnar RM, Groen JP, Manning WJ, Stuber M. Navigator-Gated Free-Breathing Three-Dimensional Balanced Fast Field Echo (TrueFISP) Coronary Magnetic Resonance Angiography. Invest Radiol. 2002; 37:637–47.
7.   Deshpande VS, Shea SM, Laub G, Simonetti OP, Finn JP, Li D. 3D magnetization-prepared true-FISP: A new technique for imaging coronary arteries. Magn Reson Med. 2001; 46:494–502.
8.   Stuber M, Botnar RM, Fischer SE, Lamerichs R, Smink J, Harvey P, Manning WJ. Preliminary report on in vivo coronary MRA at 3 Tesla in humans. Magn Reson Med. 2002; 48:425–9.
9.   Liu X, Bi X, Huang J, Jerecic R, Carr J, Li D. Contrast-enhanced whole-heart coronary magnetic resonance angiography at 3.0 t: comparison with steady-state free precession technique at 1.5 t. Invest Radiol. 2008; 43:663–8.
10. Sommer T, Hackenbroch M, Hofer U, Schmiedel A, Willinek WA, Flacke S, Gieseke J, Träber F, Fimmers R, Litt H, Schild H. Coronary MR angiography at 3.0 T versus that at 1.5 t: initial results in patients suspected of having coronary artery disease1. Radiology. 2005; 234:718–25.
11. Ibrahim TS, Lee R, Abduljalil AM, Baertlein BA, Robitaille P-ML. Dielectric resonances and B1 field inhomogeneity in UHFMRI: computational analysis and experimental findings. Magn Reson Imaging. 2001; 19:219–26.
12. Noeske R, Seifert F, Rhein K-H, Rinneberg H. Human cardiac imaging at 3 T using phased array coils. Magn Reson Med. 2000; 44:978–82.
13. Zur Y, Stokar S, Bendel P. An analysis of fast imaging sequences with steady-state transverse magnetization refocusing. Magn Reson Med. 1988; 6:175–93.
14. Fuchs F, Laub G, Othomo K. TrueFISP—technical considerations and cardiovascular applications. Eur J Radiol. 2003; 46:28–32.
15. Bi X, Deshpande V, Simonetti O, Laub G, Li D. Three-dimensional breathhold SSFP coronary MRA: A comparison between 1.5 T and 3.0 T. J Magn Reson Imaging. 2005; 22:206–12.
16. Kaul MG, Stork A, Bansmann PM, Nolte-Ernsting C, Lund GK, Weber C, Adam G. Evaluation of Balanced Steady-State Free Precession (TrueFISP) and K-space segmented gradient echo sequences for 3D coronary MR angiography with navigator gating at 3 Tesla. Fortschr Röntgenstr. 2004; 176:1560–5.
17. Lee H-L, Shankaranarayanan A, Pohost GM, Nayak KS. Improved coronary MR angiography using wideband steady state free precession at 3 tesla with sub-millimeter resolution. J Magn Reson Imaging. 2010; 31:1224–9.
18. Xie J, Lai P, Bhat H, Li D. Whole-heart coronary magnetic resonance angiography at 3.0 T using short-TR steady-state free precession, vastly undersampled isotropic projection reconstruction. J Magn Reson Imaging. 2010; 31:1230–5.
19. Yang Q, Li K, Liu X, Bi X, Liu Z, An J, Zhang A, Jerecic R, Li D. Contrast-enhanced whole-heart coronary magnetic resonance angiography at 3.0-T: a comparative study with X-Ray angiography in a single center. J Am Coll Cardiol. 2009; 54:69–76.
20. Schär M, Kozerke S, Fischer SE, Boesiger P. Cardiac SSFP imaging at 3 Tesla. Magn Reson Med. 2004; 51:799–806.
21. Zhu Y. Parallel excitation with an array of transmit coils. Magn Reson Med. 2004; 51:775–84.
22. Mueller A, Kouwenhoven M, Naehle CP, Gieseke J, Strach K, Willinek WA, Schild HH, Thomas D. Dual-source radiofrequency transmission with patient-adaptive local radiofrequency shimming for 3.0-T cardiac MR imaging: initial experience. Radiology. 2012; 263:77–85.
23. Krishnamurthy R, Pednekar A, Kouwenhoven M, Cheong B, Muthupillai R. Evaluation of a Subject specific dual-transmit approach for improving B1 field homogeneity in cardiovascular magnetic resonance at 3 T. J Cardiovasc Magn Reson. 2013; 15:68.
24. Niendorf T, Hardy CJ, Giaquinto RO, Gross P, Cline HE, Zhu Y, Kenwood G, Cohen S, Grant AK, Joshi S, Rofsky NM, Sodickson DK. Toward single breath-hold whole-heart coverage coronary MRA using highly accelerated parallel imaging with a 32-channel MR system. Magn Reson Med. 2006; 56:167–76.
25. Hays AG, Hirsch GA, Kelle S, Gerstenblith G, Weiss RG, Stuber M. Noninvasive visualization of coronary artery endothelial function in healthy subjects and in patients with coronary artery disease. J Am Coll Cardiol. 2010; 56:1657–65.
26. Terashima M, Meyer CH, Keeffe BG, Putz EJ, de la Pena-Almaguer E, Yang PC, Hu BS, Nishimura DG, McConnell MV. Noninvasive assessment of coronary vasodilation using magnetic resonance angiography. J Am Coll Cardiol. 2005; 45:104–10.
27. Ehara S, Nakamura Y, Matsumoto K, Hasegawa T, Shimada K, Takagi M, Hanatani A, Izumi Y, Terashima M, Yoshiyama M. Effects of intravenous atrial natriuretic peptide and nitroglycerin on coronary vasodilation and flow velocity determined using 3 T magnetic resonance imaging in patients with nonischemic heart failure. Heart Vessels. 2013; 28:596–605.

28. Fischer SE, Wickline SA, Lorenz CH. Novel real-time R-wave detection algorithm based on the vectorcardiogram for accurate gated magnetic resonance acquisitions. *Magn Reson Med*. 1999; **42**:361–70.

29. Cunningham CH, Pauly JM, Nayak KS. Saturated double-angle method for rapid B1+ mapping. *Magn Reson Med*. 2006; **55**:1326–33.

30. Pruessmann KP, Weiger M, Scheidegger MB, Boesiger P. SENSE: Sensitivity encoding for fast MRI. *Magn Reson Med*. 1999; **42**:952–62.

31. Stuber M, Botnar RM, Danias PG, Sodickson DK, Kissinger KV, Van Cauteren M, De Becker J, Manning WJ. Double-oblique free-breathing high resolution three-dimensional coronary magnetic resonance angiography. *J Am Coll Cardiol*. 1999; **34**:524–31.

32. Deimling M, Heid O. Magnetization prepared true FISP imaging. In: *Annual Meeting of the Society of Magnetic Resonance*. 1994th ed. San Francisco: 1994: p. 495.

33. Etienne A, Botnar RM, van Muiswinkel AMC, Boesiger P, Manning WJ, Stuber M. "Soap-Bubble" visualization and quantitative analysis of 3D coronary magnetic resonance angiograms. *Magn Reson Med*. 2002; **48**:658–66.

34. Deyo RA, Diehr P, Patrick DL. Reproducibility and responsiveness of health status measures statistics and strategies for evaluation. *Control Clin Trials*. 1991; **12**:S142–58.

35. Deshpande VS, Cavagna F, Maggioni F, Schirf BE, Omary RA, Li D. Comparison of gradient-echo and steady-state free precession for coronary artery magnetic resonance angiography using a gadolinium-based intravascular contrast agent. *Invest Radiol*. 2006; **41**:292–8.

36. Reeder SB, Wintersperger BJ, Dietrich O, Lanz T, Greiser A, Reiser MF, Glazer GM, Schoenberg SO. Practical approaches to the evaluation of signal-to-noise ratio performance with parallel imaging: Application with cardiac imaging and a 32-channel cardiac coil. *Magn Reson Med*. 2005; **54**:748–54.

37. Greil GF, Desai MY, Fenchel M, Miller S, Pettigrew RI, Sieverding L, Stuber M. Reproducibility of free-breathing cardiovascular magnetic resonance coronary angiography. *J Cardiovasc Magn Reson*. 2007; **9**:49–56.

38. Cheng L, Gao Y, Guaricci AI, Mulukutla S, Sun W, Sheng F, Foo TK, Prince MR, Wang Y. Breath-hold 3D steady-state free precession coronary MRA compared with conventional X-ray coronary angiography. *J Magn Reson Imaging*. 2006; **23**:669–73.

39. Chang S, Cham MD, Hu S, Wang Y. 3-T navigator parallel-imaging coronary MR angiography: targeted-volume versus whole-heart acquisition. *Am J Roentgenol*. 2008; **191**:38–42.

40. van Elderen SGC, Versluis MJ, Westenberg JJM, Agarwal H, Smith NB, Stuber M, de Roos A, Webb AG. Right Coronary MR Angiography at 7 T: a direct quantitative and qualitative comparison with 3 T in young healthy volunteers1. *Radiology*. 2010; **257**:254–9.

41. Zhu Y, Hardy CJ, Sodickson DK, Giaquinto RO, Dumoulin CL, Kenwood G, Niendorf T, Lejay H, McKenzie CA, Ohliger MA, Rofsky NM. Highly parallel volumetric imaging with a 32-element RF coil array. *Magn Reson Med*. 2004; **52**:869–77.

Permissions

The contributors of this book come from diverse backgrounds, making this book a truly international effort. This book will bring forth new frontiers with its revolutionizing research information and detailed analysis of the nascent developments around the world.

We would like to thank all the contributing authors for lending their expertise to make the book truly unique. They have played a crucial role in the development of this book. Without their invaluable contributions this book wouldn't have been possible. They have made vital efforts to compile up to date information on the varied aspects of this subject to make this book a valuable addition to the collection of many professionals and students.

This book was conceptualized with the vision of imparting up-to-date information and advanced data in this field. To ensure the same, a matchless editorial board was set up. Every individual on the board went through rigorous rounds of assessment to prove their worth. After which they invested a large part of their time researching and compiling the most relevant data for our readers.

The editorial board has been involved in producing this book since its inception. They have spent rigorous hours researching and exploring the diverse topics which have resulted in the successful publishing of this book. They have passed on their knowledge of decades through this book. To expedite this challenging task, the publisher supported the team at every step. A small team of assistant editors was also appointed to further simplify the editing procedure and attain best results for the readers.

Apart from the editorial board, the designing team has also invested a significant amount of their time in understanding the subject and creating the most relevant covers. They scrutinized every image to scout for the most suitable representation of the subject and create an appropriate cover for the book.

The publishing team has been an ardent support to the editorial, designing and production team. Their endless efforts to recruit the best for this project, has resulted in the accomplishment of this book. They are a veteran in the field of academics and their pool of knowledge is as vast as their experience in printing. Their expertise and guidance has proved useful at every step. Their uncompromising quality standards have made this book an exceptional effort. Their encouragement from time to time has been an inspiration for everyone.

The publisher and the editorial board hope that this book will prove to be a valuable piece of knowledge for researchers, students, practitioners and scholars across the globe.

List of Contributors

Garry Liu and Graham A Wright
Department of Medical Biophysics, University of Toronto, Toronto, ON, Canada

Rachel M Wald, Susan L Roche, Erwin N Oechslin and Andrew M Crean
Toronto Congenital Centre for Adults, Peter Munk Cardiac Centre, University Health Network, Toronto General Hospital, 585 University Avenue, 5 N-525, Toronto, ON M5G 2N2, Canada

Daniel Tobler
Department of Cardiology, University Hospital Basel, Basel, Switzerland
Toronto Congenital Centre for Adults, Peter Munk Cardiac Centre, University Health Network, Toronto General Hospital, 585 University Avenue, 5 N-525, Toronto, ON M5G 2N2, Canada

Manish Motwani and John P Greenwood
Multidisciplinary Cardiovascular Research Centre, Leeds Institute of Genetics, Health and Therapeutics, University of Leeds, Leeds, UK

Robert M Iwanochko, Flavia Verocai, Andrew M Crean and Rachel M Wald
Department of Medical Imaging, Toronto General Hospital, Toronto, Canada

Sloane McGraw, Omer Mirza, Michael A Bauml and Vibhav S Rangarajan
Section of Cardiology, Department of Medicine, University of Illinois at Chicago, 840 South Wood St. M/C 715, Suite 920 S, Chicago, IL 60612, USA

Afshin Farzaneh-Far
Division of Cardiology, Department of Medicine, Duke University Medical Center, Durham, NC, USA
Section of Cardiology, Department of Medicine, University of Illinois at Chicago, 840 South Wood St. M/C 715, Suite 920 S, Chicago, IL 60612, USA

Merlin J. Fair, Peter D. Gatehouse and David N. Firmin
National Heart & Lung Institute, Imperial College London, London, UK
Cardiovascular Magnetic Resonance Unit, Royal Brompton Hospital, Sydney Street, London SW3 6NP, UK

Edward V. R. DiBella
Utah Center for Advanced Imaging Research, University of Utah, Salt Lake City, UT, USA

Simon Greulich, Hannah Steubing, Stefan Birkmeier, Stefan Grün, Kerstin Bentz, Udo Sechtem and Heiko Mahrholdt
Department of Cardiology, Robert Bosch Medical Center, Auerbachstrasse 110, 70376 Stuttgart, Germany

Aurélien J. Trotier, William Lefrançois, Kris Van Renterghem, Jean-michel Franconi, Eric Thiaudière and Sylvain Miraux
Centre de Résonance Magnétique des Systèmes Biologiques, UMR 5536 CNRS/Université de Bordeaux, 146 rue Léo Saignat, Cedex 33076 Bordeaux, France

Christopher Schneeweis, Alexander Berger and Sebastian Kelle, Eckart Fleck and Rolf Gebker
Department of Internal Medicine/Cardiology, German Heart Institute Berlin, Augustenburger Platz 1, 13353 Berlin, Germany

Jianxing Qiu
Department of Radiology, Peking University First Hospital, Beijing, China

Bernhard Schnackenburg
Philips Research Hamburg, Hamburg, Germany

Stephen Hamshere, Cyril Pellaton, Danielle Longchamp, Tom Burchell, Saidi Mohiddin, James C. Moon, Didier Locca and Mark Westwood
Department of Cardiology, Barts Heart Centre, St Bartholomews Hospital, Barts Health NHS Trust, London EC1A 7BE, UK

Anthony Mathur, Steffen E. Petersen and Daniel A. Jones
William Harvey Research Institute, NIHR Cardiovascular Biomedical Research Unit at Barts, Queen Mary University of London, Charterhouse Square, London EC1M 6BQ, UK
Department of Cardiology, Barts Heart Centre, St Bartholomews Hospital, Barts Health NHS Trust, London EC1A 7BE, UK

Didier Locca
Service de Cardiologie et Département de Médecine
Interne, Centre Hospitalier Universitaire, Vaudois,
Lausanne, Switzerland

Jens Kastrup
Department of Cardiology, Rigshopitale, University
of Copenhagen, Copenhagen, Denmark

Daniel Z. Brunengraber
Diagnostic Cardiovascular Imaging Laboratory,
Department of Radiological Sciences, David Geffen
School of Medicine at UCLA, Los Angeles, CA,
USA

Kim-Lien Nguyen
Division of Cardiology, David Geffen School of
Medicine at UCLA and VA Greater Los Angeles
Healthcare System, Los Angeles, CA, USA
Diagnostic Cardiovascular Imaging Laboratory,
Department of Radiological Sciences, David Geffen
School of Medicine at UCLA, Los Angeles, CA,
USA
Department of Radiological Sciences, University
of California at Los Angeles, Peter V. Ueberroth
Building Suite 3371, 10945 Le Conte Ave., Los
Angeles, CA 90095-7206, USA

Peng Hu, J. Paul Finn, Fei Han and Ziwu Zhou
Department of Biomedical Physics, University of
California, Los Angeles, CA, USA
Diagnostic Cardiovascular Imaging Laboratory,
Department of Radiological Sciences, David Geffen
School of Medicine at UCLA, Los Angeles, CA,
USA
Department of Radiological Sciences, University
of California at Los Angeles, Peter V. Ueberroth
Building Suite 3371, 10945 Le Conte Ave., Los
Angeles, CA 90095-7206, USA

Ihab Ayad
Department of Anesthesiology, David Geffen School
of Medicine at UCLA, Los Angeles, CA, USA

Daniel S. Levi and Gary M. Satou
Division of Pediatric Cardiology, David Geffen
School of Medicine at UCLA, Los Angeles, CA,
USA

Brian L. Reemtsen
Division of Cardiothoracic Surgery, David Geffen
School of Medicine at UCLA, Los Angeles, CA,
USA

**Rodney De Palma, Peder Sörensson, Dinos
Verouhis, John Pernow and Nawzad Saleh**
Karolinska Institutet, Department of Medicine, Unit
of Cardiology, Karolinska University Hospital,
Stockholm, Sweden

**Mariana Bustamante, Vikas Gupta and Tino
Ebbers**
Center for Medical Image Science and Visualization
(CMIV), Linköping University, Linköping, Sweden
Division of Cardiovascular Medicine, Department of
Medical and Health Sciences, Linköping University,
Linköping, Sweden

Carl-Johan Carlhäll
Department of Clinical Physiology, Department of
Medical and Health Sciences, Linköping University,
Linköping, Sweden
Division of Cardiovascular Medicine, Department of
Medical and Health Sciences, Linköping University,
Linköping, Sweden

**Pankaj Garg, Peter P. Swoboda, James R. J.
Foley, Graham J. Fent, Tarique A. Musa, David P.
Ripley, Bara Erhayiem, Laura E. Dobson, Adam K.
McDiarmid, Philip Haaf, Ananth Kidambi, Saul
Crandon, Pei G. Chew, John P. Greenwood and
Sven Plein**
Division of Biomedical Imaging, Leeds Institute of
Cardiovascular and Metabolic Medicine (LICAMM)
& Multidisciplinary Cardiovascular Research
Centre, University of Leeds, Leeds LS2 9JT, UK

David A. Broadbent
Medical Physics and Engineering, Leeds Teaching
Hospitals NHS Trust, Leeds, UK
Division of Biomedical Imaging, Leeds Institute of
Cardiovascular and Metabolic Medicine (LICAMM)
& Multidisciplinary Cardiovascular Research
Centre, University of Leeds, Leeds LS2 9JT, UK

R. J. van der Geest
Division of Image Processing, Leiden University
Medical Centre, Leiden, The Netherlands

**Simon Veldhoen, Cyrus Behzadi, Alexander Lenz,
Frank Oliver Henes, Gerhard Adam and Peter
Bannas**
Department of Diagnostic and Interventional
Radiology and Nuclear Medicine, University
Medical Center Hamburg-Eppendorf, Hamburg,
Germany

Thorsten Alexander Bley and Simon Veldhoen
Department of Diagnostic and Interventional Radiology, University Hospital Würzburg, Bavaria, Germany

Meike Rybczynski
Department of General and Interventional Cardiology, University Medical Center Hamburg-Eppendorf, Hamburg, Germany

Lijun Zhang, Ruiyu Dou and Zhanming Fan
Department of Radiology, Beijing Anzhen Hospital, Capital Medical University, Anzhenli Avenue, Chao Yang District, Beijing 100029, China

Xiantao Song, Li Dong and Jianan Li
Department of Cardiology, Beijing Anzhen Hospital, Capital Medical University, Beijing, China

Jing An
Siemens Shenzhen Magnetic Resonance Ltd, Guangdong Shenzhen, China

Debiao Li
Biomedical Imaging Research Institute, Cedars-Sinai Medical Center, University of California, Los Angeles, USA

A. Pursnani, M. P. F. Botelho, W. Li and I. Koktzoglou
Department of Radiology, NorthShore University HealthSystem, 2650 Ridge Avenue, Evanston, IL 60201, USA
The University of Chicago Pritzker School of Medicine, Chicago, USA

Robert R. Edelman
Feinberg School of Medicine, Northwestern University, Chicago, USA
Department of Radiology, NorthShore University HealthSystem, 2650 Ridge Avenue, Evanston, IL 60201, USA

S. Giri
Siemens Medical Solutions USA, Inc., Chicago, USA

John D Groarke, Alfonso H Waller, Tomas S Vita, Marcelo F Di Carli, Ron Blankstein, Raymond Y Kwong and Michael Steigner
Cardiovascular Imaging Program, Cardiovascular Division, Department of Medicine and Department of Radiology, Brigham and Women's Hospital, Harvard Medical School, Boston, MA, USA

Gregory F Michaud
Cardiovascular Division, Department of Medicine, Brigham and Women's Hospital, Harvard Medical School, Boston, MA, USA

Riccardo Faletti, Alessandro Rapellino, Francesca Barisone, Paolo Fonio and Giovanni Gandini
Istituto di Radiologia dell'Università degli Studi di Torino, A.O. Città della Salute e della Scienza, Via Genova 3, 10126 Torino, Italy

Matteo Anselmino, Fiorenzo Gaita and Federico Ferraris
Istituto di Cardiologia dell'Università degli Studi di Torino, A.O. Città della Salute e della Scienza, Corso Dogliotti 14, 10126 Torino, Italy

Jamal N Khan, Naveed Razvi, Sheraz A Nazir, Anvesha Singh, Nicholas GD Masca, Anthony H Gershlick, Iain Squire and Gerry P McCann
Department of Cardiovascular Sciences, University of Leicester, Glenfield Hospital, Groby Road, Leicester LE3 9QP, UK
NIHR Leicester Cardiovascular Biomedical Research Unit, Glenfield Hospital, Groby Road, Leicester LE3 9QP, UK

Sahar Soleimanifard and Matthias Stuber
Department of Electrical and Computer Engineering, Johns Hopkins University, Baltimore, MD, USA

Matthias Stuber
Department of Radiology, Centre Hospitalier Universitaire Vaudois, Center for Biomedical Imaging (CIBM) and University of Lausanne, Lausanne, Switzerland

Michael Schär
Russell H. Morgan Department of Radiology and Radiological Science, Division of Magnetic Resonance Research, Johns Hopkins University, Baltimore, MD, USA
Philips Healthcare, Cleveland, OH, USA
Barrow Neurological Institute, Keller Center for Imaging Innovation, 350 W. Thomas Rd, Phoenix, AZ 85013, USA

Robert G Weiss and Allison G Hays
Department of Medicine, Division of Cardiology, Johns Hopkins University, Baltimore, MD, USA
Russell H. Morgan Department of Radiology and Radiological Science, Division of Magnetic Resonance Research, Johns Hopkins University, Baltimore, MD, USA

Index